Clinical Research
for the
Doctor *of*
Nursing Practice

Allison J. Terry, PhD, MSN, RN

Assistant Professor of Nursing
Auburn University at Montgomery
Montgomery, Alabama

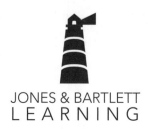

JONES & BARTLETT
LEARNING

World Headquarters

Jones & Bartlett Learning	Jones & Bartlett Learning	Jones & Bartlett Learning
40 Tall Pine Drive	Canada	International
Sudbury, MA 01776	6339 Ormindale Way	Barb House, Barb Mews
978-443-5000	Mississauga, Ontario L5V 1J2	London W6 7PA
info@jblearning.com	Canada	United Kingdom
www.jblearning.com		

Jones & Bartlett Learning books and products are available through most bookstores and online booksellers. To contact Jones & Bartlett Learning directly, call 800-832-0034, fax 978-443-8000, or visit our website, www.jblearning.com.

Substantial discounts on bulk quantities of Jones & Bartlett Learning publications are available to corporations, professional associations, and other qualified organizations. For details and specific discount information, contact the special sales department at Jones & Bartlett Learning via the above contact information or send an email to specialsales@jblearning.com.

The author, editor, and publisher have made every effort to provide accurate information. However, they are not responsible for errors, omissions, or for any outcomes related to the use of the contents of this book and take no responsibility for the use of the products and procedures described. Treatments and side effects described in this book may not be applicable to all people; likewise, some people may require a dose or experience a side effect that is not described herein. Drugs and medical devices are discussed that may have limited availability controlled by the Food and Drug Administration (FDA) for use only in a research study or clinical trial. Research, clinical practice, and government regulations often change the accepted standard in this field. When consideration is being given to use of any drug in the clinical setting, the health care provider or reader is responsible for determining FDA status of the drug, reading the package insert, and reviewing prescribing information for the most up-to-date recommendations on dose, precautions, and contraindications, and determining the appropriate usage for the product. This is especially important in the case of drugs that are new or seldom used.

Production Credits

Publisher: Kevin Sullivan	V.P., Manufacturing and Inventory
Acquisitions Editor: Amanda Harvey	Control: Therese Connell
Editorial Assistant: Rachel Shuster	Composition: Spoke & Wheel
Editorial Assistant: Sara Bempkins	Cover Design: Scott Moden
Production Manager: Carolyn Rogers	Cover Image: © Yellowj/ShutterStock, Inc.
Associate Production Editor: Katie Spiegel	Printing and Binding: Malloy, Inc.
Associate Marketing Manager: Katie Hennessy	Cover Printing: Malloy, Inc.

Library of Congress Cataloging-in-Publication Data
Terry, Allison J.
  Clinical research for the doctor of nursing practice / Allison J. Terry.
     p. ; cm.
  Includes bibliographical references and index.
  ISBN 978-0-7637-9122-3 (pbk.)
  1. Nursing--Study and teaching (Graduate)—United States—Methodology. 2. Nursing—Research—United States—Methodology. I. Title.
  [DNLM: 1. Education, Nursing, Graduate--methods. 2. Nurse Clinicians—education. 3. Nursing Research—methods. 4. Research Design. WY 18.5 T329c 2011]
  RT75.T47 2011
  610.73071'1—dc22
                              2010018354
6048
Printed in the United States of America
15 14 13 12 11   10 9 8 7 6 5 4 3 2 1

Contents

9   Data Collection   135

10   Issues Related to Survey Data Collection   151

11   Data Analysis   169

12   Writing the Research Report for Potential Publication   181

APPENDIX 12A Critique of Clinically Based Research 185

APPENDIX A Examination of Academic Self-Regulation Variances in Nursing Students 193

Michelle A. Schutt, EdD, RN

APPENDIX B Understanding the Impact of the AACN Endorsement of the DNP: A Systems Analysis Using Effects-Based Reasoning 293

Marilyn K. Rhodes, EdD, MSN, RN, CNM

APPENDIX C "Untidy": The Pre-War Policy Process for Post-War Iraq 401

Dr. Sylvia B. Gage

The Importance of Research in the Doctor of Nursing Practice Degree

1

■ OBJECTIVES

Upon completion of this chapter, the reader should be prepared to:

1 Describe the fundamental differences between a practice-oriented doctorate and the traditional research-focused doctorate.

2 Discuss the seven primary areas of content that the American Association of Colleges of Nursing (AACN) has recommended be included in all Doctor of Nursing Practice (DNP) programs.

3 Review the time line that led to the development of the DNP degree.

4 Discuss the concerns that have arisen regarding implementation of the DNP degree.

5 Review the primary areas of content of any DNP program.

6 Describe how the DNP graduate should be prepared to function as an agent for quality improvement.

7 Describe how the DNP graduate should be prepared to act as an advocate for health care through use of healthcare policy.

8 Describe how the DNP graduate should be prepared to function as an advanced practice nurse in a specialty.

9 Describe how the DNP graduate should be prepared to utilize information systems and technology.

10 Describe how the DNP graduate functions while assuming an aggregate focus.

11 Discuss the relationship of the DNP graduate's clinical scholarship to evidence-based practice.

12 Differentiate between a systematic review and the development of clinical practice guidelines.

13 Describe the process of evidence-based decision making.

14 Be familiar with websites that can provide additional information related to evidence-based practice.

INTRODUCTION TO THE DOCTOR OF NURSING PRACTICE DEGREE

The Doctor of Nursing Practice (DNP) degree is a terminal practice degree that has the goal of preparing nurses to assume leadership roles in clinical practice, clinical teaching environments, and action research arenas. It is a graduate degree that builds on the generalist foundation produced through the acquisition of a baccalaureate and master's degree in nursing (National Association of Neonatal Nurses, n.d.). The degree provides less emphasis on theoretical underpinnings and research initiation and greater emphasis on advanced clinical practice, utilization of research, and accurate evaluation of both practice and care delivery models (Association of Operating Room Nurses, 2006). According to the American Association of Colleges of Nursing (AACN), the DNP degree has tremendous momentum—whereas in 2005 eight programs were admitting DNP students and 80 institutions were considering the development of such programs, by 2006, 11 colleges were admitting students and 190 schools had programs under development. By 2007, 25 institutions were admitting DNP students (National Association of Neonatal Nurses, n.d.).

Time Line for the Development of the DNP Degree

Although the concept of a practice doctorate in nursing is not a new one, the time line for the creation of the Doctor of Nursing Practice degree extends more than 20 years. In fact, the first practice-focused nursing doctorate was offered in 1979 at Case Western Reserve University. The origins of the DNP degree can be traced back as far as the early 1900s, however, when nurses were first awarded a doctoral degree in education. Doctor of Nursing Science degree programs began to emerge by 1970. These programs required clinical competence and proficiency as well as scholarly research. Progress toward the ultimate development of the DNP degree continued as the Doctor of Nursing degree emerged in 1979 to prepare nurses who were assuming the role of the clinical leader.

The next step was the development of the Doctorate of Nursing Practice degree, which was focused on nurse practitioners. This degree was developed to prepare nurse practitioners for independent primary care roles in multiple settings. It focuses on direct care, with a concentration in research utilization to improve delivery of care, patient outcomes, and clinical systems management. The American Association of Colleges of Nursing has recommended that the DNP degree be the standard for entry into advanced practice for nurse practitioners, nurse–midwives, nurse anesthetists, and clinical nurse specialists by the year 2015. A hoped-for benefit of the DNP degree is a higher rate of reimbursement for the services for advanced practice nurses in the previously mentioned specialties (National Association of Neonatal Nurses, n.d.).

As DNP programs have developed and continue to evolve, clear differences can be discerned among these practice-oriented programs and research-focused programs. Such differences include:

- Decreased emphasis on theory in the practice doctorate
- Less content focused on research methodology, focusing instead on the evaluation and usage of research rather than the implementation of the research process
- Use of a capstone project in most DNP programs that is grounded in clinical practice and designed to solve problems in practice or to add new information to practice
- Emphasis on clinical practice improvement, innovation and testing of interventions, testing of care delivery models, evaluation of healthcare outcomes, and the expertise to provide leadership in establishing clinical excellence (American Association of Colleges of Nursing, 2006)

These differences make the Doctor of Nursing Practice degree the unique educational credential that it is, and equip the graduate with the knowledge and skills needed to be an active participant in the research process.

The Capstone Project

The previously mentioned capstone project that is used in the majority of practice-oriented doctorates is an integrative practice experience that results in a practice-focused written document that will be subjected to peer and/or professional scrutiny. It is the DNP degree's alternative to the research-focused doctorate's dissertation. The capstone project is the culmination of the student's academic experience (Rutgers College of Nursing, 2007), and should make a significant contribution to evidence-based nursing practice or indicate the solution to an existing problem in the healthcare delivery system. The capstone project is integral to the DNP degree because the hallmark of all doctoral education is the completion of a project that both illustrates the synthesis of the student's work and provides the foundation for future scholarship.

Some DNP programs prefer the capstone project to be a practice portfolio that documents the impact of practice initiatives or outcomes resulting from practice. Another frequently used format is that of a practice change initiative. This can consist of a pilot study, a program evaluation, a quality improvement project, an evaluation of a new practice model, or a consultation-type project. Although quantitative research is certainly possible for the DNP graduate and will be discussed in this text, many graduates gravitate toward qualitative research, and thus qualify for the "expedited" category if using human subjects and approaching an institutional review board. An institutional review board will usually consider a research project to qualify for the "expedited" category if it poses little risk to the human subjects involved (Auburn University at Montgomery, 2009).

A qualitative research project focused on quality improvement can frequently be an excellent choice for a DNP student's capstone project, regardless of the practice setting. This text will focus on the planning, organizing, implementing, and evaluating of the capstone project, including the intricacies of navigating through the institutional review board (American Association of Colleges of Nursing, 2006).

Other examples of DNP capstone projects that have been utilized in these programs include the submission of manuscripts for publication, involvement in a large institution-wide research project, completion of systematic reviews, and the development of evidence-based clinical practice guidelines. Systematic reviews and clinical practice guidelines will be addressed in more detail later in this chapter.

Regardless of the form it assumes, the final DNP project will be derived from the practice experience of the student and reviewed and evaluated by an academic committee, much in the way that a research-focused doctoral candidate undergoes the defense of a dissertation. The underlying theme in any project should be the use of evidence to improve practice through either healthcare delivery or patient outcomes (American Association of Colleges of Nursing, 2006). Thus, it becomes clear that the DNP program cannot be separated from the concept of evidence-based practice and its foundation in research.

Benefits of Implementing the DNP Degree

Implementing the DNP credential for advanced practice nurses may allow these nurses to become even more competent in the multiple roles of practice, faculty, and leadership. As these nurses enhance their knowledge base, they will have the ability to improve their nursing practice as well as their patient outcomes through improved healthcare delivery. Their nursing practice will also be strengthened by their enhanced leadership skills. Nurse educators have identified that the current educational curriculum is inadequate for preparation of advanced practice nurses in light of health care's increasingly complex skill set, which incorporates new knowledge in the areas of information systems, technology, healthcare policy development, and epidemiology. At least six areas of practice have been identified as being inadequately addressed in current nursing curricula for advanced practice nurses:

- Practice management
- Health policy
- Use of information technology

- Risk management
- Evaluation of evidence
- Advanced diagnosis and management of the disease process (Apold, 2008)

These can be incorporated into DNP programs to prepare the new generation of clinicians.

Concerns Regarding Implementation of the DNP Degree

As would be expected, concerns arose regarding the implementation of this new degree. A primary source of anxiety for clinicians was that of the title for the graduate of a DNP program. The DNP degree is intended to be a practice doctorate, so discussion has arisen over the use of the title of "doctor." In reality, if credentials are clearly displayed by the graduate, there should be no confusion on the part of patients, the public, or practitioners.

Advanced practice nurses who complete such a program will retain their specialized credentials, but will simply have the enhanced knowledge and leadership skills unique to the DNP program (National Association of Neonatal Nurses, n.d.).

A second concern that has been raised, particularly by practicing nurse practitioners, is the reaction of State Boards of Nursing if the DNP degree becomes the entry-level degree for nurse practitioner education. This should not be a source of anxiety for any candidate for a DNP program because no certification agency currently requires the practice-oriented doctorate as an eligibility requirement, and regulatory bodies have not drafted a plan to require all nurse practitioners in current practice to obtain the DNP degree (National Association of Neonatal Nurses, n.d.).

A third concern with very practical overtones is that of the job market for the DNP graduate. What will be the demand for DNP-prepared advanced practice nurses, and would their pay be adequate to justify the expense of the additional education? Research has shown a link between higher levels of nursing education and more positive patient outcomes, so it is believed that DNP-prepared clinicians will prove their worth through their leadership skills, honed critical thinking ability, and heightened economic and public policy knowledge, in addition to their superior clinical skills (National Association of Neonatal Nurses, n.d.).

In addition, there is a concern that nurses who have acquired the DNP credential may have difficulty finding tenure-track faculty positions, because the PhD is considered the entry-level degree for an assistant professor in academia. Although the DNP degree clearly will contribute to solving the current shortage of clinical nursing faculty, it may not initially contribute to alleviating the tenure-track faculty shortage. Because tenure provides professors with unique rights, status, and privileges in addition to implied longevity in the current position, it will be the responsibility of nursing leaders in academia to prevent the development of a subgroup of DNP faculty who are non-tenurable and are considered lesser in terms of participation in committees on university issues. The DNP graduate who opts to move into a career in academia must select his or her academic appointment carefully to ensure that the position assumed is one that enhances the recently acquired degree rather than diminishes it (Apold, 2008).

Recommended Content for DNP Programs

Because of the explosive growth in practice-oriented nursing doctoral programs, the American Association of Colleges of Nursing developed a task force that was charged with the examination of the current status of such programs. The task force recommended that practice-focused doctoral nursing programs include seven primary areas of content:

- The scientific basis for practice
- Advanced nursing practice
- Organization and system leadership/management and quality improvement
- Analytic methodologies related to practice evaluation and the application of evidence for nursing practice
- Utilization of both technology and information for the improvement and transformation of health care
- The development, implementation, and evaluation of health policy
- Interdisciplinary collaboration for improving patient healthcare outcomes as well as healthcare outcomes for the greater population (American Association of Colleges of Nursing, 2006)

Review of these areas of content will reveal the importance of the research process to the Doctor of Nursing Practice student. It is the intent of the DNP curriculum that graduates will have a broad scientific base that can be translated efficiently to influence healthcare delivery and patient outcomes. These outcomes encompass not only direct patient care, but also the needs of the family unit, the community, and ultimately, the global patient perspective. In order to be able to conceptualize new healthcare delivery models, graduates must be adept at working in both organizational and public policy arenas. The DNP graduate must be particularly proficient in quality management strategies and at functioning as a change agent at both the local organizational level and the greater policy level. He or she must be able to evaluate the cost-effectiveness of a particular aspect of care delivery and to have enough knowledge of finance and economics to design realistic, fiscally sound patient care delivery strategies. However, none of these strategies can be accomplished without the presence of a sound scientific base that can translate both effectively and efficiently into patient care delivery (American Association of Colleges of Nursing, 2006).

THE DNP GRADUATE AS AN AGENT FOR QUALITY IMPROVEMENT

The concept of the DNP graduate being an agent for quality improvement in a facility through an emphasis on systems thinking is so important that the American Association of Colleges of Nursing (AACN) considers it one of the essential hallmarks of a DNP curriculum. In fact, the AACN states that the DNP program should prepare a graduate to:

- Develop and evaluate patient care delivery approaches to meet both the current and anticipated need of patient populations; this development and evaluation process should be based on scientific findings in nursing as well as economic theory, political science, and organizational research;
- Ensure accountability for the quality of the health care delivered and the degree of safety of the patient populations with whom the graduate works;
- Use advanced communication skills and processes to lead quality improvement and patient safety initiative in a healthcare system; these advanced communication processes should include technological skills that would require the graduate to be adept with various forms of computerized communication;
- Use principles of business, finance, economics, and health policy to develop and implement plans to improve the quality of healthcare delivery; these plans may be at the practice level or the system level;
- Develop a budget for practice initiatives for improved delivery of patient care; this includes the ability to monitor the budget for efficient use of the funds;
- Analyze the cost-effectiveness of practice initiatives to improve healthcare outcomes, taking into account the risk involved to both the overall system and the patient population;
- Demonstrate sensitivity to diversity in both patients and providers, both at the cultural level and at the overall patient population level; and
- Develop and/or evaluate effective strategies for management of ethical dilemmas that can occur in the course of healthcare delivery, whether in the healthcare organization itself or within the research process. (American Association of Colleges of Nursing, 2006)

An offshoot of the incorporation of quality improvement initiatives for the DNP student is clinical prevention and population health. The AACN defines clinical prevention as health promotion and risk reduction, as well as illness prevention for both individuals and families. Population health is considered to include aggregate, community, environmental, occupational, cultural, and socioeconomic dimensions of health, with aggregates being groups of individuals who can be defined by a shared characteristic such as gender (American Association of Colleges of Nursing, 2006). The DNP graduate is focused in the areas of clinical prevention and population health in an effort to improve the overall health status of the population of the United States while continuing to integrate nursing's longstanding emphasis on health promotion and disease prevention. These foci are also consistent with the DNP graduate's focus on evidence-based practice and research because the student should be prepared to analyze epidemiological, biostatistical, occupational, and environmental data. Groundbreaking knowledge of infectious disease processes as well as disaster preparedness and triage also will be integrated into clinical prevention (American Association of Colleges of Nursing, 2006).

THE DNP GRADUATE AS AN ADVOCATE FOR HEALTH CARE THROUGH USE OF HEALTHCARE POLICY

The framework for delivery of healthcare services is provided by healthcare policy—whether through governmental regulations, institutional procedures, or the standards of a healthcare organization—and that framework can either enhance or impede healthcare delivery to patients. Although political activism and a commitment to policy development that will lead to delivery of the highest possible quality of health care for patients are integral to the role of the professional nurse, the DNP graduate will be uniquely qualified to assume a leadership role as advocate for both the public and the nursing profession. The DNP graduate will be prepared not only to design and implement new healthcare policies, but also to influence existing policies that will significantly affect the financing of health care, practice regulation, access to health care, safety in patient care, quality of care delivered, and efficacy in patient care outcomes. The DNP curriculum should prepare the graduate to analyze the policy process and competently influence policy formation. The graduate's analysis should occur from the perspectives of consumers, nursing, allied and ancillary healthcare professions, and the public, all of whom will be stakeholders in the policy development process. The graduate should be prepared to attempt to influence policy makers through participation on committees at every level, whether institutional or international, so that patients will receive improved delivery of health care and higher-level outcomes. Finally, the DNP graduate will educate all stakeholders in conjunction with serving as an advocate for both the nursing profession and patients so the public is informed regarding the need for improved patient care outcomes (American Association of Colleges of Nursing, 2006).

Accurate evaluation of healthcare policy frequently occurs most effectively through interprofessional collaboration. The modern healthcare environment is dependent on the skills of individuals from multiple professions. This means that DNP graduates must have preparation in leadership of teams as well as the establishment of interprofessional teams. Regarding interprofessional collaboration, the DNP program should prepare the graduate to:

- Use effective communication and collaborative skills in both the development and implementation of practice models; these skills should also be utilized in peer review, practice guidelines, health policy, standards of care, and production of other scholarly works;
- Lead interprofessional teams to analyze complex practice and organizational issues; and
- Use both consultative and leadership skills with intraprofessional and interprofessional teams to serve as change agents in healthcare delivery systems. (American Association of Colleges of Nursing, 2006)

THE DNP GRADUATE AS AN ADVANCED PRACTICE NURSE

A hallmark of the DNP degree is preparation to practice in a specialized area within the larger overriding umbrella of the nursing profession. Although in reality no nurse can demonstrate mastery of all advanced roles with a grasp of the knowledge required to function in each of them, DNP programs should prepare the nurse to practice within a distinct specialty that requires both expertise and an advanced knowledge base that includes legal and regulatory issues. In preparation for functioning in a specialty practice role, the DNP program will provide foundational practice competencies such as honed assessment skills and the application of biophysical, psychosocial, behavioral, sociopolitical, cultural, and economic knowledge in practice settings. The DNP graduate functioning as an advanced practice nurse utilizes a holistic perspective to assist patients, families, and communities in decision making, making positive lifestyle changes, and self-care. Because the advanced practice nurse assesses, manages, and evaluates patients at the most independent level of clinical nursing practice, the DNP student is required to take courses in advanced health physical assessment, advanced physiology and pathophysiology, and advanced pharmacology. These courses will assist the DNP graduate who is practicing as an advanced practice nurse to identify developing practice trends, identify changes occurring at the systemic level, and make improvements in the care of patient populations within their practice systems. In their function as advanced practice nurses, DNP graduates should be adequately prepared to:

- Conduct a comprehensive, systematic assessment of health and illness parameters in complex situations; because these situations may involve individual patient populations, families, communities, nations, or even global populations, the graduate must be able to incorporate cultural sensitivity in diverse scenarios.
- Use nursing science as well as other sciences to design, implement, and evaluate therapeutic interventions and the patient care outcomes that result from them. (American Association of Colleges of Nursing, 2006)

THE DNP GRADUATE AS A USER OF INFORMATION SYSTEMS AND TECHNOLOGY

The DNP graduate is distinguished by the ability to use information systems and technology to provide leadership within a healthcare system or an academic setting. The degree equips the graduate to design, select, and utilize information systems and technology to evaluate programs of healthcare delivery, outcomes of patient care, and systems of care. Incorporation of information systems and technology enables the graduate to use tools regarding budget and productivity as well as Internet-based tools to enhance patient care. The DNP graduate should be prepared to demonstrate both the conceptual ability and technical skills needed to develop and implement a plan for data extraction from databases containing practice information. Once such a plan is implemented, the graduate should be capable of categorizing the data extracted from such databases, using the appropriate computer program to generate statistics, and then accurately interpreting those statistical results. In addition, the graduate should be proficient in using information systems and technological resources as quality improvement initiatives are incorporated into the healthcare delivery system. Finally, the graduate should have knowledge of the standards and principles involved in the evaluation of patient care technology and the ethical, regulatory, and legal issues that surround such an evaluation (American Association of Colleges of Nursing, 2006).

THE DNP GRADUATE WITH AN AGGREGATE FOCUS

The DNP graduate who functions in an administrative, healthcare policy, informatics, or population-based specialty has an aggregate focus, which means the graduate directs his or her attention toward populations, systems, organizations, and state or national policies. Although these specialties may not have direct patient care responsibilities, there will still be the need for problem definition and the design of health interventions at the aggregate level. The DNP graduate who opts to have an aggregate focus will, out of necessity, be required to be competent in community assessment techniques so that aggregate health or system needs can be identified (American Association of Colleges of Nursing, 2006).

THE DNP GRADUATE'S CLINICAL SCHOLARSHIP AND EVIDENCE-BASED PRACTICE

It has been established that scholarly research is a hallmark of doctoral education. In the case of the DNP graduate, the nurse applies knowledge in the solution of a problem. This is known as the scholarship of practice in nursing. This form of scholarship highlights key activities of DNP graduates, namely, the translation of research into practice, as well as the dissemination and integration of new knowledge. Whereas research-focused nursing doctoral programs provide the research skills needed for discovery of new knowledge in the discipline, DNP programs provide the leadership skills needed for the graduate to engage in evidence-based practice. According to Pipe, Wellik, Buchda, Hansen, and Martyn (2005), evidence-based practice focuses on methods of critically appraising and applying available data and research to achieve a better understand of clinical decision making. The method integrates research evidence with clinical expertise and patient values, which means that the best available evidence will be combined with clinical judgment. This necessitates competence in knowledge application, which consists of:

- Translating research into practice
- Evaluating practice
- Improving the reliability of healthcare practice and outcomes
- Participating in collaborative research

This means DNP programs focus on applying new science and evaluating new knowledge. In addition, DNP graduates use their practice to generate evidence that will serve as parameters in guiding improvements in practice and patient care outcomes (American Association of Colleges of Nursing, 2006). Evidence in health care most frequently consists of:

- *Quasi-experimental studies*—Often used because they do not require randomization or control of all variables.
- *Descriptive research*—Considered to be a systematic analysis of an area of interest to the researcher; often uses survey instruments and does not necessarily examine causation.
- *Ex post facto studies*—These can used very effectively by the DNP graduate once a healthcare trend has been identified; they involve retrospective research that allows the cause-and-effect relationship to be discovered as variables are analyzed. Once the cause-and-effect relationship can be identified, a preventive strategy can be developed. (Hanchett, 2005)

Regarding evidence-based practice, the DNP graduate will be prepared to perform a critical appraisal of existing literature, apply relevant findings in the development of practice guidelines, design and implement processes to evaluate practice outcomes, and design, implement, and evaluate quality improvement methodologies. Ultimately, the graduate should be able to:

- Collect appropriate data to generate evidence for nursing practice
- Direct the design of databases to generate evidence for practice
- Analyze data derived from practice
- Design evidence-based nursing interventions
- Predict and analyze patient care outcomes
- Examine patterns of behavior and outcomes
- Identify gaps in the evidence for practice (American Association of Colleges of Nursing, 2006)

The relationship of the DNP graduate to evidence-based practice is illustrated by the definition of this type of practice. The American Association of Neuroscience Nurses defines evidence-based practice as the integration of the best, most accurate evidence available; nursing expertise in the field; and the values as well as preference of the individuals who are served, or the families or even communities if they assume the client role. The idea of best practices means that care concepts, interventions, and techniques are grounded in research, and therefore will promote a higher quality of client care (Mcilvoy & Hinkle, 2008). The DNP graduate addresses this concept by performing systematic reviews. This means that the findings of all methodologically sound studies that address the same research question are summarized. The systematic review treats eligible research studies as a population to be sampled and surveyed. The individual study characteristics and results will then have an abstract developed, and results will be quantified, coded, and developed into a database that can be statistically analyzed (DiCenso et al., 2000).

The systematic review can be an outstanding research tool for the DNP clinician. As a graduate of a practice-focused doctoral program, the practitioner who conducts such a review is able to make an objective assessment of the available evidence, specifically of the outcomes of particular interventions that could be implemented. The evidence will be located, evaluated, and then consolidated into a comprehensive and unbiased summary. The comprehensive nature of the review allows literature to be sorted into low and high quality. If the sheer volume of available resources is overwhelming, the quantity of literature can be reduced by:

- Reducing the time frame of the search to within the past 5 years
- Restricting the number of databases investigated
- Narrowing the focus of the study by selecting specific research methods
- Reducing the search to certain journals, although the DNP clinician should recognize that this may skew results
- Limiting searches to studies published in certain nations
- Excluding unpublished literature (also known as "gray" literature) (Forward, 2002)

The integration of the process of translating evidence into practice for the DNP clinician can best be illustrated by Carper's work, which identified four essential patterns of "knowing" in nursing: empiric, ethics, personal, and aesthetic patterns (Pipe et al., 2005). Empirical knowing was defined as relating to factual descriptions, explanations, and predictions; ethical knowing was thought to pertain to moral obligations, values, and desired results; personal knowing was defined as the genuine relationship that develops between each nurse and patient; and aesthetic knowing referred to the nurse's perception of the significant areas in the patient's behavior as well as the art involved in performing nursing skills. Evidence-based practice is believed to pertain most closely to empirical knowing, focusing on critical appraisal and application of available data and research in order to understand the process of clinical decision making more fully.

Evidence-based clinical practice guidelines developed as a means of influencing patient outcomes while bringing evidence-based practice into bedside nursing practice. Clinical practice guidelines are practice recommendations based on the analysis of the evidence available on a specific topic and a specific patient population (Mcilvoy & Hinkle, 2008). The guidelines are developed with representation from as many stakeholders as are interested in contributing, should be tested by healthcare professionals who were not involved in their development, and should be reviewed regularly and then modified as needed in order to incorporate new knowledge that is emerging in the field (DiCenso et al., 2000).

The concept of evidence-based nursing was consolidated by Flemming (1998) into five distinct stages:

1. Information needs are identified in current practice and are then translated into focused questions; the questions should be searchable while still reflecting the focus on a specific patient, clinical situation, or managerial scenario.
2. Once a focused question has been identified, it is used as a basis for a literature search so that the relevant evidence from current research can be identified.
3. The relevant evidence that has been gathered undergoes critical appraisal to determine if validity is present; the extent of the generalizability of the research will also be appraised.
4. A plan of care is developed using the best available evidence and clinical expertise, as well as the patient's perspective.
5. A process of self-reflection, audit, and peer assessment is used to evaluate implementation of the designed plan of care.

Unless the focused question is framed correctly, the DNP graduate will have difficulty implementing evidence-based practice through the translation of evidence. An accurately framed question should consist of the clinical situation being addressed, the selected intervention, and the patient care outcome (Flemming, 1998).

THE DNP GRADUATE'S PARTICIPATION IN EVIDENCE-BASED DECISION MAKING

An integral part of evidence-based practice is evidence-based decision making, and the DNP graduate is uniquely qualified to fully participate in this process. Evidence-based decision making involves combining the knowledge the DNP graduate derives from clinical practice with patient preferences and research evidence that is weighted based on its internal and external validity. It is evidence-based decision making that will allow nurses who hold a practice doctorate to actively engage with research evidence as it is accessed, appraised, and incorporated into these clinicians' professional judgment and clinical decision making. There are several components of the process of evidence-based decision making:

- Formulate a focused clinical question once there is a recognized need for additional information; the DNP clinician's capacity to fulfill a variety of roles in a facility will allow this to occur easily.
- Search for the most appropriate evidence to meet the need that has been previously identified.
- Critically appraise the evidence that has been retrieved to meet the identified need.
- Incorporate the evidence that has been critically appraised into a strategy for action.
- Evaluate the effects of decisions that are made and actions that are taken; the DNP clinician's close ties to the clinical setting will allow such evaluation to occur easily (Thompson, Cullum, McCaughan, Sheldon, & Raynor, 2004).

Each component must be fully implemented to ensure the process that is occurring is one of evidence-based decision making.

THE PROCESS OF TRANSLATING EVIDENCE INTO CLINICAL PRACTICE

As graduates of practice-focused doctoral programs, DNP students will be uniquely qualified to frequently progress through the process of reformulating evidence into clinical practice. As graduates of a practice-oriented doctoral program, these clinicians should be continually involved in the systematic review of research in preparation for designing a change in practice based on the validated evidence. Rosswurm and Larrabee's model proposed that six phases are involved in this process (1999):

- *Assessing the need for a change in practice*—Determine whether there is sufficient evidence to warrant initiating the process of changing nursing practice; this is accomplished by collecting internal data about the current practice and then comparing it to the external data (Duffy, 2004).
- *Linking the problem with nursing interventions and patient care outcomes*—Once the clinician has determined that evidence indicates a need for a change in nursing practice, he or she must identify the nursing interventions that could potentially create the change and the outcomes that would ideally result from that change.
- *Synthesizing the best evidence*—Conduct an exhaustive literature search so the literature can be weighed and examined with a critical eye; although a large body of literature may be identified, unless it

is of the highest quality, there may not be sufficient need to progress through the process of translating that evidence into practice. The DNP graduate can carry out this step through a systematic review, because once the clinical problem has been identified, it must be stated as a focused clinical question that can be answered by searching the literature. It is the focused clinical questions that will be used to select keywords and limits for the search in order to make it more precise. Potential benefits and risks to the patient must be identified prior to implementing a change in nursing practice (Duffy, 2004).

■ *Designing the practice change*—Involve stakeholders to identify strategies that will explore the original issue as much as possible and then be used to implement it into practice; often referred to as a clinical protocol, this change should take into account the practice environment, available resources, and stakeholder feedback. The less complex the new protocol, the more likely it is to be accepted by stakeholders. Conducting a pilot test of the new protocol can make the change more acceptable because it will allow stakeholders who are practitioners to influence the formation of the change to suit their needs (Duffy, 2004).

■ *Designing the practice change*—If the evidence supports changing nursing practice, begin implementation of the strategies that were identified in the previous step, evaluating each carefully to ensure they are indeed evidence-based. During this process, follow-up reinforcement of learning should occur as well as data collection of outcomes from stakeholders, analysis of the data, and interpretation of the results to determine whether the protocol was implemented as was originally intended and the effect of the new protocol on patient care outcomes (Duffy, 2004).

■ *Integrating and maintaining the change in practice*—Once the change in nursing practice has been integrated, maintain the change through development of evaluation criteria that allow for frequent reassessment of the change and the interventions that were used to implement it. Planned change principles should be used at this point, with administration providing the infrastructure and resources needed to implement the change (Duffy, 2004).

This chapter has illustrated the ever-strengthening relationship of the DNP clinician to the research process and patient care outcomes. This practitioner's educational background and capacity for fulfilling multiple roles in the nursing community prepare the DNP graduate to provide unique contributions to nursing research in all areas of the healthcare community. Subsequent chapters will break down the specific areas of the research process into reality-focused, manageable sections that can be implemented in any practice setting that is the focus of the DNP clinician.

■ LEARNING ENHANCEMENT TOOLS

1. You are a DNP graduate who is employed in a large hospital in the area of quality improvement. You have found that a large number of medication errors typically occur on a particular surgical floor when the unit admits more than six post-operative patients per shift.

    a. You are interested in developing a protocol to decrease the number of medication errors. How can this be addressed through a systematic review?

    b. After performing the systematic review, you opt to develop clinical practice guidelines.

    How should this process most appropriately occur?

2. You are a DNP graduate who is working in the area of risk management in a large medical practice. You find that evidence seems to indicate a need to manage pre-operative anxiety more effectively in the patient population in order to achieve better post-operative patient outcomes. Describe the process of translating this evidence into clinical practice.

3. You are a DNP graduate who is functioning as a clinical coordinator in a large psychiatric facility that treats primarily adolescents. You note that a few of your patients seem to achieve a more manageable level of anxiety when they practice the technique of journaling. You are interested in determining whether this would be an effective technique to use with all of the adolescent patients who are experiencing a high level of anxiety. How would you want to frame the focused question regarding this clinical situation to accurately implement evidence-based nursing?

    a. You have developed the focused question, implemented the literature search, and begun the critical appraisal of the research evidence. You determine that validity is present, but the degree of generalizability to other patient populations will be smaller than you had originally envisioned. What should you do?

    b. You develop a plan based on the individual patient's input, available evidence, and clinical expertise.

    The plan is implemented and performance is evaluated using a combination of audits and peer assessment. The evaluation indicates that the plan was not as effective as you had hoped it would be. What should you do?

4. You are a DNP graduate who is functioning in an education position in a large teaching medical center that is university-affiliated. You are concerned that the IV catheter insertion technique that is currently being used with new registered nurses is not as effective as other methods.

    a. How would you perform a systematic review of the evidence on this subject?

    b. Once the systematic review of the evidence is completed, how would you design new clinical practice guidelines for the facility?

■ RESOURCES

American Association of Colleges of Nursing. (2006). DNP roadmap task force report. Retrieved September 25, 2009, from www.aacn.nche.edu/DNP/pdf/Essentials.pdf

Lenz, E. (2005). The practice doctorate in nursing: An idea whose time has come. *Online Journal of Issues in Nursing, 10*(3). Retrieved September 25, 2009, from www.medscape.com/viewarticle/514543

Marion, L., O'Sullivan, A., Crabtree, K., Price, M., & Fontana S. (2003). Curriculum models for the practice doctorate in nursing. *Topics in Advanced Practice Nursing eJournal.* Retrieved from www.medscape.com/viewarticle/500742

Mundinger, M. (2005). Who's who in nursing: Bringing clarity to the doctor of nursing practice. *Nursing Outlook, 53,* 173–176.

PEW Health Professions Commission. (1995). *Reforming health care workforce regulation: Policy considerations for the 21st century.* San Francisco: Pew Health Professions.

Wall, B., Novak, J., & Wilkerson, S. (2005). Doctor of Nursing Practice program development: Reengineering health care. *Journal of Nursing Education, 44*(5), 396–403.

■ WEBSITES FOR ADDITIONAL INFORMATION ON EVIDENCE-BASED PRACTICE

Agency for Health Care Research and Quality. www.ahrq.gov

EPIQ (Effective Practice, Informatics, and Quality Improvement). www.health.auckland.ac.nz/population-health/epidemiology-biostats/epiq

Evidence-Based Nursing. http://ebn.bmj.com

The Ovid Experience. www.ovid.com

The Cochrane Collaboration. www.cochrane.org

The Joanna Briggs Institute. www.joannabriggs.edu.au/about/home.php

TRIP (Turning Research into Practice). www.tripdatabase.com/index.html

■ REFERENCES

American Association of Colleges of Nursing. (2006). *The essentials of doctoral education for advanced nursing practice.* Retrieved September 26, 2009, from www.aacn.nche.edu/DNP/pdf/Essentials.pdf

Apold, S. (2008). The Doctor of Nursing Practice: Looking back, moving forward. *Journal for Nurse Practitioners, 4*(2), 101–107.

Association of Operating Room Nurses. (2006). *AORN white paper: Doctor of Nursing Practice.* Retrieved September 25, 2009, from http://www.aorn.org/docs/assets/F2DD0BBA-EA36-235F-8C197F312749F608/Ref_Doctor_of_Nursing_Practice_-_REVISED.pdf

Auburn University at Montgomery. (2009). *Institutional review board.* Retrieved March 26, 2010 from http://www.aum.edu/indexm_ektid8178.aspx

DiCenso, A., Ciliska, D., Marks, S., McKibbon, A., Cullum, N., & Thompson, C. (2000). *Evidence-based nursing.* Retrieved September 29, 2009, from www.cebm.utoronto.ca/syllabi/nur/print/whole.htm

Duffy, M. (2004). Resources for building a research utilization program. Retrieved September 30, 2009, from www.medscape.com/viewarticle/495915_print

Flemming, K. (1998). Asking answerable questions. *Evidence Based Nursing, 1,* 36–37.

Forward, L. (2002). A practical guide to conducting a systematic review. *Nursing Times, 98*(2), 36.

Hanchett, M. (2005). Infusion nursing's greatest barrier: The lack of evidence to support evidence-based practice. *Topics in Advanced Practice Nursing.* Retrieved October 1, 2009, from www.medscape.com/viewarticle/507908_print

Mcilvoy, L., & Hinkle, J. (2008). What is evidence-based neuroscience nursing practice? *Journal of Neuroscience Nursing.* Retrieved September 25, 2009, from http://findarticles.com/p/articles/mi_hb6374/is_6_40/ai_n31179123

National Association of Neonatal Nurses. (n.d.). *Understanding the Doctor of Nursing Practice (DNP): Evolution, perceived benefits and challenges.* Retrieved September 25, 2009, from www.nann.org/pdf/DNPEntry.pdf

Pipe, T., Wellik, K., Buchda, V., Hansen, C., & Martyn, D. (2005). Implementing evidence-based nursing practice. *MedSurg Nursing.* Retrieved September 25, 2009, from http://ajm.sagepub.com/cgi/reprint/22/3/148.pdf

Rosswurm, M., & Larrabee, J. (1999). A model for change to evidence-based practice image. *Journal of Nursing Scholarship, 31*(4), 317–322.

Rutgers College of Nursing. (2007). *DNP Program in Nursing handbook for students.* Retrieved September 25, 2009, from www.nursing.rutgers.edu/files/DNPHandbook07.pdf

Thompson, C., Cullum, N., McCaughan, D., Sheldon, T., & Raynor, P. (2007). Nurses, information use, and clinical decisions making—the real world potential for evidence-based decisions in nursing. *Evidence Based Nursing, 7,* 68–72.

Developing the
Researchable Problem

2

■ OBJECTIVES

Upon completion of this chapter, the reader should be prepared to:

1 Discuss the elements needed to formulate a research question, specifically discussing the PICO process of developing a research question.

2 Utilize sample scenarios to formulate suitable research questions.

3 Discuss the development of a testable hypothesis.

4 Describe the different categories of hypotheses: research vs. statistical, directional vs. nondirectional.

5 Determine when it would be most appropriate to utilize a research question and when it would be most appropriate to utilize a hypothesis.

6 Discuss the difference between a directional hypothesis and a nondirectional hypothesis.

7 Discuss the difference between a research hypothesis and a statistical hypothesis.

8 Discuss the relationship of a hypothesis to the theoretical framework.

9 Distinguish between the conceptual framework and the theoretical framework.

10 Describe the different categories of nursing theories: grand, midrange, and microrange.

11 Describe the difference between inductive reasoning and deductive reasoning.

12 Discuss the process of selecting an appropriate theoretical framework.

SELECTION OF THE RESEARCH PROBLEM AND DEVELOPMENT OF THE RESEARCH QUESTION

The selection of the **research problem** is arguably the most important step in the research process, for if the problem is not viable and therefore testable, the entire process may be implemented in vain, wasting valuable man-hours and financial resources while generating nothing more than frustration for the researcher. For the DNP clinician, the research problem must above all relate to some area of practice. The germ of the idea can come directly from patients or colleagues, or more indirectly from the auditing process if the clinician functions in quality management or nursing administration (Fitzpatrick, 2007).

The DNP clinician must select a research problem that will contribute to evidence-based practice and to the development of either a **hypothesis** or a **research question**. The development of hypotheses and their proper usage will be discussed in the next section. According to Cluett (2002), four components will indicate that the researcher has developed a research question that is rooted in an evidence-based practice problem:

- The patient group or patient condition is clearly identified.
- There is an issue or intervention that is being investigated, such as a method of patient care or a specific diagnostic test.
- There is a specified way for a baseline measurement to be made as well as a method for comparison.
- An outcome or result is indicated.

In order for the researcher to keep these elements in mind while developing the research question, Cluett (2002) has suggested using the acronym PICO:

- P = the specified patient or target population
- I = the issue or intervention being investigated
- C = the comparison being made
- O = the outcome that may be the result

An example of an acceptable evidence-based practice question would be: Does use of a pain scale reduce the patient's experience of pain post-operatively? In this case,

- P = Patient is undergoing a surgical procedure.
- I = Patient is taught how to measure pain using a pain scale.
- C = The pain level without using a pain scale is compared to the pain level when using a pain scale.
- O = The patient has verbalized or indicated experience of post-operative pain.

The impetus for a researchable problem frequently may arise from a clinical situation the researcher notes. In addition, the DNP clinician may make an observation in his or her daily practice and wonder whether the clinical issue is coincidental or fact-based. A researchable problem may arise from reading journal articles in the DNP graduate's field of practice. Research articles typically state areas for further study that have arisen from that particular manuscript. Often an article will state that a recommendation is made for replication of the original study with a different population of patients or using a different type of methodology (Beyea, 2000). As potential researchable problems arise during the course of a typical practice-oriented day, the researcher should maintain a pocket-sized notebook specifically to jot down such thoughts. At the end of the day, additional details can be recorded and then Internet search engines can be used to review the literature that is readily available on the topic. This will aid in the decision of whether the problem is manageable for the researcher, practical to implement in the form of research, and of sufficient interest to the researcher to be the focus of a lengthy project (Van Cott & Smith, 2009).

The researcher should also consider several practical concerns while formulating the research question:

- Is the research question one that could be easily understood by readers who are not nurses? This will help ensure the research report can be formulated into an article that could be published, because the broader the audience, the more likely that publication will occur. Furthermore, the nature of the practice-oriented doctorate incorporates elements of multiple fields of study, including management, economics, finance, and psychology, to name only a few. It is important to strive to appeal to the wide audience of professionals who practice in these areas.
- Is the answer to the research question not immediately obvious? If the answer is clearly obvious, the problem has no researchable basis.
- Can the research question be answered in the time available to the researcher? If the question requires an indeterminately long period of time to be answered, it will not be practical as a researchable problem.
- Can the research question be answered using the financial and personnel resources available to the researcher? If the question would require more money and personnel than the researcher has available, it is not practical as a researchable problem (Learning Domain, 2009). The researcher must be brutally honest regarding his or her own skills and resources—if the project would require hiring additional personnel to fill in knowledge gaps, and funds for such personnel are lacking, the researcher must strongly consider either phrasing the research question in a different manner or selecting a new topic.

APPROPRIATE USE OF A RESEARCH QUESTION

A research question is most often used instead of a hypothesis when an **exploratory** or **descriptive study** is being undertaken. This type of qualitative research design is frequently used when there is a lack of literature in an area of interest to the researcher. The descriptive findings that are often generated in qualitative studies can provide the basis for further research that will utilize hypotheses. As previously mentioned, the sole intention of exploratory research designs is to make the researcher more familiar with the phenomena being investigated so that additional, more precise research questions can be generated as well as hypotheses. These studies can be utilized when the researcher is working with a new phenomenon that has never been thoroughly investigated. Compare this research design to descriptive studies, which are intended to more accurately represent a phenomenon that may have already undergone some previous investigation so that additional research questions and potentially even hypotheses can be generated (Manheim, Rich, & Willnat, 2002). Recognizing that a research question should be written for an exploratory research design when the phenomenon being studied is one that has never been thoroughly investigated before, an acceptable research question could be, "Is the incidence of substance abuse greater in hospice nurses who have experienced cancer in their own families than in hospice nurses who have no first-hand experience with the disease?" Note that there is no attempt to predict any relationship that might exist, although the question is specific enough to provide direction for the study.

APPROPRIATE USE OF A HYPOTHESIS

As previously mentioned, research questions are typically used when an exploratory or descriptive research design is being undertaken. For the most part, hypotheses should be developed for all other types of research projects. Hypotheses can be considered to be a prediction that will help the researcher seek a solution to the research problem. Specifically, a hypothesis is a statement about the relationship between two or more variables, with variables being the properties the researcher is studying. Variables are designated as either the **independent variable** or the **dependent variable**. The independent variable leads to the effect produced in the dependent variable. For example, if the researcher is studying the effect of caffeine intake and test anxiety in students, caffeine intake would be the independent variable leading to the effect, which in this case would be test anxiety or the dependent variable. The dependent variable is actually the one the researcher is primarily concerned with understanding more thoroughly. It is important to understand that although the researcher recognizes that variability in the dependent variable is assumed to depend on changes in the independent variable, there is no implication that a causal relationship is occurring (LoBiondo-Wood & Haber, 2002).

DEVELOPING A TESTABLE HYPOTHESIS

Once the researcher has formulated a researchable problem and has determined that a hypothesis is more appropriate for the research project than a research question, the next step in the research process for the DNP clinician involves developing the testable hypothesis. According to LoBiondo-Wood and Haber (2002), hypotheses serve three purposes for the researcher:

- To provide a connection between theory and the real world of the patient
- To advance knowledge of the researcher through potential new discoveries
- To provide direction for a research project by identifying a possible anticipated outcome of the research

Hypotheses are generated by either **dependent variable** or **deductive reasoning**. If trial and error is used to construct a theory, the hypotheses may be produced by inductive generalization. Hypotheses generated inductively can be prominent in exploratory research, which can be used to construct theories, but they do not help explain phenomena. Once a theory has been stated relating variables in a logical system, hypotheses can be derived from the theory by deductive reasoning (Manheim et al., 2002).

Several characteristics make an acceptable hypothesis, one of which is a relationship statement, which identifies the predicted relationship between the variables. For example, a possible hypothesis for a research project could be "High school students who do not drink caffeinated sodas have a lesser degree of test anxiety in comparison to high school students who drink at least two caffeinated sodas daily." This is an acceptable hypothesis because it makes a predictive statement about the variables, specifically, that caffeine use in high school students has an effect on their level of test anxiety. Note that the direction of the predicted relationship is also specified, in this case, using the phrase "lesser degree" (LoBiondo-Wood & Haber, 2002). Furthermore, an appropriate hypothesis should specify the variables being investigated, the population being studied, and the predicted outcome.

Perhaps the most important characteristic of an acceptable hypothesis is its testability by the researcher. This means that the variables of the hypothesis can be observed, measured, and analyzed. Specifically, this indicates that once the data are collected and analyzed accurately, the hypothesis will be either supported or not supported. Once the hypothesis is tested, the outcome proposed by the hypothesis either will be congruent with the actual outcome that occurs or will be different. A hypothesis can fail to achieve testability if the researcher has not predicted the anticipated outcome, has not utilized observable or measurable variables, or has failed to use objective phrases in wording the hypothesis (LoBiondo-Wood & Haber, 2002).

If a research problem was proposed at the beginning of the research report, the hypothesis should directly respond to that problem. The variables of the hypothesis should be understandable to the reader. A criterion that is related to testability is the idea of the hypothesis being stated in such a way as to be clearly supported or not supported. Although the more evidence provided the more likely it is for a hypothesis to be accepted, hypotheses are ultimately never proven (LoBiondo-Wood & Haber, 2002).

A hypothesis can be formulated in such a way as to be directional or nondirectional. A **directional hypothesis** specifies the predicted direction of the relationship between the independent and dependent variables. Some proponents of directional hypotheses argue that researchers naturally have expectations about the outcomes of their research, and thus may be potentially biased. An example of a directional hypothesis would be "An oncology floor staffed with at least 75 percent registered nurses is positively related to patients verbalizing a decreased level of pain and nausea." A hypothesis that is deductive and is derived from a **theoretical framework** is usually directional. This means that the theory will provide the rationale for proposing that a relationship between variables will have a particular outcome. If there is no theoretical framework to provide rationale, a **nondirectional hypothesis** may be more appropriately utilized. Even if a theoretical framework is used as a base for a nondirectional hypothesis, it usually is not as fully developed as a directional hypothesis would be. A nondirectional hypothesis indicates the existence of a relationship between variables but does not specify the predicted direction. An example would be, "There will be a difference in the level of anxiety reported by nursing faculty who participate in a weekly focus group on current research." Researchers who favor the nondirectional hypothesis believe that this format is more objective and impartial than the directional hypothesis (LoBiondo-Wood & Haber, 2002).

Just as a hypothesis can be categorized as directional or nondirectional, it can also be categorized as a **statistical hypothesis** or a **research hypothesis**. A research hypothesis is also called a **scientific hypothesis**. The research hypothesis consists of a statement about the expected relationship among the variables and indicates what the outcome of the study is expected to be. If statistically significant findings are obtained for a research hypothesis, the hypothesis is supported. The statistical hypothesis is also called the **null hypothesis**, and states that there is no relationship between the independent and dependent variables. If a statistically significant relationship emerges between the variables at a specific level of significance, the null hypothesis is rejected and consequently the research hypothesis is accepted. An example of a null hypothesis would be, "There will be no difference in the level of anxiety reported by nursing faculty who participate in a weekly focus group on current research and those nursing faculty who do not participate in such a focus group" (LoBiondo-Wood & Haber, 2002).

LoBiondo-Wood and Haber (2002) have provided specific steps that would indicate whether a research question or a hypothesis should be developed, and if a hypothesis is most appropriate, the type of hypothesis to formulate:

1. The literature review and theoretical framework are examined to determine the concepts to be studied.
2. The primary purpose of the study is determined as well as the research problem.
3. If the primary purpose is exploratory, descriptive, or hypothesis-generating, then research questions should be generated.
4. If the primary purpose is to test causal or associative relationships, then hypotheses should be generated.

An additional characteristic of a sound hypothesis is its consistency with an existing body of knowledge and its basis on sound scientific rationale. The reader of the research study should be able to trace the flow of an idea from the researchable problem to the research question or hypothesis, which also has a direct route to the literature review and the theoretical framework (LoBiondo-Wood & Haber, 2002). The **theoretical** or **conceptual framework** will be discussed in more detail later in this chapter, and the literature review that will generate the theoretical framework will be discussed in Chapter 3. To reiterate, at this point in the research process, the DNP clinician should have:

- Selected a researchable problem that is realistic based on available resources, both financial and personnel, and on the accessible patient population
- Sketched out a rough enough outline of what is being investigated so as to determine if an exploratory or descriptive research design is needed
- Determined whether a research question or a hypothesis is more appropriate for the project

The next step in the process will be to determine a theoretical framework for the project, and that will guide the wording of the hypothesis, assuming that a hypothesis is more appropriate for the project than a research question. The theoretical framework will assist the DNP clinician in determining whether the hypothesis should be directional or nondirectional, statistical, or research in nature.

USE OF A THEORETICAL OR CONCEPTUAL FRAMEWORK

It is important to recognize the link that exists among nursing theory, practice, and research. Just as nursing theory guides nursing practice, it is practice that tends to generate the questions that will ultimately form research questions or hypotheses, and it is research that will aid in the development of guidelines for practice. The terms *conceptual framework* and *theoretical framework* are frequently used interchangeably, although it is important to remember that whereas a concept is a mental image of an idea, theories are made up of interrelated concepts. For example, anxiety is a concept, and a theory could use the concepts of testing and anxiety to attempt to predict how test anxiety can fluctuate in junior year nursing students. The different categories of nursing theories will be discussed briefly in the following paragraphs prior to discussing the process of selecting a theoretical framework to guide the research project.

Nursing literature frequently uses the terms *grand theory, midrange theory,* and *microrange theory* to categorize nursing theories. A **grand theory** is the most abstract level of theory that establishes a knowledge base for nursing. Such a theory tends to include concepts such as "person," "health," and "environment." Grand theories include those proposed by the great nursing theorists such as Dorothea Orem, Martha Rogers, and Imogene King, to name only a few (LoBiondo-Wood & Haber, 2002). In comparison, **midrange theories** incorporate nursing practice and research into ideas that are integral to the discipline. Finally, a low-level **microrange theory** could actually be synonymous with a hypothesis. It contains concrete concepts that are linked to form a statement that will be examined in practice and research. The beauty of the microrange theory is that DNP clinicians, because of their unique relationship to both practice and research due to the nature of the practice doctorate, are in a position every day to generate such low-level theories (LoBiondo-Wood & Haber, 2002).

Once the DNP clinician understands the types of nursing theories that make up theoretical frameworks, the next step in the research process involves selection of a framework that is appropriate for the research project and will provide direction and organization for the study. In order to select the appropriate framework, the researcher must determine whether inductive or deductive reasoning will be used throughout the process. It is the choice of inductive or deductive reasoning that will determine whether a conceptual framework or a more structured theoretical framework should be used to guide the project. If the DNP clinician chooses to use inductive reasoning when developing his or her research project, he or she will need to start with the details of experience with nursing practice and moving toward a general picture. In comparison, deductive reasoning can also be used to develop the project. This involves starting with the general picture or theory and moving toward a direction for nursing practice (LoBiondo-Wood & Haber, 2002).

LoBiondo-Wood and Haber (2002) developed a decision tree that can be broken down to provide direction for the novice researcher on how to decide whether a conceptual or theoretical framework is more appropriate for the research project:

1. The researcher must initially decide whether deductive or inductive reasoning will be used to guide and organize the project:

   - Is the goal to create a structure that will guide the research? In this case, deductive reasoning is being used, and a conceptual framework should be utilized.
   - Is the goal to identify a structure that will guide the research? In this case, deductive reasoning is still being used, but a theoretical framework should be utilized instead.
   - Is the goal to begin to collect data to address a research question or hypothesis? In this case, inductive reasoning is being used, and a framework does not have to be specified at this point because it will be based on the data collected and the literature review.

2. If a theoretical framework is judged to be most appropriate for this project, then the researcher must select the type of theory that will serve as the basis of the framework: grand, midrange, or microrange.

   Once the type of reasoning that will guide the project has been determined, the researcher needs to specify a framework and determine whether a conceptual or theoretical framework will be used. If he or she decides that inductive reasoning will be used and there is not a need to specify the type of framework to be used at this point, then the researcher should proceed with the literature review. It is that step that will be the focus of the next chapter.

■ LEARNING ENHANCEMENT TOOLS

1. You are a DNP graduate who is functioning in a management position. You want to find out if using 8-hour shifts rather than 12-hour shifts in an intensive care unit will lead to a decreased number of medication errors. Formulate a research question for this inquiry, specifying each element of the PICO acronym.

2. You are a DNP graduate who is functioning in a nurse manager position. You want to find out if using a differently designed medication cart will lead to a decreased number of medication errors on a medical-surgical floor. Formulate a research question for this inquiry, specifying each element of the PICO acronym.

3. You are a DNP student who is interested in performing a research project on nurses' perceptions of nurse co-workers who continue to function in their current job role while undergoing treatment for cancer.

   a. Do you think that a research question or a hypothesis would be more appropriate for this study? Give the rationale for your answer.

   b. Write either a research question or a hypothesis for this project based on your answer.

   c. As the researcher, you opt to use a hypothesis for this research project. Write both a directional and a nondirectional hypothesis for the project.

   d. Write a statistical hypothesis for the research project.

4. You are a DNP student who is interested in performing a research project on whether cancer patients' level of pain is affected by being cared for by nurses who use prayer as their primary coping method.

   a. Do you think that a research question or a hypothesis would be more appropriate for this study? Give the rationale for your answer.

   b. Write either a research question or a hypothesis for this project based on your answer.

   c. As the researcher, you opt to use a hypothesis for this research project. Write both a directional and a nondirectional hypothesis for the project.

   d. Write a statistical hypothesis for the research project.

5. You are a DNP student who is interested in performing a research project on whether the children of hospice nurses tend to engage in substance abuse to a greater extent than the children of nurses who work in other areas of patient care.

   a. Do you think that a research question or a hypothesis would be more appropriate for this study? Give the rationale for your answer.

   b. Write either a research question or a hypothesis for this project based on your answer.

   c. As the researcher, you opt to use a hypothesis for this research project. Write both a directional and a nondirectional hypothesis for the project.

   d. Write a statistical hypothesis for the research project.

6. a. Read the passage and determine if research questions or hypotheses are embedded in the material. Do you think that they were appropriate for the selection?

   b. If not, explain your answer and write new ones for the material, writing both directional and nondirectional hypotheses, as well as research and statistical hypotheses.

   c. Can you determine if inductive or deductive reasoning was the basis for the study's organization? Examine your answer.

   d. Can you identify a conceptual or theoretical framework that was utilized?

   e. If you can identify a framework, do you think that the conceptual or theoretical framework that was used was appropriate for the type of study performed? Explain your answer.

> The recent paradigm shift in higher education has directly impacted nursing academia. The shift from teacher-centered teaching to learner-centered learning has resulted in a nursing educational environment that is student-driven "where the faculty guides the individual development of students as needed" (Billings & Halstead, 2005, p. xiii). Nurse educators must consider the unique needs of the individual student and the theoretical constructs of self-directed learning, self-regulation, and learning motivation and the use of educational strategies and support methods to promote and enhance student integration of content value and progression toward intrinsic motivation. Academic learning activities focus on the development of critical thinking skills, autonomous decision making, clinical competence, case management skills, and teaching strategies focused on health promotion and disease management (Billings & Halstead, 2005; Cowman, 1998; Keating, 2005; Magena & Chabeli, 2005; Välimäki, Itkonen, Joutsela, Koistinen, Laine, Paimensalo, Siiskonen, Suikkanen, Ylitörmänen, Ylönon, & Helenius, 1999).
>
> Multiple studies on academic self-regulation have been conducted in nursing education (Bahn, 2007; Birks, Chapman, & Francis, 2006; Cooley, 2008; Delaney & Piscopo, 2004; Hudson, 1992; Mansouri, Soltani, Rahemi, Nasab, Ayatollahi, Nekooeian, 2006; McEwan & Goldenberg, 1999; Mullen, 2007; Nilsson & Stomberg, 2008; Smedley, 2007; Thompson, 1992; Tutor, 2006; Välimäki, Itkonen, Joutsela, Koistinen, Laine, Paimensalo, Siiskonen, Suikkanen, Ylitörmänen, Ylönon, & Helenius, 1999; Zuzelo, 2001); however, a review of the literature revealed that no study has been conducted in nursing education to determine the presence or absence of academic motivation differences between groups of nursing students.

■ RESOURCES

Alligood, M., & Marriner-Tomey, A. (2002). *Nursing theory: Utilization and application.* St. Louis, MO: Mosby.

Barrett, E. (2002). The nurse theorists: 21st-century updates—Callista Roy. *Nursing Science Quarterly, 15,* 308–310.

Clarke, P., Killeen, M., Messmer, P., & Sieloff, C. (2008). Practitioner as theorist: A reprise. *Nursing Science Quarterly, 21,* 315–321.

Cody, W. (ed.). (2006). *Philosophical and theoretical perspectives for advanced nursing.* Sudbury, MA: Jones and Bartlett.

Fawcett, J. (2002). The nurse theorists: 21st-century updates—Jean Watson. *Nursing Science Quarterly, 15,* 214–219.

Fawcett, J. (2003). The nurse theorists: 21st century updates—Martha E. Rogers. *Nursing Science Quarterly, 16,* 44–51.

Fawcett, J. (2004). *Contemporary nursing knowledge: Analysis and evaluation of nursing models and theories.* Philadelphia: F.A. Davis Company.

Fawcett, J. (2007). Envisioning nursing in 2050 through the eyes of nurse theorists: King, Neuman, and Roy. *Nursing Science Quarterly, 20,* 108.

Fawcett, J. (2005). *Analysis and evaluation of contemporary nursing knowledge: Nursing models and theories.* Philadelphia: F.A. Davis Company.

Fitzpatrick, J., & Whall, A. (2005). *Conceptual models of nursing: Analysis and application.* Upper Saddle River, NJ: Pearson Prentice Hall.

Leininger, M., & McFarland, M. (eds.). (2006). *Culture care diversity and universality: A worldwide nursing theory.* Sudbury, MA: Jones and Bartlett.

Madrid, M. (1997). *Patterns of Rogerian knowing.* New York: NLN Press.

Neumann, B., & Fawcett, J. (2002). *The Neumann systems model.* Upper Saddle River, NJ: Prentice Hall.

Pilkington, F. (2003). Conceptual models of nursing: International in scope and substance? The case of the Roy adaptation model. *Nursing Science Quarterly, 16,* 315–318.

Pilkington, F. (2007). Envisioning nursing in 2050 through the eyes of nurse theorists: Katie Eriksson and Margaret Newman. *Nursing Science Quarterly, 20,* 200.

Pilkington, F. (2007). Envisioning nursing in 2050 through the eyes of nurse theorists: Leininger and Watson. *Nursing Science Quarterly, 20,* 8.

Pilkington, F. (2007). Envisioning nursing in 2050 through the eyes of nurse theorists: Rosemarie Rizzo Parse and Martha E. Rogers. *Nursing Science Quarterly, 20,* 307–308.

Polifroni, E., & Welch, M. (1999). *Perspectives on philosophy of science in nursing.* Philadelphia: Lippicott.

Powers, B., & Knapp, T. (2006). *Dictionary of nursing theory and research.* Philadelphia: Springer.

Reed, P. (2002). What is nursing science? *Nursing Science Quarterly, 15,* 51–60.

Reed, P. (2004). Conceptual models of nursing: International in scope and substance? The case of the Neumann systems model. *Nursing Science Quarterly, 17,* 50–54.

Renpenning, K., & Taylor, S. (2003). *Self care theory in nursing.* Philadelphia: Springer.

Sitzman, K., & Eichelberger, L. (2004). *Understanding the work of nurse theorists: A creative beginning.* Sudbury, MA: Jones and Bartlett.

■ WEBSITES

Clayton State University School of Nursing Theory Link Page. http://nursing.clayton.edu/eichelberger/nursing.htm

University of San Diego. http://nursing.sdsu.edu

NurseScribe. www.enursescribe.com

■ GLOSSARY

conceptual framework Creates a structure that guides the research project.

deductive reasoning Thought process in which reasoning moves from the general to the specific, using theory to produce a hypothesis.

dependent variable The variable of interest in a hypothesis; the variable that is influenced by the independent variable.

descriptive study Describes a specific population of research subjects.

directional hypothesis Specifies the predicted direction of the relationship between the independent and dependent variables.

exploratory study: Type of research design that explores a phenomenon in order to provide additional insight for the researcher.

grand theory Most abstract level of theory that establishes a knowledge base for nursing.

hypothesis Statement of the proposed relationship between the dependent variable (variable of interest) and the independent variable (variable influencing the dependent variable).

independent variable The variable in a hypothesis that influences the dependent variable.

inductive reasoning Thought process in which reasoning moves from specific to general; used when the researcher collects data to address a research question or hypothesis.

microrange theory Synonymous with a hypothesis; considered to be concrete concepts that are linked so as to form a statement that can be examined in practice and research.

midrange theory Incorporates nursing practice and research into ideas that are integral to nursing.

nondirectional hypothesis Indicates the existence of a relationship between variables, but does not specify the predicted direction.

null hypothesis States that there is no relationship between the dependent and independent variables in a research study.

research hypothesis Statement regarding the expected relationship between the dependent and independent variables; synonymous with the scientific hypothesis.

research problem Issue that will be investigated by the researcher and will generate either a research question or a hypothesis.

research question   Most frequently used in an exploratory or descriptive research study; a research question rooted in an evidence-based practice problem identifies the patient group or patient condition, provides an issue or intervention that is being investigated, specifies a way for a baseline measurement to be made as well as a method for comparison, and indicates an outcome or result.

scientific hypothesis   Synonymous with the research hypothesis.

statistical hypothesis   Synonymous with the null hypothesis.

theoretical framework   Identifies a structure that will serve to guide the research project.

■ REFERENCES FOR GLOSSARY

LoBiondo-Wood, G., & Haber, J. (2002). *Nursing research: Methods, critical appraisal, and utilization.* St. Louis, MO: Elsevier.

University of Maryland Medical Center—Nursing Research Council. (n.d.) *Glossary of research terms.* Retrieved October 14, 2009, from http://www.umm.edu/nursing/docs/glossary_research_terms.pdf

■ REFERENCES

Beyea, S. (2000). Getting started in nursing research and tips for success. *AORN Journal.* Retrieved October 4, 2009, from http://findarticles.com/p/articles/mi_m0FSL/is_6_72/ai_68534735

Cluett, E. (2002). Evidence-based practice. In E. Cluett & R. Bluff (eds.), *Principles and practice of research in nursing and midwifery (pp. 33–53).* London: Churchill Livingstone.

Fitzpatrick, J. (2007). Finding the research for evidence-based practice. *Nursing Times, 103*(17), 32–33.

Learning Domain. (2009). *Module 2: Stating the research problem.* Retrieved October 4, 2009, from http://www.learningdomain.com/module_2.stating.problem.doc

LoBiondo-Wood, G., & Haber, J. (2002). *Nursing research: Methods, critical appraisal, and utilization.* St. Louis, MO: Elsevier.

Manheim, J., Rich, R., & Willnat, L. (2002). *Empirical political analysis: Research methods in political science.* New York: Addison Wesley Longman.

Terry, A. (2006). *An analysis of Alabama's RN workforce: 2006.* Retrieved October 6, 2009, from www.abn.state.al.us

Van Cott, A., & Smith, M. (2009). Nursing research: Tips and tools to simplify the process. *Dermatology Nursing.* Retrieved October 4, 2009, from http://findarticles.com/p/articles/mi_hb6366/is_3_21/ai_n31950871

Conducting a
Literature Review

3

■ OBJECTIVES

Upon completion of this chapter, the reader should be prepared to:

1 Discuss the process of critically analyzing data sources.

2 Identify databases that may be useful in locating data sources to include in a literature review.

3 Identify the purpose of the literature review.

4 Discuss important characteristics of a research article's Introduction section.

5 Discuss important characteristics of a research article's Methods section.

6 Discuss important characteristics of a research article's Discussion/Conclusion section.

7 Describe the importance of reliability to the research appraiser.

8 Describe the importance of statistical significance to the research appraiser.

9 Discuss the importance of external validity to the research appraiser.

10 Discuss the difference between a primary data source and a secondary data source.

PURPOSE OF THE LITERATURE REVIEW

As mentioned in the previous chapter, the reader of a research study should be able to trace the flow of an idea from the researchable problem to the research question or hypothesis, which also has a direct route to the **literature review** and the theoretical framework. This chapter will discuss the development of the literature review. A literature review is literally an account of what has been published on a topic by researchers, critically appraising each data source included for its relevance rather than simply summarizing what the author originally stated. The literature review is guided by the research question or the hypothesis. A literature review should discuss conceptual theories or models from nursing as well as other fields that will be used to examine the problem at hand. Because the review will reveal inconsistencies or unanswered questions about a subject, a correctly formulated literature review will allow for the research question or hypothesis to be further refined, if necessary (LoBiondo-Wood & Haber, 2002).

Apart from merely seeking out the literature that is available on a topic, the literature review must be formed using the researcher's critical appraisal skills. This means the researcher is able to apply principles of analysis to identify unbiased research studies, accurately assessing the data sources so that the strengths and weaknesses of each are discussed. If the literature review is developed appropriately, the reader should find it to be relevant, appropriate, and useful. The review should never deteriorate into simply a list summarizing one document after another (Taylor & Procter, 2009).

Ultimately, the purpose of the literature review is to establish the value of previous research on the study topic. The literature review should:

- Address a question not investigated in the literature previously and generate new research questions
- Fill in a knowledge gap that has been found to exist in previously conducted research or reveal the existence of a knowledge gap in the field for the first time
- Test an existing model under previously untested conditions or using a different patient population
- Correct for errors in previously conducted research, or reveal existing errors for the first time
- Resolve research findings that appear to be contradicting each other and determine the accuracy of reported findings (Taylor & Procter, 2009)

STRUCTURING THE LITERATURE REVIEW

A literature review most commonly uses one of three formats. First is a discussion and evaluation of previous research beginning in chronological order. This would be used when the DNP researcher is utilizing studies that are evaluated beginning with the earliest published report and moving chronologically until the most recently reported is discussed. Second is a literature review organized around a central concept. An example of this type of organization would be when the researcher is studying the patient's pain experience as the overall research concept. The literature review would then organize studies according to instruments used to operationalize or measure the degree of pain the patient experienced, treatments utilized for relief of pain, and the long-term effects of chronic pain. Finally, the literature review can be organized to first discuss an evaluation of studies that apply to the general research topic, and then move toward the more narrowly defined research topic of the researcher (O'Sullivan & Rassel, 1999). This could be used if a researcher first evaluated studies on the topic of the patient's pain experience and then moved to the more narrow focus of the experience of pain in cancer patients under the age of 21. In addition to these types of reviews, a derivation of a literature review that is frequently utilized is a meta-analysis. This consists of the use of quantitative procedures to statistically combine the results of studies. A small meta-analysis is considered to use no more than 50 articles (American Psychological Association, 2010).

As the author is developing the literature review, locating sources, and beginning the process of initial evaluation of data sources, he or she should consider:

- Are there gaps in the knowledge available on this subject? If so, identify the specific areas that are lacking. This will generate new research questions and potentially new research studies.
- Are there areas of further study that have been identified by other scholars that may serve as sources of additional research for a DNP researcher?
- How could these areas of further study impact the research project currently underway?
- Do potential relationships exist between concepts that would generate additional researchable hypotheses?
- How have other researchers defined and measured key concepts that will be used in the current research project? Do these definitions and measurements appear to be accurate and reliable?
- Have other researchers used data sources, including topic-specific websites, that the DNP researcher was not aware of?
- What key words can be identified to help guide the researcher's search for information?
- How does the current research project relate to the work already generated by other researchers? (F.D. Bluford Library, n.d.)

CRITICAL APPRAISAL OF THE LITERATURE

Because of the nature of the DNP researcher's practice-oriented doctoral program, the DNP student must be particularly scrupulous in ensuring that each source included as part of the literature review contributes in some manner to evidence-based nursing practice. In order to ensure that the literature review is the result of a critical appraisal on the part of the researcher, Taylor and Procter (2009) have developed a series of questions the researcher should ask him- or herself regarding each data source undergoing critical evaluation:

- Has the author clearly formulated a problem statement? If not, is it at least clearly implied?
- Is the problem's significance established in terms of scope, severity, and relevance to the nursing profession?
- Could the defined problem have been approached more effectively from another perspective? If so, what perspective could have been selected?
- If the data source is a research study, what was the author's research design? Was the design appropriate for the type of research study implemented?
- What is the theoretical framework? Was it appropriate, or should a conceptual framework have been used instead?
- Is there a relationship between the theoretical or conceptual framework and research question or hypothesis, or is a disconnect evident?
- If a research study is being evaluated, can the study population, interventions, and outcomes be clearly identified?
- How accurate and valid are the measurements utilized—do they measure what they were intended to measure? Would the same results be obtained if the study was replicated?
- Is the analysis of the data that was performed in the study both accurate and relevant to the research question or hypothesis?
- Are the conclusions appropriately based on the analysis of the data?
- How does the data source contribute to the understanding of the problem under scrutiny, and how does it contribute to evidence-based practice?
- What are the strengths as well as the limitations of the research article? Do the limitations outweigh any benefits derived from the implementation of the research?
- How does the data source relate to the researcher's research question or hypothesis?

COLLECTING DATA SOURCES

As the DNP researcher begins the process of searching out data sources that will be critically appraised for possible inclusion in the literature review, he or she should initially ensure that the topic that is the central focus of the research question or hypothesis is absolutely clear. The researcher should

remain focused on the practice-related topic as well as the basic patient population being studied.

Next, the researcher should identify terms that are unique to the study. For
example, if the study uses the research question "Is the incidence of substance
abuse greater in hospice nurses who have experienced cancer in their own
families than in hospice nurses who have no first-hand experience with the disease?," then the unique terms that will be researched will be *substance abuse*,
hospice, and *nurses*. As the researcher uses these terms to initiate a computerized search for data sources, broad-spectrum medical/nursing databases
should initially be utilized, such as Cumulative Index to Nursing and Allied
Health Literature (CINAHL), Index Medicus (MEDLINE), and Educational
Resources Information Center (ERIC). This will provide the researcher with
a large volume of articles that can then undergo critical appraisal. In addition,
the use of multiple databases increases the researcher's access to multiple
sources, allows for searching of the key terms selected, provides for ease of
document retrieval, and increases the credibility of the search (LoBiondo-Wood
& Haber, 2002).

Initiating the Process of Critical Appraisal

A crucial skill that the DNP researcher must practice as part of the process of
formulating a literature review that contains credible data sources is that of critical appraisal of the research. Wooten and Ross (2005) recommend breaking a
journal article down into its component parts in order to appraise it efficiently.
Initially, the DNP researcher should look for a journal article that is contained
in a publication that is peer-reviewed. This means the study underwent a pre-
publication review by experts in the specialty field to ensure the information
it contained was both unbiased and accurate. The researcher must identify
whether the source is primary or secondary. A **primary source** is one that was
written by the person who either developed a theory or conducted the research
being reported. A **secondary source** is written by someone other than the person who developed the theory or conducted the research (LoBiondo-Wood &
Haber, 2002). A literature review should contain a majority of primary sources.

Next, the DNP researcher should look at the authors' qualifications. Are
the authors' credentials appropriate for the topic being researched? Have they
published other studies on similar subjects? For example, if the research is
written using a population of intensive care patients, is the author a nurse
with an intensive care practice background? If not, the author may lack credibility. Also, look at any funding sources the author used. Can it be determined
if the research is biased in such a way as to reflect favorably on the funding
organization?

Critical Appraisal of the Abstract

Once the DNP researcher has determined that the article in question is included in a peer-reviewed journal and that the author has sufficient qualifications to generate the research, he or she should take a cursory look at the study's **secondary source**, bearing in mind that the study cannot be accurately evaluated based on its abstract alone. The researcher should read the abstract to find a summary of the purpose; problem under investigation; participants; procedures utilized including a brief mention of the sample size, outcome measures, data gathering procedures, and research design; as well as results and the author's conclusions (American Psychological Association, 2010). This abstract appraisal may indicate the need to pursue a more detailed review of the article or may show that the article is not needed for inclusion in the literature review (Wooten & Ross, 2005).

Critical Appraisal of the Introduction

The next step in the critical appraisal of the literature involves breaking down the article into its individual parts that form the true "skeleton" of the research report: the introduction, methods, results, and discussion and/or conclusions. The **introduction** section should include the author's research question or hypothesis that clearly states the population being studied, the intervention being proposed, the comparison that will occur, and the expected outcome. The study should be based on research that has previously been conducted on the same topic or one very similar, so there should also be a discussion of previously conducted studies and a review of their findings. A well-crafted introduction should tell the reader:

- *Why the problem is important*—The reader should be able to understand the importance of the topic both to the individual nurse and to the nursing profession.
- *How the study relates to previous work in the area*—This will show a clear connection with the theoretical or conceptual framework.
- *If other aspects of the study have been reported prior to this study, how this report differs from the previous reports*—The study should be able to indicate what it will provide to the reader that other studies have not.
- *How the study relates to previous work in the area*
- *The relationship of the hypotheses and research design to each other.*
- *The theoretical and practical implications of the study that have been identified* (American Psychological Association, 2010).

If the introduction section doesn't include a clearly stated research question or hypothesis, the novice researcher should consider it a poor addition to his or her own literature review for the project (Wooten & Ross, 2005).

Critical Appraisal of the Methods Section

When the DNP student begins appraisal of the **methods** section of an article, he or she will find that this is arguably the most important section in a research report, because it should contain the author's description of exactly what was done in the research as well as how it was implemented. It is the methods section that tells the DNP student about the reliability of the research being scrutinized—if this study were replicated, would the same results be achieved? If not, then the research has a very low degree of reliability and should not be included in the literature review.

The methods section should include a concise description of the procedure for data collection. If the author designed an instrument for data collection, such as a questionnaire or other tool that participants used during the research, then a copy should be included in this section. If statistical calculations are needed to make this section's description of the author's procedures more clear, were they included? This section should also include a detailed description of the population of research subjects, including how they were selected. Major demographic characteristics, level of education, socioeconomic status, and topic-specific characteristics should be included, such as number of years actively licensed as a registered nurse. Participant characteristics may help the researcher determine the extent to which findings can be generalized, or applied, to other populations (American Psychological Association, 2010).

The methods section should include a discussion of the technique used to determine sample size and randomization of subjects, if probability sampling was utilized. If nonprobability sampling was utilized and this randomization of subjects did not occur, the author should clearly state this and the reasoning for opting not to randomize. The methods section should also contain criteria for including subjects in the study population. Was the population studied large enough to validate the research on the problem being studied? If the author presented findings on a population of randomized subjects that yielded a group of five participants, the results of the research, and possibly the credibility of the researcher, will very likely be called into question. The methods section should include information on any agreements that were made with participants as well as any incentives they received for participating. This can include a tangible incentive such as receiving a payment as well as a more esoteric incentive such as awarding continuing education units.

The procedures used for data collection should be described, such as administration of questionnaires, online surveys, or interviews, or conducting of focus groups, as well as any training that was provided to researchers implementing the study. If data are missing, such as would occur if participants failed to complete every question in a questionnaire, procedures designed to deal with the missing information should be discussed (American Psychological Association, 2010). The author should include information on the procedure used to approach an **institutional review board (IRB)** if there was manipulation of human subjects, the agreement made with the IRB, the procedures used to meet ethical standards, and safety monitoring methods instituted (American Psychological Association). In addition, the author should be able to describe the design of the study. Polit and Hungler (2000) describe several characteristics of an acceptable design for a research project:

- The research design should suit the research question or the hypothesis; for example, if the researcher is interested in investigating four variables or areas being studied, then four groups of participants should be used.
- The design should not be biased; if groups of study participants are formed in a nonrandom manner, the threat of bias is always present. Therefore, the article's authors should state how the threat of bias was handled.
- The statistical procedures for analysis of the findings should be appropriate for the research design. If a quantitative research design was selected, were statistics used for analysis appropriate for such a design, or were the statistics primarily descriptive, such as might be used for a qualitative design?

The study should state if subjects were manipulated or randomly selected to specific groups. If control groups were used, they should be described, as well as any interventions that were applied (American Psychological Association, 2010). If the DNP student feels that the methods section presents nebulous details that don't describe how the research was implemented, the article should not be utilized as a reputable source in the literature review (Wooten & Ross, 2005).

Critical Appraisal of the Results Section

After a detailed appraisal of the methods section, the DNP student should move to a review of the research article's **results** section. This is a presentation of the author's findings. If the author used a hypothesis as part of the research study, he or she should be able to state that the hypothesis was accepted or rejected on the basis of statistically significant findings. This means it can be shown that the findings the author obtained are not likely to have resulted from chance at a specific degree of probability. If the hypothesis was rejected, it should be due to a nonsignificant outcome, meaning the findings were shown to possibly result from chance. The study should include all results obtained, even if they do not support the author's original hypothesis or are contrary to the research question. If findings are presented in the form of charts or tables, they should be scrutinized to determine if they are congruent with the rest of the research report. All participants should be accounted for at the conclusion of the study, including those who chose to opt out of the study before its conclusion. When participants choose not to complete a research project it is known as attrition. The author should present findings that have statistical significance, but they should also have clinical significance in some way. This will be particularly important to the DNP student who is preparing a research project that relates to evidence-based practice. The results section should include some measure of the effect size generated in order for the reader to grasp the importance of the study's findings. If serious consequences occurred after interventions were applied, these should be detailed in this section (American Psychological Association, 2010). If the author appears to contradict his or her own findings, the DNP researcher should not include this source in the literature review (Wooten & Ross, 2005).

Critical Appraisal of the Discussion/Conclusions Section

The DNP student should analyze the **discussion** and **conclusions** section of the article. Findings should be traced back in a logical manner to the research question or hypothesis that was investigated. The researcher should evaluate the author's interpretation of findings carefully, looking for feasibility and clinical significance. The discussion and conclusions section should allow the researcher to evaluate and interpret the implications of the results presented in the previous section. If hypotheses were not supported, explanations should be offered. Are the findings meaningful to the audience originally targeted? Were unexpected findings revealed during the course of the study? Were the findings that were uncovered of insufficient magnitude as to be meaningful to readers? The author should include any potential limitations of the research project as well as the generalizability or external validity of the findings. These would include any problems with bias, sample size or inability to random sample, or the type of study design utilized. The author should be able to discuss how the research could be improved upon were it to be replicated (American Psychological Association, 2010).

Critical Appraisal of References

Finally, the DNP researcher should determine whether adequate references were included to provide sufficient credibility, or if the author repeatedly cited his or her own work. The reference list should contain predominantly research published in recent years using primary sources, unless the reference is considered to be a classic in the field. In the reference list, the author should include information on the data source author (or editor in the case of an edited book), publication date of the document, as well as the title of the data source (American Psychological Association, 2010). The DNP researcher also should review any footnotes, tables, or figures included to determine the accuracy and appropriateness of information included. In particular, tables and figures should be reviewed for readability—do they require the reader to review numerous directions and footnotes in order to understand the data presented?

An integral part of the critical appraisal of the articles and other data sources being considered for inclusion in a literature review is the review of the report's treatment of informed consent, confidentiality, and the mandates of the IRB that were used if the research involved manipulation of human subjects. The following chapter discusses the ethics involved in implementing research that involves human subjects and the correct approach to applying to an IRB for a review of a proposed research protocol.

■ BOX 3-1

Checklist for the Critical Appraisal of Data Sources to Determine Suitability for Inclusion in Literature Review

---

1. Abstract
   - Problem being investigated
   - Characteristics of participants
   - Sample size
   - Outcome measures
   - Procedures for data-gathering
   - Research design
   - Findings
     - Confidence intervals
     - Statistical significance levels
   - Conclusion
     - Implications
     - Application to clinical practice

2. Introduction
   • Importance of the problem
   • Review of previous researchers' relevant work
     – Relationship of current research study to previously conducted research
     – Differences between current research study and previously conducted research
   • Hypothesis
   • Research question
   • Conceptual framework
   • Theoretical framework
3. Method
   • Participant characteristics
     – Eligibility criteria
     – Exclusion criteria
     – Demographic characteristics
   • Sampling procedures
     – Settings and location of sampling
     – Agreements made with participants/incentives offered
     – Institutional review board
       ○ Results of review by institutional review board
       ○ Changes made in study to accommodate institutional review board
       ○ Monitoring procedures implemented
     – Determination of sample size
       ○ Desired sample size
       ○ Actual size used
     – If systematic sampling plan implemented, sampling method used
     – Percentage of sample approached that ultimately participated in research
     – Description of self-selection process if such occurred
   • Measures used for data collection
     – If coding was needed, such as for a survey, procedure for coding data
     – Number of coders used
     – Qualifications of coders if used
     – Intercoder reliability
   • Training required of data collectors
   • Research design utilized
     – Experimental
     – Nonexperimental
     – Quasi-experimental
4. Results
   • Total number of participants
   • Periods of recruitment of participants
   • Discussion of problems with statistical assumptions and/or data distributions

(continues)

■   **BOX 3-1 (continued)**

Checklist for the Critical Appraisal of Data Sources to Determine Suitability for Inclusion in Literature Review

- Statistics and data analysis
  - Missing data
    - Possible causes
    - Methods for addressing missing data
  - Statistical software program used for analysis
  - Statistical outcome reported
    - Means
    - Standard deviations
    - Other estimates of precision
    - Other descriptive statistics
    - If inferential statistics reported
      - Direction
      - Magnitude
      - Degrees of freedom
      - *P* value
5. Discussion/Conclusion
   - If research question used, answer derived
   - If hypotheses used, support or nonsupport for each
   - Explanations for the support or nonsupport for all hypotheses
   - Comparison of results derived to work of previous researchers
   - Report of threats to internal validity, including bias
   - Report of precision of measures used
   - Report of weaknesses or limitations noted
   - External validity (generalizability) of findings, including populations to which results could be generalized
   - Implications for further research or policy development

American Psychological Association. (2010). *Publication manual of the American Psychological Association.* Washington, DC: American Psychological Association.

■ **WEBSITES FOR LOCATING SOURCES FOR A LITERATURE REVIEW**

Administration on Aging's Statistics on Aging Population. www.aoa.gov/aoaroot/ aging_statistics/index.aspx

Agency for Healthcare Research and Quality Grants On-Line Database. www.gold.ahrq.gov

AHRQ Patient Safety Network. www.psnet.ahrq.gov/index.aspx

American Association of Colleges of Nursing. www.aacn.nche.edu

American Hospital Association. www.aha.org

Association of periOperative Registered Nurses Patient Safety First Resources. www.aorn.org

Berkeley Systematic Reviews Group. www.medepi.net/meta

Bureau of Economic Analysis. www.bea.gov

Bureau of Labor Statistics. http://stats.bls.gov

Centers for Disease Control and Prevention Emergency Preparedness and Response Site. www.bt.cdc.gov

Centers for Medicare and Medicaid Services. www.cms.hhs.gov

ClinicalTrials.gov. http://clinicaltrials.gov

DataWeb Collaboration Site. www.thedataweb.org

Department of Defense Patient Safety Center. http://dodpatientsafety.usuhs.mil

FedStats. www.fedstats.gov

Health Resources and Services Administration Bureau of Health Professions: Nursing. www.bhpr.hrsa.gov/nursing

Interagency Collaborative on Nursing Statistics. www.iconsdata.org

International Nursing Coalition for Mass Casualty Education. http://www.nursing .vanderbilt.edu/incmce

International Pharmaceutical Abstracts. http://library.dialog.com/bluesheets/html/ bl0074.html

Joanna Briggs Institute Site for Evidence Based Nursing. www.joannabriggs.edu.au/ about/eb_nursing.php

Kaiser Family Foundation State Health Policy. www.kff.org/statepolicy/index.cfm

Lippincott's NursingCenter. www.nursingcenter.com

MedlinePlus Patient Safety Page. www.nlm.nih.gov/medlineplus/patientsafety.html

Medscape Patient Safety Resources. www.medscape.com/resource/patientsafety

National Center for Education Statistics. http://nces.ed.gov

National Center for Health Statistics. www.cdc.gov/nchs/Default.htm

National Center for Research Resources. www.ncrr.nih.gov

National Committee on Vital and Health Statistics. www.ncvhs.hhs.gov/sssmemb.htm

National Database of Nursing Quality Indicators. www.nursingquality.org

National Institute of Nursing Research. www.ninr.nih.gov

National League for Nursing, Nursing Education Research. www.nln.org/research/index.htm

National Quality Forum. www.qualityforum.org

New York Academy of Medicine. www.nyam.org

Nursing Education Research, Technology, and Information Management Advisory Council. www.nln.org/aboutnln/nertimac.htm

Nursing Information & Data Set Evaluation Center. www.ncbi.nlm.nih.gov/pubmed/10184814

Online Journal of Issues in Nursing. American Nurses Association. www.nursingworld.org/ojin

Pan American Health Organization. www.paho.org

PDR Electronic Library. www.micromedex.com/products/pdrlibrary

Rand Public Health Preparedness Database. www.rand.org/health/centers/preparedness

Sigma Theta Tau International Honor Society of Nursing. www.nursingsociety.org

State Data Center Program. www.census.gov/sdc

TRIP Database. www.tripdatabase.com

U.S. Department of Homeland Security. www.dhs.gov/xprepresp/committees/editorial_0566.shtm

VA National Center for Patient Safety. www.patientsafety.gov

Virginia Henderson International Nursing Library. www.nursinglibrary.org

White House site for latest federal government statistics. www.whitehouse.gov

World Health Organization WHO Patient Safety. www.who.int/patientsafety/en

■ LEARNING ENHANCEMENT TOOLS

1. A DNP researcher is concerned with studying the reaction of elementary school age children to the death of a parent. Choose a format for the structure of the literature review, select the key terms to utilize during the review, and select the sources that would be used to search for appropriate articles from the list included in *Websites for Locating Sources for a Literature Review*.

2. A DNP researcher is concerned with studying the organizational behavior changes that occur in nursing staff when nursing students undergo a clinical experience on the medical unit. Choose a format for the structure of the literature review, select the key terms to utilize during the review, select the sources that would be used to search for appropriate articles from the list included in *Websites for Locating Sources for a Literature Review,* and discuss how the process of critical appraisal of the data sources will be implemented.

■ GLOSSARY

abstract Brief summary of the process of implementing a research study.

conclusion A section of a research article that should allow the researcher to evaluate and interpret the implications of the results presented in the previous section.

discussion A section of a research article in which the findings are traced back in a logical manner to the research question or hypothesis that was investigated. The section should allow the researcher to evaluate and interpret the implications of the results presented in the previous section.

institutional review board (IRB) An entity established within an agency to review research involving human subjects to ensure participants are treated within ethical guidelines.

introduction A section of a research article that should include the author's research question or hypothesis, which clearly states the population being studied, the intervention being proposed, the comparison that will occur, and the expected outcome.

literature review Literally an account of what has been published on a topic by researchers.

methods A section in a research article that should contain the author's description of exactly what was done in the research as well as how it was implemented.

primary source One that was written by the person who either developed a theory or conducted the research being reported.

results A section in a research article that presents the author's findings.

secondary source One that was written by someone other than the person who developed the theory or conducted the research.

■ REFERENCES FOR GLOSSARY

LoBiondo-Wood, G., & Haber, J. (2002). *Nursing research: Methods, critical appraisal, and utilization.* St. Louis, MO: Elsevier.

O'Sullivan, E., & Rassel, G. (1999). *Research methods for public administrators.* New York: Longman.

Polit, D., & Hungler, B. (2000). *Essentials of nursing research: Methods and applications.* Philadelphia: Lippincott.

Wooten, J., & Ross, V. (2005). *How to make sense of clinical research.* Retrieved October 18, 2009, from http://www.modernmedicine.com/modernmedicine/article/articleDetail.jsp?id=142654

■ REFERENCES

American Psychological Association. (2010). *Publication manual of the American Psychological Association.* Washington, DC: Author.

LoBiondo-Wood, G., & Haber, J. (2002). *Nursing research: Methods, critical appraisal, and utilization.* St. Louis, MO: Elsevier.

F.D. Bluford Library, North Carolina State University. (n.d.). *How to do a literature review.* Retrieved October 19, 2009, from www.library.ncat.edu/ref/guides/literaturereview03.htm

O'Sullivan, E., & Rassel, G. (1999). *Research methods for public administrators.* New York: Longman.

Polit, D., & Hungler, B. (2000). *Essentials of nursing research: Methods and applications.* Philadelphia: Lippincott.

Taylor, D., & Procter, M. (2001). *The literature review: A few tips on conducting it.* Retrieved October 18, 2009, from www.utoronto.ca/writing/litrev.html

Wooten, J., & Ross, V. (2005). *How to make sense of clinical research.* Retrieved October 18, 2009, from http://www.modernmedicine.com/modernmedicine/article/articleDetail.jsp?id=142654

Ethics in Clinical Research

4

■ OBJECTIVES

Upon completion of this chapter, the reader should be prepared to:

1 Describe the principle of autonomy and its relationship to the DNP researcher.

2 Describe the principle of beneficence and its relationship to the DNP researcher.

3 Describe the principle of justice and its relationship to the DNP researcher.

4 Discuss the rights of an individual who provides informed consent for participation in a research study.

5 Discuss the conditions that must be fulfilled before an institutional review board (IRB) can approve a research proposal.

6 Discuss the research categories that may qualify for an expedited review by an IRB.

7 Discuss the research categories that may qualify for an exempt review by an IRB.

8 Describe the basic sections of the average IRB application form that must be completed before a proposal can be submitted.

9 Describe how informed consent differs from confidentiality.

10 Describe the Privacy Rule and the Common Rule.

11 Discuss the importance of de-identified data.

12 Discuss the expectations of IRBs regarding identified risks to human subjects as research participants.

13 Discuss common pitfalls that can develop during the process of working with an IRB.

14 Discuss the IRB requirement of the development of a Data and Safety Monitoring Plan.

ETHICAL PRINCIPLES

The greatest amount of attention given to ethical and legal considerations regarding research occurred immediately after World War II during the trials of war criminals. The American Medical Association was asked to develop a code of ethics for research that would provide standards for judging the crimes committed by physicians who conducted experiments on prisoners in concentration camps. This request resulted in the Nuremberg Code, which defined the terms *voluntary, legal capacity, sufficient understanding,* and *enlightened decision* (LoBiondo-Wood & Haber, 2002).

Autonomy

One of the main ethical principles that should be engrained into all researchers is that of autonomy and the responsibilities it brings the researcher. Because so many research projects that DNP researchers implement will utilize human subjects, it is imperative that these researchers have an understanding of the ethical principles that are important to research. **Autonomy** is the ethical principle related to informed consent. This provides a person with the right to make an informed decision about whether to participate in a research study. Potential participants must be told about any risks that could occur during the course of a research study and must be allowed to decide whether to enter the study without coercion.

Beneficence

In comparison, **beneficence** is the ethical principle that guides healthcare providers to act in the best interest of the research participant. It is the principle of beneficence that provides the participant with protection from harm. This can be achieved through monitoring the research participant's response during the study once informed consent is given.

Justice

Finally, recruitment of research subjects is governed by the principle of **justice**. This principle affects recruitment of research subjects. It mandates that research participants be selected from multiple groups rather than only from a pool of those most likely to be coerced, such as subjects with severe physical or mental illness or those who are economically disadvantaged (American Association of Critical Care Nurses, 1999).

INFORMED CONSENT

Although autonomy, beneficence, and justice are the ethical principles that should govern the conduct of the DNP student who is engaged in research that involves human subjects, it is informed consent that ensures that these principles are observed when this type of research is implemented. **Informed consent** ultimately implies that the potential participant's ratio of risk to benefits has been clearly identified. Potential risks could consist of physical harm, pain, embarrassment, loss of privacy, and loss of time, to name only a few, whereas potential benefits could consist of participating in a treatment that could relieve a physical or psychological problem.

Informed consent is given when a person with the capacity to make decisions exercises the power to make a choice without force, fraud, deceit, or any type of coercion. Such an individual is usually an adult with decision-making capacity, although in some states a legally emancipated minor who makes decision for themselves can provide informed consent. If the individual is not capable of providing informed consent, the person's family member or their legal representative can provide informed consent for the person.

RIGHTS OF PARTICIPANTS IN A RESEARCH STUDY

Specific guidelines regarding the informed consent process must be followed in order for federal funding to be provided to implement research projects. In addition, there are certain federal regulations that stipulate that participants in a research study have specific rights. These include:

- The right to be informed of both the nature and the purpose of the research;
- The right to receive an explanation of the procedures that will be followed and any drug or device that will be used during the research;
- The right to receive a description of any risks or discomfort that may occur during the course of the research;
- The right to receive any explanation of benefits that may be expected from the research;
- The right to receive a disclosure of any procedure, drug, or device that could be used during the research that could benefit the participant, as well as their potential risks and benefits;
- The right to receive information on forms of treatment available to the participant after the research project is concluded, if complications occur during the study;

- The right to ask questions regarding the research study or any procedure involved in it;
- The right to be told that consent to participate in the research may be withdrawn at any time, and that the participant may withdraw from the project without consequences;
- The right to receive a copy of any signed and dated written consent form that was issued during the course of the study; and
- The right to decide to consent to participate or not in the research without any type of force, fraud, deceit, duress, coercion, or other influence being applied to pressure the subject (American Association of Critical Care Nurses, 1999)

The principal investigator of the research project is ultimately responsible for obtaining informed consent. However, it is the ethical responsibility of all researchers involved in the project to assure that informed consent has been obtained in an appropriate manner. Problems with informed consent can arise based on the type of research being conducted. The Code of Federal Regulations does not require written consent for surveys unless the information that is collected is recorded in a manner that allows participants to be identified and disclosure of the information could lead to criminal or civil liability for participants or damage the reputation of participants. Research that consists of field experiments or observation of participants in a covert manner presents the greatest challenge to the researcher regarding informed consent. In both of these types of studies, the researcher's need to observe participants in spontaneous behavior is not compatible with the provision of informed consent. Implementing these types of research studies could lead the primary investigator to be labeled as engaging in unethical research practices (Singleton & Straits, 1999).

CONFIDENTIALITY

It is important for the DNP researcher to recognize that informed consent is not synonymous with **confidentiality**. Although **privacy** can be considered to be a person's ability to control the access of other people to information about him- or herself, confidentiality refers to protection of such information so that researchers will not disclose records that identify individuals. Regardless of the sensitivity of the information gathered during the course of a research study, the ethical investigator will guarantee the confidentiality of the data collected from human subjects. A researcher may collect anonymous information in an attempt to avoid problems with confidentiality. This means that no records are kept on the identity of subjects and data cannot be traced back to a specific person. However, some research designs do not lend themselves to confidentiality; in this case, the researcher must be capable of auditing his or her own records to ensure that information was collected accurately and reported correctly (O'Sullivan & Rassel, 1999).

In order to ensure confidentiality, the researcher can remove subjects' names and any other identifying information as early in the research project as possible. In addition, the investigator can code subjects' identities so that such information is not divulged during any part of the research report. This is frequently done in field research, which may require more creativity in order for data to be de-identified. If other researchers or organizations request information from the primary investigator, the researcher should never release information that contains sensitive material without the research subjects' permission (Singleton & Straits, 1999).

HIPAA COMPLIANCE

There are various aspects of compliance with the Health Information Portability and Accountability Act that the DNP researcher must clearly grasp. These include an understanding of the Privacy Rule, Protected Health Information, and release of information with prior authorization.

The Privacy Rule and the Common Rule

As the DNP researcher engages in practice-oriented research, along with informed consent and confidentiality, he or she must be cognizant of the requirements of the Health Information Portability and Accountability Act (HIPAA). A researcher can gain access to medical records only through a privacy review conducted by an **institutional review board (IRB)**. The Privacy Rule was implemented as the first phase of HIPAA in 2004. It defined patient rights regarding individual health information and established protection for access to and release of a patient's medical records. HIPAA also mandates the creation of privacy boards whose sole authority is to review individual privacy rights. Privacy boards operate similar to IRBs. In comparison, an IRB derives its authority from the Federal Policy for the Protection of Human Subjects, also known as the Common Rule. The Common Rule is similar to the Privacy Rule, although it applies only to federally funded research (Artnak & Benson, 2005).

Protected Health Information

If the DNP researcher opts to utilize what HIPAA refers to as **protected health information** in his or her research project, the researcher opts to use information about an individual's health status, the provision of health care, or payment for health care that can be linked to the person. The investigator should recognize that the legislation considers this type of information to fall into one of three categories:

- No consent form is required, but the researcher must sign a restricted use agreement.
- No consent form is required, but review by an IRB or privacy board is required.
- Individual authorization is necessary.

There are cases when an IRB or a privacy board can allow a researcher access to protected health information without authorization. For example, if the medical record in question contains de-identified information, no individual privacy protection is required. De-identified data means that all information that could identify an individual has been removed (Artnak & Benson, 2005).

Data that Cannot Be Released Without Prior Authorization

The researcher should further recognize that there are specific data elements that cannot be released during the course of a research project without prior authorization from the subject in question. These include:

- Name of the research participant
- Geographic areas smaller than a state, except for the first three digits of the ZIP code
- Dates of birth, dates of death, dates of admission, or ages greater than 89 years
- Driver's license or automobile license numbers
- Social security numbers
- Medical records numbers
- Health plan numbers
- Account numbers
- Telephone numbers
- Fax numbers
- E-mail addresses
- License numbers, such as nurse's license or medical license
- Vehicle identification numbers

- Medical device or serial numbers
- Internet URLs
- Internet IP addresses
- Biometric information
- Any additional information that would allow the re-identification of subject information (Lavin, 2006)

INSTITUTIONAL REVIEW BOARDS

Ultimately, the components of informed consent are overseen by an institutional review board (IRB). This was mandated in 1991 when a federal policy for the protection of human subjects in research activities was published. This policy required that every institution that receives federal funding for research involving human participants must create an IRB and appoint its members. Federal guidelines require that an IRB be composed of at least five members, with one of the five being a person not associated with the facility. This means that a facility's IRB must review all research that involves human subjects either conducted at the facility or sponsored by the facility. Most healthcare research conducted in the United States currently is approved by an IRB because, in addition to the federal requirement for an IRB to be in place in order for funding to be awarded, many private funding agencies and most biomedical journals require an IRB to approve research that is conducted. Also, most universities and healthcare institutions require IRB approval in order to avoid liability as research is implemented (Olsen & Mahrenholz, 2000).

An institution's IRB looks for certain conditions to be fulfilled before a research proposal can be approved. These consist of:

- Minimal identified risks to human subjects
- Equitable selection of human subjects
- Appropriate documentation of informed consent from all participants
- Appropriate monitoring of data to ensure safety of subjects
- Provision for ensuring privacy of human subjects and confidentiality of data gathered (O'Sullivan & Rassel, 1999)

Evaluation of a Research Proposal

An IRB will usually evaluate a proposal on the basis of several areas. Because the rights of the human subjects involved are considered to be paramount, the consent form utilized will be scrutinized. The board will determine if the consent form addresses concerns such as deception of the participants, presentation of the purpose of the research, obvious or hidden costs to the subjects, benefits and risks to the participants, protection of confidentiality, the contact person if participants have questions, and what will be done with the results generated by the study. The board will also look carefully at the conditions under which subjects are excluded from and included in the research study. Approval of a project will be denied if there is an indication that the subjects believe they will receive a special benefit merely by participating, such as students who believe they will be given extra points in a class if they participate in a research project for their professor (Kamienski, 2000).

Most IRBs also have concerns regarding recruitment of participants for a research study. They usually are adamant that permission to approach a subject regarding possible participation be obtained by someone other than the researcher. This means that someone such as a co-worker in the potential subject's work area could approach the person regarding the possibility of participation, and then the researcher would follow up with a conversation with the subject regarding an explanation of the research and approach the person with an invitation to participate. This area must be well planned before sending a proposal to the IRB in order to avoid a denial (Kamienski, 2000).

Expedited Reviews by an IRB

A facility's IRB has the capacity to award a research proposal an **expedited review** if the risk to research subjects is considered to be at a minimal level. This shortens the length of the review process because usually only one member of the IRB will review the project to ensure protection of human subjects (Stone, 2003). Receiving an expedited review can still require a researcher to obtain informed consent, however. It should always be the goal of the DNP researcher to obtain an expedited review from an IRB. Research categories that may be eligible for an expedited review may include:

- Collection of hair and nail clippings in a manner that does not disfigure the human subject
- Collection of excreta and external secretions including perspiration
- Recording of information on human subjects who are at least 18 years old, using noninvasive procedures that are considered to be routine in clinical practice
- Collecting voice recordings
- Study of data, documents, records, pathological specimens, or diagnostic data that are already in existence (LoBiondo-Wood & Haber, 2002)

Exempt Review by an IRB

Some research projects may be considered to be **exempt** from an IRB review. According to the federal guidelines generated by the Department of Health and Human Services, there are five categories that can qualify research as being exempt from IRB review:

- Research in educational settings such as universities
- Research involving surveys and tests in which the participant cannot be identified
- Research involving collection of existing data if sources are either publicly available or have already been de-identified
- Research conducted by or subject to approval by federal agencies that are designed for the good of the general public
- Research related to the taste and quality of food

Although the DNP researcher may be reasonably certain that his or her research proposal will be exempt from a full review by an IRB, an application must still be completed and submitted; the IRB will make the final decision (Stone, 2003).

IRB Application

Regardless of the type of review the researcher is hoping for, whether a full review, expedited, or exempt, an application must still be completed and submitted, and the IRB will make the final decision. Usually the facility's application form can be downloaded from the institution's website. The researcher must bear in mind that often these forms are not formatted in a way that allows them to be saved once their blanks are filled in. Therefore, it may be more convenient for the researcher to type the proposal in a word processor and then copy and paste the information into the form. This is particularly helpful if the IRB requires changes and thus subsequent submissions of the form.

Initially the IRB application usually requires a brief statement of the study's hypothesis, research question(s), and purpose. In addition, a statement of the objectives of the research project will usually be required. Information will then be requested regarding the subjects to be utilized in the study. This will include who they are, how they will be recruited, copies of any letters or advertisements that will be used in recruitment, how many contacts will be made with each subject and the length of each contact, as well as any payment that will be given to participants. The board will be particularly interested in the inclusion of subjects from vulnerable populations, such as children, infants, prisoners, or the mentally handicapped. If the study site is a college and the study involves students whose grade could be affected by the research project, these students would be considered a vulnerable population (Kamienski, 2000).

As the application process progresses, the researcher should plan to produce copies of the informed consent to be utilized, a concise and accurate description of what the researcher will be doing to the subjects or with the subjects, and a copy of instruments that will be used in the research, including surveys, questionnaires, and any interview questions. The researcher should also be prepared to detail the procedures that will be used to maintain confidentiality. If the researcher plans to use deception of the subjects, he or she should be prepared to describe in detail why this is necessary and how subjects will be debriefed after completion of the project. The researcher should have a contingency plan to alter the proposal if the IRB denies the proposal based on his or her use of deception. A similar plan should be in place if the researcher proposes to ask the participants questions or perform procedures that might cause participants stress or anxiety or disturb participants emotionally. Again, the IRB will be concerned by this request and will want to know why this is necessary and what the researcher intends to do to provide counseling and treatment to participants who become upset. As previously mentioned, a statement of the risk-to-benefit ratio will be needed to round out the complete proposal (Kamienski, 2000).

Pitfalls of the IRB Process

There are some common pitfalls that can sidetrack even the most seasoned researcher if not avoided when approaching the time of IRB review. For example, failure to be consistent throughout all of the documentation can circumvent the process. This means that the application, protocol narrative, consent forms, and any other documents must contain information with consistent details. In addition, the researcher can easily overlook the need to provide "layman's" language in the informed consent document, which should be written at no higher than a sixth- to eighth-grade reading level for adult participants. Because every IRB must include at least one member who is not a researcher affiliated with the sponsoring facility, the primary investigator should bear in mind that his or her protocol should be written using language that can be easily understood by nonnursing personnel. It can be considered a general standard that no IRB will approve a protocol that cannot be easily understood by its members (Colt & Mulnard, 2006).

IRB Review Criteria

As has been previously mentioned, specific criteria must be met in order for an IRB to determine that a protocol can be approved for the recruitment and participation of human subjects. If the DNP researcher is already familiar with the criteria and how an IRB will typically interpret them, he or she can develop an IRB application that presents information that meets the board's concerns and thus avoids repetitive requests for protocol modifications. For example, clearly it is the overriding mission of an IRB to ensure that risks to subjects are minimized to the greatest extent possible. This means that questions the IRB may ask regarding risks of research and board members' expectations regarding minimizing these risks include:

- *Do the protocol's eligibility criteria adequately minimize the identified risks to subjects?* A protocol will never be approved by an IRB if the board determines there are risks to the human subjects that have not been minimized to the greatest extent possible. Such a situation would violate the overall mission of the IRB if it were allowed to persist.
- *Do the protocol's eligibility criteria adequately monitor the identified risks to subjects?* The protocol must describe explicitly the monitoring procedures the researchers have initiated in order to make certain the subjects are continually exposed to the lowest level of both risk and discomfort possible during the course of the study.
- *Are the proposed procedures justified, reasonable, and as comfortable as possible for the participants?* This also includes being as convenient for the participants as possible. For example, if a particular protocol that will involve cancer patients could produce nausea and a monitoring procedure has been developed to determine that nausea either is not being produced or is at a very minimal level, the protocol should state that the procedure would be implemented as much as possible during the patient's regularly scheduled clinic appointments. This will prevent the patient from having to schedule extra appointments, thus potentially also avoiding extra expense.
- *Are the research personnel both qualified and adequately trained to implement the study procedures?* Most IRBs now require all of the personnel who will be implementing research utilizing human subjects to undergo and document their participation in standardized training on the ethical principles of research and the regulations that pertain to such research.

- *Are the identified risks to subjects reasonable in relation to the anticipated benefits?* Many IRBs identify assessment of the risk/benefit ratio of the research study to be the most important ethical consideration of the entire project. The researcher should clearly identify if there are characteristics of the proposed subject population that will increase their risks as research participants (Pech, Cob, & Cejka, 2005).

Data and Safety Monitoring Plan

If, in fact, a research protocol identifies that more than minimal risk to human subjects will be present during a research project, most IRBs will subsequently require the researcher to present a data and safety monitoring plan. This will be a description of how the primary investigator will monitor the research data in order to respond quickly to any adverse events or unanticipated problems that occur during the study, to ensure participant safety. A thorough description of the monitoring process should be prepared because accrual of preliminary data may indicate that the research design should be changed, information provided to subjects should be altered, or the project lacks sufficient validity and should be terminated (Pech, Cob, & Cejka, 2005).

In addition to concerns regarding the ratio of risks to benefits to the human subjects involved in the research, an IRB will also pose questions to the researcher regarding the level of confidentiality available to the participants. The researcher should be prepared with a plan to supply this information to avoid becoming sidetracked by the need to supply unanticipated data. The IRB will be concerned with determining:

- Will the location of the data collection allow subjects sufficient privacy? If information collected will be especially sensitive, the IRB will expect privacy to be provided by interviewing participants in a secured room, for example.
- *How will data be stored?* The researcher should determine where collected data will be stored and the precautions that will be implemented to prevent personnel not involved in the research study from having access to the sensitive information.
- *How will data be recorded?* The researcher should be prepared to describe the process by which data will be recorded, whether anonymously or by coded response. If the data will be coded, the researcher should be able to state where the codebook will be stored, who will have access to it, and when the identifiers for the information will be destroyed (Pech, Cob, & Cejka, 2005).

Formula for Success

In summary, Colt and Mulnard (2006) have developed a formula for success for researchers attempting to navigate through the IRB review and approval process:

- Use simplified language that is easy for anyone to understand.
- Provide rationale for the research project as well as the choice of design and the degree of risk to potential participants.
- Emphasize the multiple ways that protection of subjects is provided throughout the project.
- Provide complete and detailed information in all areas of the required documentation.
- Achieve consistency of the information provided in each section and across all documents utilized in the research study.

As previously mentioned, the institutional review board can have a great influence on the research design for a study, because the board's concerns regarding monitoring procedures can signal that the design may need to be changed somewhat or completely substituted with another design. The next chapter will discuss research designs, specifically those that are appropriate for quantitative research projects.

■ GLOSSARY

autonomy Ethical principle related to informed consent. This provides a person with the right to make an informed decision about whether to participate in a research study.

beneficence Ethical principle that guides healthcare providers to act in the best interest of the research participant. It is the principle of beneficence that provides the participant with protection from harm.

confidentiality Protection of information so that researchers will not disclose records that identify individuals.

exempt Research involving human subjects that falls into a category that is not deemed necessary for review by an institutional review board.

expedited review Usually only one member of the IRB will review the project to ensure protection of human subjects; shortens the length of the review process.

informed consent Ultimately implies that the potential participant's ratio of risks to benefits has been clearly identified.

institutional review board Reviews all research that involves human subjects either conducted at a facility or sponsored by that facility.

justice Ethical principle governing recruitment of research subjects. It mandates that research participants be selected from multiple groups rather than only from a pool of those most likely to be coerced, such as subjects with severe physical or mental illness or those who are economically disadvantaged.

privacy A person's ability to control other people's access to information about him- or herself.

protected health information Information about an individual's health status, the provision of health care, or payment for health care that can be linked to the person.

■ LEARNING ENHANCEMENT TOOLS

1. Discuss autonomy, beneficence, and justice and how these principles should relate to the conduct of a DNP researcher and his or her research participants.

2. You are the principal investigator for a research project that will study the anxiety level of nursing students who are undergoing testing for their state nursing licensure examination. Discuss all of your responsibilities regarding informed consent for this project.

3. You are developing a research proposal that will go before an institutional review board and are hoping for an expedited review. How can you format your proposal to be more likely to receive an expedited review?

4. You are developing a research proposal that will go before an institutional review board and are hoping for either an expedited or an exempt review. Discuss how the categories that will require an expedited review will differ from the categories that require an exempt review.

5. You are preparing a proposal for submission to an institutional review board. Describe the various parts that you anticipate being included in the request for information from the IRB.

6. You have submitted a research proposal to an institutional review board. The IRB has concerns regarding the ratio of risks to benefits for research participants. As the researcher, describe how you would respond to the IRB's concerns and how you would keep the risk level minimal for participants.

7. As the primary investigator, you have submitted a proposal to an IRB. The board returns the proposal to you with the stipulation that a Data and Safety Monitoring Plan must be developed and implemented. Why would such a stipulation be given, and how can you meet the board's expectation?

■ RESOURCES

Belmont Report. http://ohsr.od.nih.gov/guidelines/belmont.html

Collaborative Institutional Training Initiative. www.citiprogram.org

Ethical and Regulatory Aspects of Clinical Research. www.bioethics.nih.gov/hsrc/index.shtml

HIPAA Privacy Rule. www.hhs.gov/ocr/hipaa

HRSA Protecting Human Subjects Training. www.hrsa.gov/humansubjects

Human Participant Protections Education for Research Teams. http://main.uab.edu/show.asp?durki=75243

NIH Office of Human Subjects Research. http://ohsr.od.nih.gov/about/index.html

Office for Human Research Protection (OHRP), U.S. Department of Health and Human Services. www.hhs.gov/ohrp

Office of Research Integrity (ORI), U.S. Department of Health and Human Services. http://ori.hhs.gov

Teaching the Responsible Conduct of Research in Humans. www.medsch.ucla.edu/public/korenman

■ IRB WEBSITES THAT OFFER INVESTIGATOR GUIDANCE

Duke University. http://irb.mc.duke.edu

Johns Hopkins Medicine. http://irb.jhmi.edu

Stanford University. http://humansubjects.stanford.edu

University of California-San Francisco. www.ucsf.edu

University of Minnesota. www.research.umn.edu/irb

University of Pittsburgh. www.irb.pitt.edu

University of Wisconsin-Madison (School of Medicine and Public Health). http://info.gradsch.wisc.edu/research/compliance/humansubjects/hsirbs/index.html

■ REFERENCES FOR RESOURCES AND WEBSITES

Artnak, K., & Benson, M. (2005). Evaluating HIPAA compliance: A guide for researchers, privacy boards, and IRBs. *Nursing Outlook, 53*, 79–87.

Pech, C., Cob, N., & Cejka, J. (2005). Understanding institutional review boards: Practical guidance to the IRB review process. *Nutrition in Clinical Practice.* Retrieved November 4, 2009, from http://ncp.sagepub.com/cgi/content/full/22/6/618

Scheetz, L., & Oman, K. (2008). Research, quality improvement, and institutional review boards: What's the deal? *Journal of Emergency Nursing, 34*(1), 3–5.

▪ REFERENCES

American Association of Critical Care Nurses. (1999). *Ethics in critical care nursing research*. Retrieved October 28, 2009, from http://www.aacn.org/wd/practice/content/research/ethics-in-critical-care-nursing-research.pcms?menu=practice

Artnak, K., & Benson, M. (2005). Evaluating HIPAA compliance: A guide for researchers, privacy boards, and IRBs. *Nursing Outlook, 53*, 79–87.

Colt, H., & Mulnard, R. (2006). Writing an application for a human subjects institutional review board. *Chest, 130*, 1605–1607.

Kamienski, M. (2000). Tips on navigating your research proposal through the institutional review board. *Journal of Emergency Nursing, 26*(2), 178–181.

Lavin, R. (2006). HIPAA and disaster research: Preparing to conduct research. *Disaster Management & Response, 4*(2), 32–37.

LoBiondo-Wood, G., & Haber, J. (2002). *Nursing research: Methods, critical appraisal, and utilization*. St. Louis, MO: Elsevier.

Olsen, D., & Mahrenholz, D. (2000). IRB-identified ethical issues in nursing research. *Journal of Professional Nursing, 16*(3), 140–148.

O'Sullivan, E., & Rassel, G. (1999). *Research methods for public administrators*. New York: Longman.

Pech, C., Cob, N., & Cejka, J. (2005). Understanding institutional review boards: Practical guidance to the IRB review process. *Nutrition in Clinical Practice*. Retrieved November 4, 2009, from http://ncp.sagepub.com/cgi/content/full/22/6/618

Singleton, R., & Straits, B. (1999). *Approaches to social research*. New York: Oxford University Press.

Stone, P. (2003). HIPAA in 2003 and its meaning for nurse researchers. *Applied Nursing Research, 16*(4), 291–293.

Designing a Clinically Based Quantitative Capstone Research Project

5

## 6

■ OBJECTIVES

Upon completion of this chapter, the reader should be prepared to:

1 Describe the origin of quantitative research.

2 Define the categories of quantitative research.

3 Describe the advantages and limitations of using a quantitative research design.

4 Discuss the basic differences in experimental, non-experimental, and quasi-experimental research designs.

5 Discuss the advantages and limitations of using a randomized controlled trial research design.

6 Discuss the advantages and weaknesses of using a pre-test–post-test research design.

7 Discuss the advantages and weaknesses of using a nonrandomized clinical trial.

8 Describe the special challenges posed to the researcher who opts to utilize the Solomon four-group research design.

9 Discuss the advantages and limitations of using a cross-sectional survey research design.

10 Discuss the advantages and limitations of using a longitudinal study with cohorts.

11 Describe the special challenges posed to the researcher who opts to utilize a case control study as a research design.

12 Describe the various types of time series designs that are available for use as a research design.

13 Discuss threats to internal validity that can occur.

14 Describe ways to minimize threats to internal validity when developing a research design.

15 Discuss threats to external validity that can occur.

16 Describe ways to increase external validity when developing a research design.

BASIC TYPES OF QUANTITATIVE RESEARCH

A clinically based capstone research project could potentially focus either on an individual patient or on groups of patients, although quantitative research focuses on patient groups. Quantitative research is concerned with patterns that are unique to a population of patients, and can be particularly useful for investigating the effectiveness of an intervention. The roots of quantitative research are in **positivism**, which maintains that there is an objective reality in the world that can be quantified in some way so that observation or measurement can occur (Seers & Critelton, 2001).

As a research classification, quantitative research consists of two broad categories: experimental studies and non-experimental or observational studies. **Observational studies** are further delineated into:

- Cross-sectional surveys
- Longitudinal studies using cohorts, or groups of subjects who are followed over a period of time
- Case control studies

Experimental studies include the following subgroups:

- Clinical trials
- Randomized controlled trials
- Pre-test–post-test designs (Seers & Critelton, 2001)

A variation on the two major categories of research designs is the quasi-experimental category. Each type will be discussed according to its strengths, weaknesses, and relevance to the DNP researcher.

ADVANTAGES AND LIMITATIONS OF QUANTITATIVE RESEARCH

Quantitative research allows the investigator to establish correlational and causal relationships between variables. When the researcher is able to analyze statistics and test a theoretically derived hypothesis using a quantitative research design, he or she can present logical outcomes that have scientific validation. When the researcher uses a quantitative research design, data can be gathered using an objective approach to observing and reporting either a phenomenon that occurs or the behavior of the research subjects. This will allow the investigator to scientifically select the instrument to be used and gather the data without becoming emotionally involved with the participants or the overall research project. Therefore, the statistical significance of the hypothesis is maintained as the primary focus of the project. In addition, the researcher is able to identify the potential risks to research subjects early in the project so that complications can be minimized before the study progresses any further (Palmer, 2009).

On the negative side, conducting quantitative research may yield a lack of subjective data about human interactions that would be necessary to answer research questions pertaining to social, internal, or holistic phenomena. When a purely quantitative research design is used, the project cannot include the establishment of human emotions, habits, perceptions, or experiences that could expose personal variables related to the research subjects that could influence the final outcome of the project. For example, patients' perceptions of treatments require a level of understanding that is more complex than a quantitative research design can produce. In addition, because the relationship between the researcher and the research subjects is detached and clinical in nature, participants may receive a negative impression of the overall project and the intent of the researcher (Palmer, 2009).

EXPERIMENTAL RESEARCH DESIGNS

A design is considered to be **experimental** if the research subjects are randomly assigned to treatment groups and to control or comparison groups, with the comparison group receiving either no treatment or simply standard treatment.

Randomized Controlled Trial

One example of an experimental research design is the **randomized controlled trial** mentioned in the previous section. This is considered the strongest design to provide healthcare professionals with information regarding the benefits of a specific healthcare intervention; this might be the primary reason for a DNP researcher to decide to use this as a research design. The trial is a true experiment in which research subjects are randomly selected to be in the **experimental group** and receive a new intervention or to be in the **control group** and either receive a standard intervention or no intervention at all. The two main strengths of the randomized controlled trial are:

- The random selection of participants to be in one group or the other
- The longitudinal nature of the study, which means participants are followed forward in time to determine if a specific outcome occurred

In comparison, the main disadvantages of using such a design would be:

- The cost involved in conducting a lengthy randomized controlled trial
- The extensive follow-up period required to determine if research subjects actually experienced an outcome
- The possibility that participants who agreed to take part in a trial may be different from those to whom the research would be applied (Roberts & Dicenso, 1999)

According to Seers and Critelton (2001), randomization and the use of a control group are essential features of this type of research design. The control group is needed for comparison purposes, and the randomization is needed to ensure that the experimental and control groups are as similar as possible except for exposure to the intervention or treatment. Randomization also is needed to protect from selection bias, because it ensures that both known and unknown factors are distributed in a uniform way among the groups. **Selection bias** is considered to be a threat to the research design's internal validity, meaning the ability to infer that the independent variable causes a specific change in the dependent variable (Manheim, Rich, & Willnat, 2002).

Bias can also be kept to a minimal level during a randomized controlled trial through the use of blinding. **Blinding** occurs when neither the research subject nor the person assessing the outcome of the treatment is aware of the group to which the client belongs. Under ideal circumstances, no one involved with the research project would be aware of the group assignment of the participants. A double blind trial occurs when both the research subject and the person assessing the outcome are blind to the treatment group assignment (Seers & Critelton, 2001).

The long-term implications of such requirements mean that in order to use such a research design, a DNP student must be able to guarantee:

- Randomization can occur.
- Sufficient numbers of research participants can be used to allow for both an experimental and a control group.
- An adequate budget is present to allow for a lengthy project requiring extensive follow-up.
- Participants are willing to be followed to determine if they experienced an outcome.
- The research subjects can be readily located.

The commitment to such a project may be greater than the student's available time or resources.

Pre-Test–Post-Test Designs

Pre-test–post-test designs look at the outcome of interest before the application of an intervention and then after an intervention. This type of research design suffers from a fundamental weakness, making it difficult to attribute causation to the intervention when there is no randomization and control group. This opens up the possibility that some other factor has affected the outcome of the research study. However, the DNP researcher should recognize that occasionally this research design is the only practical method of assessing the impact of an intervention. For example, if the researcher is assessing the respiratory status of a critically ill patient before and after the addition of a new type of ventilator to the treatment regimen, the pre-test–post-test design would be a practical choice. Despite its obvious weakness, the pre-test–post-test design can be strengthened by using a control group that also has a pre-test and a post-test, using more than one pre-test in both groups, and using multiple time points for assessing the outcomes in both groups (Seers & Critelton, 2001).

A variation of the pre-test–post-test design is the **Solomon four-group design**. The researcher opting for this research design can examine both the main effects of testing and the interaction of testing and the application of an intervention. The four-group design uses two groups that receive the intervention and two groups that do not. Only one treatment group will be administered a pre-test, but all four groups will receive the post-test. A primary advantage of this type of research design is its ability to assess the presence of pre-test sensitization; this means that the post-test measure could be affected not only by the treatment or intervention, but also by exposure to the pretest. However, the Solomon four-group design has some fundamental weaknesses as well. For example, it requires a large number of research participants. In addition, it can be difficult for the researcher to introduce the treatment or intervention at exactly the same time for both groups. Finally, the researcher may find it difficult to randomize subjects to only one of the four groups (McGahee & Tingen, n.d.).

Subgroups of Clinical Trials

As previously mentioned, subgroups of clinical trials can be used as a type of experimental research design. An example of this would be a **nonrandomized clinical trial**. This type of research design would be used when randomization is not feasible or ethical, or when there is insufficient evidence to justify the difficulty and expense of a randomized clinical trial. This could be an option for a DNP researcher who does not have the time, manpower, or budgetary resources to implement a randomized clinical trial. Nonrandomized clinical trials may also be referred to as "quasi-experimental" or "non-equivalent control group" designs because the characteristics of research participants in groups that were not randomized will not be equivalent. Quasi-experimental designs will be discussed later in the chapter. This failure to ensure randomization is the primary weakness of this type of research design; therefore, an estimation of the intervention's effects can be biased if the group differences in the participant characteristics are not controlled for when the data are analyzed (Hooked on Evidence, n.d.).

NON-EXPERIMENTAL RESEARCH DESIGNS

A research design is considered to be non-experimental if there is systematic collection of data but no use of control groups or randomization of subjects and no use of statistical controls.

Cross-Sectional Surveys

A primary non-experimental research design is the **cross-sectional study**. This is a study undertaken at a specific point in time. There is no follow-up of the research subjects. Data are usually collected using a questionnaire, which is increasingly being administered via the Internet. Survey responses are usually made from a pre-arranged list and most questions are closed-ended. Although the primary advantage of cross-sectional surveys is their ability to reach large numbers of people quickly, such a research design can be difficult for the clinically based DNP student to implement. A major disadvantage of the cross-sectional survey is that there may be missing data in the responses, because respondents frequently may choose to answer only specific questions and may leave blank questions they don't understand or that require a maximal amount of effort to answer.

The response rate of the cross-sectional survey is always going to be a major concern for the DNP researcher. The higher the response rate, the more clarity is contained in the overall "snapshot" provided by the research design; therefore, questions must be worded to be as clear as possible. The more open questions are to interpretation, the more likely respondents are to be confused by them, and the more frequently the questions will be skipped. According to Seers and Critelton (2001), a response rate of less than 40 percent can make the responses questionable in terms of how representative they are of the target population. Such a low response rate could mean that respondents were motivated by a specific set of factors unknown to the researcher. The representativeness of a cross-sectional survey can be increased if a randomized sample is used when distributing the survey instrument. Representativeness means that the characteristics of the sample of subjects closely approximate those of the larger population of potential respondents. Ultimately, the cross-sectional survey can be an effective research design for the DNP student who has access to a specific population, such as the employees of a facility, but may be difficult to utilize with an ever-changing patient population (Seers & Critelton, 2001).

Longitudinal Studies Using Cohorts

A **longitudinal study** is often used to focus on causative agents because it follows a group of people over time. A **cohort** is the group of research subjects the researcher follows over time. If the researcher chooses, the cohort can be sampled over multiple points in time. The DNP researcher could use this type of research design to address a question regarding potential harm to a patient in a clinical situation when it would be unethical to perform a randomized controlled trial. For example, it would unethical to randomize research subjects who have cardiac disease to take an excessive amount of a specific medication in order to measure the impact on the subjects' cardiovascular systems. However, the researcher could certainly follow a group of cardiac patients over time to determine their compliance with their medication regimen and the changes that occurred to their cardiovascular systems over time.

The major drawback to the use of longitudinal studies using cohorts is the time and expense involved, both of which can be major concerns for the clinically based DNP researcher with a limited budget, little personnel support, and multiple deadlines. In addition, longitudinal studies suffer from **attrition**. This is the loss of research subjects that occurs during the course of the research study, making follow-up difficult (Seers & Critelton, 2001).

Case Control Studies

When the researcher chooses a **case control study** as the research design, research subjects are selected because they have some condition of interest. A control group made up of participants who do not have the disease or condition will be selected and typically will match the cases selected on demographic variables such as age, gender, and location. The case participants and the control participants will be questioned regarding factors that could have potentially caused the condition of interest, then the case participants and control group's exposure to each factor being studied will be compared. For example, if the researcher is examining the relationship between stress and cardiovascular disease, cases selected may be people who have experienced an acute myocardial infarction and been treated for stress with anti-anxiety agents. Control participants selected could be patients who are simultaneously undergoing treatment for both cardiac disease and stress. Control participants would be matched to the case participants according to age, gender, clinical diagnosis, and significant historical data.

The primary advantage to use of case control studies as a research design is that it can be quickly and easily implemented—major advantages for the DNP researcher—and also allow assessment of causation. It can be particularly useful when the condition being studied is rare, or when there is a lengthy amount of time between exposure to the potential causative conditions and the resulting outcome (Seers & Critelton, 2001). In comparison, there are several drawbacks attached to use of this research design:

- The difficulty in obtaining control subjects who are very similar to the case participants in all of the factors being investigated
- The objection of healthy patients to participation in a research project that is disease-focused (Seers & Critelton, 2001)
- Difficulty in establishing that exposure to the causative factors actually occurred before the outcome
- Difficulty in obtaining accurate information about exposure to the potentially causative agent that has occurred in the past, because participants' memory may be sketchy and medical records may be incomplete and inaccurate (Roberts & Dicenso, 1999)

QUASI-EXPERIMENTAL RESEARCH DESIGNS

A variation on the previously discussed categories of research designs is the quasi-experimental category. A research design is considered to be quasi-experimental if the research subjects are not randomly assigned to groups, although there may still be a control or comparison group. Although subjects are not randomly assigned, either they can be randomly sampled or all of the relevant cases can be used. In addition, statistical controls are used instead of the random assignment of subjects. A quasi-experimental research design can be used instead of an experimental design when an experimental design is not feasible or perhaps even ethical, or when a true experiment cannot be conducted in a real world situation. Data analysis may have to occur on the basis of archival information alone, randomization of subjects may not be an option, and there may be no pre-test data available. A quasi-experimental design should also be utilized when an experimental design has become flawed due to attrition in the treatment group.

One-Group Post-Test-Only Design

A primary quasi-experimental research design is the one-group post-test-only design. Similar to a case study, this research design does not use a pre-test baseline or a comparison group, and thus it is difficult to arrive at valid conclusions about the effects of a treatment because only post-test information is available. This type of research design is not recommended for the DNP student who wants to be able to draw conclusions about the outcome resulting from application of a specific intervention (Garson, 2009).

Nonequivalent Control Group Design

This type of quasi-experimental design is used in research projects conducted in field settings. It looks very similar to a true experiment except for a lack of random assignment to groups. The essential problem with the nonequivalent control group design is the difficulty the researcher can have in assuming that the experimental and comparison groups are similar when the study is initiated. The design also requires the researcher to contend with multiple threats to the internal validity of the study. This means there will be competing explanations for the results that are obtained. Such threats to internal validity will include:

- **Selection**—This results from the way in which research subjects were chosen for the project, particularly if precautions were not utilized to achieve a **representative sample**.
- **History**—A specific event occurring either inside or outside the experimental setting has an effect on the dependent variable.
- **Maturation**—The natural developmental changes such as the aging process that would occur to research subjects over the course of time and are unrelated to the research project being conducted.
- **Testing**—The effect of taking a pre-test on the subject's post-test score. Taking a pre-test may improve the research subject's score on the post-test, and thus the result of the differences between post-test and pre-test scores may not be an outcome of the application of an intervention but may instead be the result of the experience gained through the testing process.
- **Instrumentation**—This threat to internal validity occurs when there are changes in the way variables are measured or the techniques used for observation that will cause changes in the measurements that are obtained.

- **Mortality**—The loss of study subjects from the time of administration of the pre-test to the time of administration of the post-test. If the subjects who remain in the study are vastly different from the subjects who opt to remove themselves from the project, the results obtained will most likely be affected (LoBiondo-Wood & Haber, 2002).

The DNP researcher who opts to use this research design must be prepared to minimize the threats to internal validity to the greatest extent possible. This may be difficult if the researcher does not have the budgetary resources for training all data collectors to minimize the threat of instrumentation or if an insufficient number of subjects are available to minimize the threat of mortality as subjects leave the study.

Time Series

The **time series** research design involves the collection of data over an extended period of time and the introduction of an experimental treatment during the data collection process. A primary advantage of the time series is that the extended time perspective greatly increases the likelihood that changes that occur can be attributed to the introduction of the treatment or intervention that is being implemented (Polit & Hungler, 2000). There are multiple variations on this research design:

- **Simple interrupted time series design**—This is a one-group pre-test–post-test design that utilizes multiple pre-tests and post-tests. Trends noted in multiple pre-tests can be compared to trends noted in multiple post-tests to determine whether post-intervention improvement is the result of a maturation effect that would have led to improvement anyway. This could be a possible research design for the DNP researcher who has access to a group of research subjects in a clinical setting for an extended period. Because there is no control group, however, the researcher cannot assess other threats to internal validity such as history. As with the nonequivalent control group design, other threats to internal validity that may occur include selection bias, instrumentation bias, and testing (Garson, 2009).
- **Interrupted time series with a nonequivalent no-treatment comparison group**—This is a two-group pre-test–post-test design using an untreated control group, but with the addition of multiple pre-tests and post-tests. A comparison group is used, so even though randomization does not occur, the same threats to validity can occur but they usually

can be more easily disproved. The main challenge with this research design is the need to show that the two groups used were equal on all of the variables that were important to causation prior to the introduction of treatment. This may be difficult for the researcher who has little knowledge of the status of the research subjects prior to initiation of the treatment intervention (Garson, 2009).

- **Interrupted time series with multiple replications**—This interrupted time series has the treatment intervention and removal of the treatment occurring multiple times according to a schedule; the design is strengthened when the researcher times these interventions and removals randomly. The difficulty associated with this design is its assumption that the researcher is dealing with the effect of an intervention that dissipates before the next intervention is applied without a cumulative effect. This would not be an effective research design to use when the researcher is working with, for example, the effects of some pain medications or psychiatric drugs that may be cumulative over time (Garson, 2009).
- **Interrupted time series with switching replications**—This research design uses two groups, each serving as either the treatment or comparison group on an alternating basis. This is accomplished through multiple applications of the treatment intervention and removal of the treatment. Although this design requires a high level of control over the research subjects by the researcher, it is a strong design that can rule out threats to validity. The main difficulty encountered with use of this research design is that it is ineffective when the treatment intervention has been introduced gradually or when the effect of the treatment intervention does not dissipate easily. This means that this design probably would not be effective when a research project involves the effects of chemotherapy, because these effects would not dissipate easily and are typically administered in a cycle of treatments (Garson, 2009).

External Validity

The importance of internal validity and threats that must be minimized already has been discussed. However, **external validity** must also be considered. This pertains to the generalizability of the results obtained. A study will have little external validity if it is so specific to a certain population that its results cannot be applicable to anyone else. Like internal validity, there are specific threats to external validity that also must be minimized by the researcher to the greatest extent possible. These include:

- *External validity*—Post-test scores of pre-tested subjects may not be representative of the unpre-tested population of subjects if the subjects are pre-test–sensitized to the effects of the intervention or treatment being applied.
- *Interaction of selection and experimental treatment*—If the process of selection has been biased, a test group may be produced that responds to the independent variable in ways not typical of the larger population of subjects.
- *Reactive effects of experimental arrangements*—This occurs when the conditions of the experiment are not representative of real-world situations.
- *Multiple-treatment interference*—If multiple treatments are applied simultaneously, changes may occur that are different from what would occur if one treatment were used alone.
- *Irrelevant responsiveness of measures*—The measures being used may include irrelevant components that indicate change has occurred when in fact it has not.
- *Irrelevant replicability of treatments*—Researchers may fail to include the part of the intervention or treatment actually responsible for creating change each time the research subjects are exposed to it (Manheim, Rich, & Willnat, 2002).

As the DNP student continues to decide on a research design for the research project, he or she must investigate qualitative research designs as well as quantitative designs. The following chapter will review the qualitative designs.

FIGURE 5-1 Decision tree to determine whether a quantitative research design is appropriate.

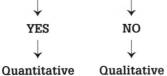

Am I trying to establish causation or correlation?

YES   NO

Quantitative   Qualitative

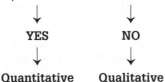

Do I want to know about the benefits of a specific healthcare intervention?

YES   NO

Quantitative   Qualitative

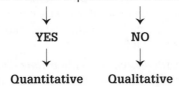

Do I need to know about human interaction, emotions, or experiences to answer a question about social phenomena?

YES   NO

Quantitative   Qualitative

■ GLOSSARY

attrition Loss of research subjects that occurs during the course of the research study.

bias Any influence that is capable of distorting the results of a research study.

blinding Occurs when neither the research subject nor the person assessing the outcome of the treatment is aware of the group to which the client belongs.

case control study Type of observational, non-experimental research design.

cohort A group of subjects who are followed over a period of time.

control group Research participants in an experiment who do not receive the treatment or intervention; it will be compared to the experimental group whose participants do receive the intervention.

cross-sectional study Based on observations obtained at a single point in time.

experimental group Research participants in an experiment who receive the treatment or intervention; it will be compared to the control group whose participants do not receive the intervention.

experimental study Research subjects are randomly selected to be in the experimental group and receive a new intervention or to be in the control group and receive either a standard intervention or no intervention at all.

external validity The generalizability of results obtained to other populations.

history Type of threat to the internal validity of a research design; occurs when a specific event either inside or outside the experimental setting has an effect on the dependent variable.

instrumentation This threat to internal validity occurs when there are changes in the way variables are measured or in the techniques used for observation that will cause changes in the measurements that are obtained.

internal validity The ability to infer that the independent variable in a research project is truly related to the dependent variable. A threat to internal validity means there are competing explanations for the results obtained in a research project.

interrupted time series with a nonequivalent no-treatment comparison group This is the two-group pre-test–post-test design using an untreated control group, but with the addition of multiple pre-tests and post-tests.

interrupted time series with multiple replications This interrupted time series has the treatment intervention and removal of the treatment occurring multiple times according to a schedule. The design is strengthened when the researcher times these interventions and removals randomly.

interrupted time series with switching replications This research design uses two groups, each serving as either the treatment or comparison group on an alternating basis. This is accomplished through multiple applications of the treatment intervention and removal of the treatment.

longitudinal study Study designed to collect data at more than one point in time.

maturation Threat to internal validity of a research design; refers to the natural developmental changes such as the aging process that would occur to research subjects over the course of time and are unrelated to the research project being conducted.

mortality This threat to internal validity is the loss of study subjects from the time of administration of the pre-test to the time of administration of the post-test. If the subjects who remain in the study are vastly different from the subjects who opt to remove themselves from the project, the results obtained will most likely be affected.

nonrandomized clinical trial Used when randomization is not feasible or ethical, or when there is insufficient evidence to justify the difficulty and expense of a randomized clinical trial.

observational study A type of non-experimental research design.

positivism A school of thought that maintains there is an objective reality in the world that can be quantified in some way so that observation or measurement can occur.

pre-test–post-test design Looks at the outcome of interest before the application of an intervention and then after an intervention.

randomized controlled trial The strongest design to provide healthcare professionals with information regarding the benefits of a specific healthcare intervention.

representative sample A sample whose key characteristics closely resemble those of the larger population.

selection bias Type of threat to internal validity resulting from the way in which research subjects were chosen for the project, particularly if precautions were not utilized to achieve a representative sample.

simple interrupted time series design A one-group pre-test–post-test design that uses multiple pre-tests and post-tests.

Solomon four-group design Uses two groups that receive the intervention and two groups that do not. Only one treatment group will be administered a pre-test, but all four groups will receive the post-test.

testing Threat to the internal validity of a research design used in a research project; refers to the effect of taking a pre-test on the subject's post-test score. The result of the differences between post-test and pre-test scores may not be an outcome of the application of an intervention but may instead be the result of the experience gained through the testing process.

time series This research design involves the collection of data over an extended period of time and the introduction of an experimental treatment during the data collection process.

■ LEARNING ENHANCEMENT TOOLS

1. Describe the ideal conditions under which a DNP researcher could utilize a randomized controlled trial as a research design.

2. Describe the ideal conditions under which a DNP researcher could utilize a non-randomized clinical trial as a research design.

3. Describe the ideal conditions under which a DNP researcher could utilize a pre-test–post-test research design.

4. Develop a set of criteria you would use in critiquing an experimental research design used in a research project. Describe why you selected each criterion and how you would implement each one.

5. You are a DNP researcher who is considering using a cross-sectional survey as a research design for a project involving administrators' training in disaster preparedness. You are employed in a 425-bed acute care hospital that is affiliated with a large university. Describe what you can do to make the survey as representative as possible.

6. Describe the ideal conditions under which a DNP researcher could utilize a longitudinal research design using a cohort.

7. Develop a set of criteria you would use in critiquing a non-experimental observational research design that is used in a research project. Describe why you selected each criterion and how you would implement each one.

8. Outline a plan for a research study that would effectively fit use of a case control study as a research design.

9. Develop a set of criteria you would use in critiquing a quasi-experimental research design used in a research project. Describe why you selected each criterion and how you would implement each one.

10. Outline a plan for a research study that would effectively fit use of one-group post-test only as a research design.

11. Outline a plan for a research study that would effectively fit use of nonequivalent control group as a research design.

12. You are planning to use a quasi-experimental research design for your research project. Explain how you can reduce the threats to internal validity as you implement the design.

13. Describe the ideal conditions under which a DNP researcher could utilize a time series research design.

14. Describe the circumstances under which a DNP researcher would choose to utilize the following research designs:

   a. Simple interrupted time series design

   b. Interrupted time series with a nonequivalent no-treatment comparison group

   c. Interrupted time series with multiple replications

   d. Interrupted time series with switching replications

15. You are planning to use a quasi-experimental research design for your research project. Explain how you can reduce the threats to external validity as you implement the design.

■ RESOURCES

Bordens, K., & Abbott, B. (2008). *Research design and methods: A process approach.* New York: McGraw-Hill.

Crawford, L. (2003). *What is research and why do we do it?* Retrieved August 22, 2005, from http://courseroom.capella.edu/webct/ RelativeReosurceManager/44535266/area.1117721431399_1423855340/ topic.1117721580396_712469535/attachments.46158618/Crawford.rtf;JSESSIONID =DL3kN9vryYp3QCSipncMAwEaJv9ZHwuYFKSOxEhPOu5NHq13drsy! -336469518!NONE!1124825060764?fileContentID=46158624

Creswell, J. (2008). *Research design: Qualitative, quantitative, and mixed methods approaches.* Thousand Oaks, CA: Sage Publications.

Endacott, R. (2007). Clinical research 1: Research questions and design. *Accident and Emergency Nursing, 15*(2), 106–109.

Fontana, J. (2004). A methodology for critical science in nursing. *Advances in Nursing Science, 27*(2), 93–101.

Halcomb, E., & Andrew, S. (2005). Triangulation as a method for contemporary nursing research. *Nurse Researcher, 13*(2), 71–82.

Hopwood, N. (2004). Research design and methods of data collection and analysis: Researching students' conceptions in a multiple method case study. *Journal of Geography in Higher Education, 28*(2), 347–353.

Leedy, P., & Ormrod, J. (2009). *Practical research: Planning and design.* Upper Saddle River, NJ: Prentice-Hall.

Russell, C. (2005). Interpreting research in nephrology nursing: Evaluating quantitative research reports. *Nephrology Nursing Journal, 32*(1), 61–64.

Sandelowski, M. (2000). Focus on research methods: Combining qualitative and quantitative sampling, data collection, and analysis techniques in mixed-method studies. *Research in Nursing & Health, 23*, 246–255.

Shadish, W., Cook, T., & Campbell, D. (2002). *Experimental and quasi-experimental designs for generalized causal inference.* Boston: Houghton-Mifflin.

Verschuren, P. (2001). Case study as a research strategy: Some ambiguities and opportunities. *International Journal Social Research Methodology, 6*(2), 121–139.

■ REFERENCES

Garson, D. (2009). *Research designs.* Retrieved November 25, 2009, from http://faculty.chass.ncsu.edu/garson/PA765/design.htm

Hooked on Evidence. (n.d.). *Hooked on evidence study design type definitions.* Retrieved November 23, 2009, from www.hookedonevidence.com/formsubmit/ popups/designtypedef.cfm

LoBiondo-Wood, G., & Haber, J. (2002). *Nursing research: Methods, critical appraisal, and utilization.* St. Louis, MO: Mosby.

Manheim, J., Rich, R., & Willnat, L. (2002). *Empirical political analysis: Research methods in political science.* New York: Addison Wesley Longman.

McGahee, T., & Tingen, M. (n.d.). The use of the Solomon four-group design in nursing research. *Southern Online Journal of Nursing Research, 9*(1), 1–7.

Palmer, J. (2009). Nursing research: Understanding the basics. *Plastic Surgical Nursing, 29*(2), 115–121.

Polit, D., & Hungler, B. (2000). *Essentials of nursing research: Methods and applications.* Philadelphia: Lippincott.

Roberts, J., & Dicenso, A. (1999). Identifying the best research design to fit the question. Part 1: Quantitative design. *Evidence-Based Nursing, 2,* 4–6.

Seers, K., & Critelton, N. (2001). Quantitative research: Designs relevant to nursing and healthcare. *Nursing Times, 6*(1), 487–500.

Designing a Clinically Based Qualitative Capstone Research Project

■ OBJECTIVES

Upon completion of this chapter, the reader should be prepared to:

1 Discuss the principles that function as the basis of qualitative research.

2 Describe the advantages and limitations of using a qualitative research design.

3 Discuss the specific challenges faced by the researcher who is engaged in qualitative research involving sensitive issues.

4 Discuss the differences between qualitative and quantitative research.

5 Discuss the use of ethnography as a qualitative research design.

6 Differentiate between an etic perspective and an emic perspective.

7 Discuss the use of phenomenology as a qualitative research design.

8 Differentiate between descriptive and interpretative phenomenology.

9 Discuss the use of grounded theory as a qualitative research design.

10 Describe the characteristics of a core variable.

11 Discuss the use of life history as a qualitative research design.

12 Differentiate between an interview guide and a life history grid.

13 Discuss the use of ethnomethodology as a qualitative research design.

14 Describe the key features of an ethnomethodological research design.

15 Delineate the limitations known to be associated with an ethnomethodological research design.

BASIC TYPES OF QUALITATIVE RESEARCH

A clinically based capstone project can use a qualitative research design when the DNP researcher is concerned mainly with the process being implemented rather than the outcomes being achieved or products being utilized. The qualitative researcher is concerned with how research subjects make sense of their lives, experiences, and structures in their own world and the meaning that these experiences and structures have for them. This indicates that qualitative research frequently is descriptive because the researcher is concerned with the process, meaning, and understanding that can be gained. Hoepfl (1997) broadly defines qualitative research as any type of research that uses a means other than statistical procedures or some method of quantification to generate findings.

In qualitative research, the researcher is the primary instrument for data collection as well as data analysis. Data collection frequently occurs through fieldwork, which means the researcher goes on-site to the location of research subjects so behavior is recorded in its natural setting. In addition, data is frequently recorded using field notes. These are free-flowing descriptions of research subjects, activities, and setting that can also include sketches or maps. Recognizing that writing extensive field notes can be very difficult during participant observations, some researchers advocate writing brief notes to serve as a memory aid after the conclusion of the observation while full field notes are being constructed (Hoepfl, 1997). A valuable source of information for the qualitative researcher can be document analysis. This can include letters, diaries, and newspaper articles in addition to the standard reports and official records. Some researchers have used journal entries and memos to supplement interviews with research participants (Hoepfl, 1997).

Regardless of the format of the research design selected, the researcher engaged in qualitative research most often is interested in inductive research. This means the researcher builds hypotheses and theories from details derived from the collection of data from the research subjects. The researcher will be interested in the generation of new hypotheses rather than the testing of hypotheses (Siegle, n.d.).

The basic difference between qualitative and quantitative research can be best described in terms of their philosophical bases. Qualitative research is based on principles of phenomenology, which acknowledges the individual qualities of each research subject while exploring human responses and the influence of society on each person's perception of reality. In comparison, quantitative research is based on the principles of positivism, as was previously noted in Chapter 5. Knowing that quantitative research is the best approach to use in order to establish the existence of a cause-and-effect relationship between variables, it is logical that positivism seeks to conduct research that is both objective and measurable so that a direction for a hypothesis will emerge. Therefore, it becomes clear that qualitative research can be a logical choice when the researcher is interested in issues other than a cause-and-effect relationship between variables (Palmer, 2009). The researcher engaged in quantitative research is concerned with the following:

- What knowledge exists about a problem that will allow a hypothesis to be formulated and then tested?
- What concepts are available for testing the hypothesis?
- How can the concepts be operationalized or measured?
- What scientific theory can explain the data as they currently exist?
- How can the results be interpreted and then reported to be of interest to the nursing community initially and then to stakeholders for health care in general? Are there implications that could be of interest to stakeholders in other fields as well? Do the results have global implications?

In contrast, the researcher engaged in qualitative research is primarily concerned with:

- What do research subjects know about their culture that can be discovered by the researcher?
- What concepts do research subjects use to classify their experiences?
- How do these subjects define the concepts they use to classify their experiences? Where do the subjects derive the information they use to formulate their definitions of the concepts?
- Is there a folk theory that subjects are using to explain their experiences? What is the basis of the folk theory once it is identified?
- How can the researcher translate the subjects' cultural knowledge into a cultural description that will be of interest to the nursing community initially and then to stakeholders for health care in general? Is there an aspect of the cultural description that will be of interest to stakeholders in other fields as well? Does the cultural description have global implications? (Siegle, 2009)

Key (1997) summarized the differences between qualitative and quantitative research, which can be seen in **Table 6-1**.

TABLE 6-1 Differences Between Qualitative and Quantitative Research

Characteristic	Qualitative Research	Quantitative Research
Philosophical origin	Phenomenology, symbolic interaction	Positivism, logical empiricism
Goal of investigation	Understanding, description, discovery, generation of hypothesis	Prediction, control, description, explanation, confirmation, testing of hypotheses
Design characteristics	Flexible, evolving	Predetermined, structured
Setting	Natural, familiar	Unfamiliar, artificial
Sample utilized	Small, not randomized, not necessarily representative of the larger population; may use purposeful sampling in which information-rich cases are selected for in-depth study (Hoepfl, 1997)	Large, randomized, representative of the larger population
Data collection	Researcher serves as the primary instrument, with interviews and observations as data collection methods; interviews used can consist of informal and conversational, semi-structured, or standardized using open-ended questions (Hoepfl, 1997)	Instruments used include scales, tests, surveys and questionnaires; computers used for administration of online instruments
Mode of analysis	Inductive, by the researcher	Deductive, by statistical methods

Source: Key (1997).

ADVANTAGES AND LIMITATIONS OF QUALITATIVE RESEARCH

A primary advantage of qualitative research stems from its subjective nature. The data gathered is unique to the individual research subject's perspective, so the subject is given the opportunity to express feelings and perceptions in an environment that is nonjudgmental. Qualitative research allows a connection to be established between phenomena being studied and research subjects' perceptions of those phenomena. Another advantage of qualitative research is its flexibility. It allows the DNP researcher to be prepared to adjust the study in response to obstacles that arise during the study and to alter the established course of the project so that new research questions can be developed and other methods for data collection established as needed. Qualitative research can also provide a realistic description of how a research subject relates to his or her environment as well as to the interventions being implemented in the study. This means that a research question regarding the reason why a patient is not responding as expected to treatment could be solved through qualitative research. It can use subjective information and observations of research participants to describe the natural setting of the variables being studied, and thus may produce more comprehensive information than could be generated through quantitative research. Qualitative research also lends itself particularly well to academia because questions regarding how students respond to a specific teaching strategy can be resolved using a qualitative research design (Palmer, 2009).

Although qualitative research can be a rich source of untapped data for the DNP researcher, its potential limitations must be considered as well. It sometimes has been viewed in a negative light because of its reliance on subjective data and the difficulty involved in channeling perceptions or emotions into data that are measurable. The very subjective data that can describe the **context** of the variables being considered can make it difficult to prevent researcher-induced bias. Results may be questioned in terms of validity and credibility. The primary limitation attached to this type of research design is the potential lack of logical reasoning and statistical analysis required by a scientific field such as health care. A qualitative study places a great deal of reliance on the knowledge and reliability of the researcher and the relationship that he or she establishes with research subjects during the course of the project. If the researcher becomes too emotionally involved with research subjects, a threat to the research may develop as subjects begin to feel vulnerable during interviews. This means that some types of qualitative research designs may require greater scrutiny by an institutional review board than the researcher originally anticipated in order to prevent the research subjects from feeling that their privacy is being overly invaded (Palmer, 2009). In addition, the DNP researcher who opts to use a qualitative research design will find that there are few guidelines regarding when to conclude the data collection process. This may lead to overextension of the sampling procedure to such an extent that the boundaries of the research project are expanded inappropriately (Hoepfl, 1997).

Even greater challenges can emerge for the qualitative researcher who opts to engage in research that involves sensitive issues. Dickson-Swift, James,

Kippen, and Liamputtong (2007) found specific issues would arise for the researcher who selects a particularly sensitive topic:

- The researcher must recognize that he or she is actually entering the life of the research subject; when this process occurs at a time of crisis and involves extensive interviews, the researcher must be able to show both discretion and respect for the subject's willingness to disclose extremely personal information.
- The researcher must be able to develop rapport with the research subject from the first encounter; participant disclosure will be increased if there is a strong rapport between the researcher and the participant.
- Researcher self-disclosure may occur to facilitate disclosure by the research subject, but may cause the researcher to feel vulnerable.
- The researcher may feel the need for reciprocity, or the desire to give something back to the subject to acknowledge what the person has given to the researcher. This can lead to the development of a social relationship with the research subject.
- A researcher who is hearing many life stories of traumatized research subjects may begin to feel desensitized and distant from his or her feelings.
- The researcher may begin to develop emotional attachments to research subjects and thus may continue to think about research subjects after completing data collection.
- The researcher who performs data collection in a setting such as subjects' homes may feel physically vulnerable if the setting causes him or her to feel unsafe or emotionally vulnerable when the setting leads to a great amount of self-disclosure.
- The researcher may ultimately feel guilt related to collecting sensitive data and may wrestle with questions regarding exploitation of research subjects.

The researcher who chooses to select a sensitive topic must be prepared before initiating the study to address these challenges to avoid spending valuable time struggling with a project that is not viable.

QUALITATIVE RESEARCH DESIGNS

There are various qualitative research designs that the DNP researcher can select from in formulating the capstone project. These include ethnography, phenomenology, grounded theory, life history, and ethnomethodology.

Ethnography

When a researcher selects **ethnography** as the research design for a study, he or she is primarily concerned with the need to learn about a culture from the people who actually are immersed in it every day. The term *culture* can be used to mean not only a population of people with common ethnicity, but also a society, a community, or an organization. Ethnography entails intensive involvement with the participants being studied through immersion in their world via fieldwork. The researcher uses participant observation and in-depth interviews to discover the meanings that participants have for their knowledge, behaviors, and activities (Ploeg, 1999). Informants are interviewed multiple times, and they are asked to identify other informants who would be useful to the researcher and are representative of the community being studied. This is referred to as **chain sampling**. This would occur, for example, when the informant being interviewed by the DNP researcher in an area of hospital administration suggests the researcher speak with members of another subdivision of the same department who are involved in similar activities. It is most typical for the researcher who uses ethnography as a research design to live in the culture being studied for an extensive period of time, so the DNP researcher could easily study the employees of the hospital where he or she is employed.

If the research is primarily concerned with how members of the culture being studied perceive their own world, this is referred to an **emic perspective**. This would be used, for example, when the research centers around nurses employed in a specific area of a hospital and their perception of their own unit. If the research is more concerned with the way non-members perceive and interpret the behaviors of members of the culture, this is an **etic perspective** (Garson, 2008). This would be appropriate when the research focuses on non-nurses employed by the hospital or even volunteers associated with the hospital on a frequent basis and their perception of the behaviors of the nurses in a specific area of the hospital. The context of the culture is particularly important in ethnography, whether social, political, or economic. This means that this design easily could be utilized by a DNP researcher who is interested in studying hospital employees, whether nurses or administrative employees (Ploeg, 1999).

Phenomenology

The researcher who decides to use a phenomenological approach to a study is primarily interested in accurately describing the lived experiences of the research subjects rather than formulating theories or models of the phenomenon being studied. In-depth interviews are most frequently used as the primary means of data collection (Ploeg, 1999). The role of the researcher is often that of a facilitator to encourage the respondent to talk freely. This means the only interview questions are those that promote clarification of an area or further exploration of an issue. Data analysis occurs through interpretation of the interview material as meaningful information is identified and categorized into themes (Balls, 2009).

A phenomenological research design may be approached from two perspectives: descriptive phenomenology or interpretative phenomenology. **Descriptive phenomenology** uses a concept known as **bracketing** to maintain researcher objectivity. This consists of setting aside the researcher's knowledge of the experience being investigated and approaching the data without preconceived ideas about the phenomenon being studied (Balls, 2009). Some researchers who advocate the descriptive phenomenological approach opt to not conduct a detailed literature review before beginning the study and to not format specific research questions other than the desire to describe participants' lived experiences as they relate to the topic of the project. The descriptive approach also proposes that there are aspects to any participant's lived experience that are common to anyone who has that experience. These aspects are referred to as **universal essences** (Lopez & Willis, 2004). The descriptive approach could be used by a DNP researcher interested in describing the lived experiences of parents whose children are hospitalized with a chronic illness.

In comparison, **interpretative phenomenology** proposes that the researcher cannot eliminate preconceptions about a phenomenon and, in fact, it is those experiences that are used to interpret the experiences of other people (Balls, 2009). The interpretative approach proposes that a person's reality is influenced by the world in which he or she lives to such an extent that his or her choices are confined by the specific conditions of his or her daily existence. The DNP researcher who uses an interpretative phenomenological approach would interpret the narratives of participants to determine the historical, social, and political forces that are shaping their experiences. This approach does not prohibit the use of a conceptual framework, and in fact allows a theoretical approach to be used to add focus and to assist in decisions about sampling, subjects, and research questions. If the researcher opts to utilize a framework, he or she has a responsibility to show that the framework did not bias the participant narratives and to demonstrate how the framework was used in data interpretation and in the generation of findings. The DNP researcher could use the interpretative approach to study the lived experiences of nurse managers in a hospital that is undergoing a buyout by another corporation. The interpretative approach would investigate the historical, social, and political forces that are influencing the managers' experiences (Lopez & Willis, 2004).

Grounded Theory

The researcher who opts to use grounded theory is interested in utilizing theory that is derived from everyday experiences. The researcher attempts to explain a specific social situation by identifying the guiding principle underlying it (Byrne, 2001). Rather than developing a theory and then seeking out evidence to support that theory, the researcher using grounded theory as a research design gathers data and then develops an explanatory theory derived from the data (Walker & Myrick, 2006). Research topics that would lend themselves well to use of grounded theory by a DNP researcher would be interaction between client and nurse, the process of discharge planning, interaction between physician and nurse, or the management styles utilized by nurse managers.

The sources of data acquired through grounded theory will include any resource that provides information about the social interaction being investigated. The grounded theory underlying the social interaction being investigated will be determined by the researcher through the **constant comparative method**, which means that data will be analyzed concurrently throughout the process of data collection as the researcher searches for a **core variable** that will be the foundation for formulation of the grounded theory. The core variable that is sought by the researcher typically:

- Recurs on a frequent basis
- Links various data
- Has greater implications for development of formal theory
- Develops detail in the research
- Includes people from various backgrounds (Byrne, 2001)

The researcher using a grounded theory design begins to analyze the data through a process known as coding, initially examining the data line by line and then comparing and contrasting to create categories. These categories are used to develop the theory, which emerges as the researcher implements **data reduction**. Data reduction occurs as information relevant to the topic is filtered and information that is not relevant to the topic is discarded. Data will be collected using the process of **data saturation**—data are collected until no additional new information is located (Byrne, 2001). Grounded theory as a research design lends itself well to being used by a researcher who functions in a quality assurance–type area and is already familiar with the root-cause-analysis investigative process.

Life History

The researcher who opts to utilize life history as a research design is interested in exploring, discovering, and understanding the lives of participants, with research subjects actively reconstructing their lives as they tell their stories. The researcher is able to explore a variety of the participants' experiences and relationships and examine changes over time as lifelong data are collected. The researcher who uses the life history design views research subjects as collaborative partners. Each participant will be guided through his or her life history by the researcher and encouraged to reflect on memories and insights into behaviors. The life history approach is intended to provide an understanding of how past events and relationships influence current phenomena and how people instill meaning into their lives. As the design is implemented, context is determined. This is the subject's worldview that influences how his or her life is lived and interpreted and allows the subject to assign meaning to his or her life events, thoughts, experiences, and relationships. Context is crucial as the researcher attempts to understand how the subject views an event in his or her life or a specific experience (Haglund, 2004).

Some researchers advocate use of an interview guide as well as a life history grid when utilizing the life history research design. The **interview guide** can be particularly useful in obtaining institutional review board approval because it ensures the interviewer will ask all participants similar questions. The interview guide for the life history design should move in chronological order, including contexts that are particularly important to the participants, and should include both open-ended questions and follow-up questions. Multiple one-hour interviews should be scheduled with participants, with the first interview scheduled when the research subject initially gives consent and the second interview scheduled immediately after the first interview. This will allow the researcher to begin the interview with questions that are the least personal and reserve more sensitive questions for subsequent interviews. The **life history grid** is important as a tool for the researcher because it adds details during the analysis so that life patterns can be diagrammed. It allows the researcher to organize the participant's life events, correlate events in the life history, and summarize the written record. The grid can be used to identify patterns of experiences to understand the stories that research subjects have narrated about their lives. If the researcher opts to complete the grid during the course of the interviews, it may serve to engage the participant in the research process (Haglund, 2004).

The life history research design could be used effectively by the researcher who is interested in exploring and understanding the lives of nurses who served in World War II, for example. This type of design, because of its inclusion of contextual data, participants' interpretations, as well as emotional responses, may provide a depth of understanding that would be difficult to match with other, less effective designs (Haglund, 2004).

Ethnomethodology

The researcher who utilizes ethnomethodology as a research design is concerned with how members of a social group (such as a specific area of a hospital, for example) perceive, define, and ultimately classify the ways in which they perform their daily activities (such as patient care duties) and the meaning the members assign to these activities. Ethnomethodology is used to show how group members produce order within their own ranks so that cultural activities are interpreted and understood. A DNP researcher could use this research design to study the practices that are culturally unique to nursing, such as the giving of reports from nurse to nurse or the pinning ceremony that is implemented at the successful graduation from a nursing program (Harper, 2008).

The researcher who opts to use ethnomethodology as a research design believes that social order is made up of patterns of behavior and interactions that can be chaotic; however, members produce order from this chaos mentally by interpreting rules to guide their social actions. This belief can be considered in light of the socialization of a new nurse in nursing practice, within which the nurse learns accepted and expected attitudes. As the nurse's practice becomes more routine, the attitudes influencing the practice will become so incorporated into the nurse's psyche that he or she will no longer have to interpret the underlying reasons for specific aspects of practice (Harper, 2008).

Ethnomethodological ethnography has specific unique features that must be considered by the researcher who is considering using it as a research design:

- *Taken for granted assumptions*—The routine activities undertaken by the members of a group, including the expectations of what should happen in the course of a normal day.
- *Common-sense knowledge and procedures*—The knowledge used by the group members to make sense of their world; for a DNP researcher, this could consist of the body of knowledge that all nurses share.
- *Typification*—The way group members classify objects or experiences; this could include the terminology nurses use to classify the acuity levels of their patients.
- *Accounting*—All of the activities group members use to make sense of their world; for the DNP researcher, this would consist of how nurses use their "taken-for-granted assumptions," "common-sense knowledge," and experience to make decisions.

- *Indexicality*—This means that actions and verbal statements depend on the context of the situation for their meaning.
- *Reflexivity*—The relationship between a description of how an event occurred and the circumstances of an event; for the DNP researcher, this could consist of a nurse describing the behaviors associated with different levels of anxiety and also describing patients who exhibited these behaviors.

In addition to these key features that must be considered by the researcher who decides to use ethnomethodological ethnography as a research design, certain limitations also are associated with such a design. For example, the design does not address the external constraints imposed upon research subjects that will limit their choices, both in action and in thought patterns. This type of design will not be effective for a researcher who needs to explain the cause of research subjects' behaviors, primarily because the design's intention is to describe the interpretive practices used by subjects rather than the causes of action. However, for the DNP researcher interested in exploring how nurses rationalize their decisions relating to daily nursing activities that are so routine that they require no thought, it can be a very effective design for a research project (Harper, 2008).

SELECTING A QUALITATIVE RESEARCH DESIGN

Hoepfl (1997) has described a basic process for selecting the most appropriate qualitative research design for a study. The researcher who is attempting to decide on a design should systematically:

- Decide on a focus for the study; this will allow the researcher to establish boundaries and decide on types of data to include and exclude as data collection occurs.
- Determine whether the qualitative research paradigm characteristics fit with the overall goals of the research; this will allow the researcher to determine early in the research process if in fact a qualitative design meets the needs of the research project.
- Decide where data will be collected and whom the data will be collected from, incorporating factors such as confidentiality issues.
- Determine how data collection will proceed; for example, the first phase of data collection may consist of open-ended participant observation, while the next phase might consist of more focused interviews.

- Decide on instrumentation that will be needed beyond simply using the researcher as the human instrument; this will help the researcher decide if additional time needs to be incorporated into the project to allow for the design of an instrument.
- Decide how detailed and specific research questions will be and how accurately and detailed the data will be recorded.
- Decide on procedures for data analysis.
- Address the logistics of data collection; interviews will need to be scheduled, personnel for data collection may need to be recruited, and a budget will need to be planned.
- Plan how the issues of reliability and validity will be addressed.

As the DNP student continues to decide on a research design for the research project, mixed framework research designs must be investigated in addition to the quantitative and qualitative designs. Mixed framework designs are research designs that incorporate elements of both of the previously discussed categories of research. Chapter 7 will review the mixed framework designs.

■ GLOSSARY

bracketing Setting aside the researcher's knowledge of the experience being investigated and approaching the data without preconceived ideas about the phenomenon being studied.

chain sampling Informants are asked to identify other informants who would be useful to the researcher and are representative of the community being studied.

constant comparative method Data will be analyzed concurrently throughout the process of data collection as the researcher searches for a core variable that will be the foundation for formulation of the grounded theory.

context The subject's worldview that influences how his or her life is lived and interpreted and allows the subject to assign meaning to his or her life events, thoughts, experiences, and relationships.

core variable The foundation for formulation of the grounded theory. The core variable that is sought by the researcher typically recurs on a frequent basis, links various data, has strong implications for development of formal theory, develops a great deal of detail, and includes people from various backgrounds.

data reduction Occurs as information relevant to the topic is filtered and information not relevant to the topic is discarded.

data saturation Data are collected until no additional new information can be located.

descriptive phenomenology A form of phenomenological research design that proposes there are aspects to any participant's lived experiences that are common to anyone who has that experience.

emic perspective Research primarily concerned with how members of a culture being studied perceive their own world.

ethnography Research primarily concerned with the need to learn about a culture from the people who actually are immersed in it every day.

etic perspective Research concerned with the way that non-members perceive and interpret the behaviors of members of the culture.

interpretative phenomenology Proposes that the researcher cannot eliminate preconceptions about a phenomenon and, in fact, it is those experiences that are used to interpret the experiences of other people.

interview guide Used as part of life history research design; should move in chronological order, including contexts that are particularly important to the participants, and should include both open-ended questions and follow-up questions.

life history grid Allows the researcher to organize the participant's life events, correlate events in the life history, and summarize the written record.

■ LEARNING ENHANCEMENT TOOLS

1. Describe the ideal conditions under which a DNP researcher could utilize ethnography as a research design.

   a. Describe a study that has an ethnographic research design and an emic perspective.

   b. Describe a study that has an ethnographic research design and an etic perspective.

2. Describe the ideal conditions under which a DNP researcher could utilize a phenomenological research design.

   a. Describe a study that has a phenomenological research design and a descriptive perspective.

   b. Describe a study that has a phenomenological research design and an interpretative perspective.

3. Describe the ideal conditions under which a DNP researcher could utilize grounded theory as a research design.

   a. Describe an outline for a research study that would use grounded theory as a research design and would require the researcher to implement both data saturation and data reduction.

   b. Describe an outline for a research study that would use grounded theory as a research design. Discuss how the researcher would implement the constant comparative method and how the core variable would be derived.

4. Describe the ideal conditions under which a DNP researcher could utilize life history as a research design.

   a. Describe an outline for a research project using life history as a research design. Formulate an interview guide for the project.

   b. Describe an outline for a research project using life history as a research design. Formulate a life history guide for the project.

5. Describe the ideal conditions under which a DNP researcher could utilize ethnomethodology as a research design.

6. Discuss how the DNP researcher using an ethnomethodological research design could incorporate all of the key features of such a design into a research project.

7. How can the DNP researcher who is interested in using an ethnomethodological research design plan to circumnavigate the limitations that are known to be associated with such a design?

8. You are a DNP researcher who has chosen to perform qualitative research with rape victims who arrive at your hospital's emergency department. Discuss specific ways in which you can cope with the challenges posed by performing research on such a sensitive topic while consistently remaining cognizant of the needs of your research subjects.

■ RESOURCES

Alexander, B. (2005). Performance ethnography: The reenacting and inciting of culture. In N. K. Denzin & Y. S. Lincoln (eds.), *The Sage handbook of qualitative research* (3rd ed., pp. 411–441). Thousand Oaks, CA: Sage.

Annells, M. (2007). What's common with qualitative nursing research these days? *Journal of Clinical Nursing, 16*(2), 223–224.

Balls, P. (2009, August 13). *Phenomenology in nursing research: Methodology, interviewing and transcribing.* Retrieved April 12, 2010, from http://www.nursingtimes.net/nursing-practice-clinical-research/phenomenology-in-nursing-research-methodology-interviewing-and-transcribing/5005138.article

Birch, M., & Miller, T. (2000). Inviting intimacy: The interview as therapeutic opportunity. *International Journal of Social Research Methodology, 3*, 189–202.

Crist, J., & Tanner, A. (2003). Interpretation/analysis in hermeneutic interpretative phenomenology. *Nursing Research, 52*(3), 202–205.

Dickson-Swift, V., James, E., Kippen, S., & Liamputtong, P. (2006). Blurring boundaries in qualitative health research on sensitive topics. *Qualitative Health Research, 16*, 853–871.

Hubbard, G., Backett-Milburn, K., & Kemmer, D. (2001). Working with emotions: Issues for the researcher in fieldwork and teamwork. *International Journal of Social Research Methodology, 4*, 119–137.

Johnson, B., & Clarke, J. (2003). Collecting sensitive data: The impact on researchers. *Qualitative Health Research, 13*, 421–434.

LeVasseur, J. (2003). The problem of bracketing in phenomenology. *Qualitative Health Research, 13*, 408–420.

Madison, D. (2005). *Critical ethnography: Method, ethics, and performance.* Thousand Oaks, CA: Sage Publications.

Rager, K. (2005). Self-care and the qualitative researcher: When collecting data can break your heart. *Educational Researcher, 34*, 23–27.

Smith, C., & Gallo, A. (2007). Applications of performance ethnography in nursing. *Qualitative Health Research, 17*, 521–527.

Sque, M. (2000). Researching the bereaved: An investigator's experience. *Nursing Ethics, 7*, 23–33.

Stubblefield, C., & Murray, R. (2002). A phenomenological framework for psychiatric nursing research. *Archives of Psychiatric Nursing, 16*(4), 149–155.

■ REFERENCES

Balls, P. (2009, August 13). *Phenomenology in nursing research: Methodology, interviewing and transcribing.* Retrieved April 12, 2010, from http://www .nursingtimes.net/nursing-practice-clinical-research/phenomenology-in-nursing -research-methodology-interviewing-and-transcribing/5005138.article

Byrne, M. (2001, June). Grounded theory as a qualitative research methodology. *AORN Journal*, June 2001. Retrieved December 9, 2009, from http://findarticles .com/p/articles/mi_m0FSL/is_6_73/ai_75562157/

Dickson-Swift, V. James, E., Kippen, S., & Liamputtong, P. (2007). Doing sensitive research: What challenges do qualitative researchers face? *Qualitative Research, 7*, 327–353.

Garson, D. (2008). *Ethnographic research.* Retrieved December 9, 2009, from http://faculty.chass.ncsu.edu/garson/PA765/ethno.htm

Haglund, K. (2004). Conducting life history research with adolescents. *Qualitative Health Research, 14*, 1309–1319.

Harper, P. (2008). Ethnomethodological ethnography and its application in nursing. *Journal of Research in Nursing, 13*, 311–322.

Hoepfl, M. (1997). Choosing qualitative research: A primer for technology education researchers. *Journal of Technology Education, 9*(1). Retrieved December 7, 2009, from http://scholar.lib.vt.edu/ejournals/JTE/v9n1/hoepfl.html

Key, J. (1997). *Research design in occupational education.* Retrieved December 7, 2009, from http://www.okstate.edu/ag/agedcm4h/academic/aged5980a/5980/ newpage110.htm

Lopez, K., & Willis, D. (2004). Descriptive versus interpretative phenomenology: Their contributions to nursing knowledge. *Qualitative Health Research, 14,* 726–735.

Palmer, J. (2009). Nursing research: Understanding the basics. *Plastic Surgical Nursing, 29*(2), 115–121.

Ploeg, J. (1999). Identifying the best research design to fit the question. Part 2: Qualitative designs. *Evidence Based Nursing, 2,* 36–37.

Siegle, D. (n.d.). *Qualitative versus quantitative.* Retrieved December 7, 2009, from http://www.gifted.uconn.edu/siegle/research/Qualitative/qualquan.htm

Walker, D., & Myrick, F. (2006). Grounded theory: An exploration of process and procedure. *Qualitative Health Research, 16,* 547–559.

Designing a Clinically Based Mixed Method Capstone Research Project

7

■ OBJECTIVES

Upon completion of this chapter, the reader should be prepared to:

1 Describe the underlying premise of a mixed method research design.

2 Discuss the principles that function as the basis of a mixed method research design.

3 Describe the advantages and limitations of using a mixed method research design.

4 Discuss the importance of triangulation and complementarity in deciding to implement a mixed research design.

5 Describe the two primary types of mixed method research subtypes.

6 Discuss the types of across-stage mixed method research designs.

7 Discuss the various classifications of mixed method research designs.

8 Describe the specific types of mixed research designs.

9 Describe how timing plays a part in selecting the type of mixed research design to be implemented.

10 Describe how weighting plays a part in selecting the type of mixed research design to be implemented.

11 Describe how mixing plays a part in selecting the type of mixed research design to be implemented.

12 Discuss how concurrent timing is used in a mixed research design.

13 Discuss how sequential timing is used in a mixed research design.

14 Describe what occurs during the stages of the mixed research process.

15 Discuss the specific skills that a researcher will need in order to implement a mixed research study.

INTRODUCTION TO MIXED METHODS RESEARCH

The DNP researcher who chooses to use a **mixed method** approach to his or her research design is interested in essentially combining the qualitative and quantitative methods. When the strengths of the two methods are combined, the researcher can achieve a broader perspective than would have been possible using only one type of research method. However, use of a mixed method approach entails the researcher having a thorough understanding of the fine points of both quantitative and qualitative research to avoid generating and ultimately reporting inaccurate findings (Palmer, 2009).

Researchers who promote the mixed method approach to research base their ideas on the compatibility thesis as well as pragmatism. The **compatibility thesis** is essentially the idea that the quantitative and qualitative research methods can be compatible and can be used together in a research study. **Pragmatism** adherents believe that a researcher should use any approach or combination of approaches that will function the best in a real-world situation, regardless of assumptions of paradigms or philosophies. Out of these ideas can come the fundamental principle of mixed research, which is that the research should use a combination of research methods that have complementary strengths but without overlapping weaknesses (University of South Alabama, n.d.).

ADVANTAGES AND LIMITATIONS OF MIXED METHOD RESEARCH

As with use of qualitative and quantitative research alone, mixed method research has specific advantages and limitations that must be considered as the researcher plans the study. The advantages and limitations, as might be expected, are very similar to those that were reviewed in the chapters on quantitative and qualitative research. The limitations should be addressed specifically in the early stages of the planning process so as to minimize their effect on the study.

Advantages of mixed method research can include:

- The use of pictures and narrative to add meaning to numbers.
- Can be used to study large numbers of people.
- May have higher credibility than use of quantitative research or qualitative research alone.
- May generate statistically significant results.
- Data analysis could be performed with statistical software.
- Can generate numerical data.
- May be able to show a cause-and-effect relationship.

- Can be used to study a small number of cases in depth.
- Can be used to describe complex phenomena.
- Can be used to test a grounded theory.
- Can answer a broader and more complex range of research questions because the researcher is not confined to use of a single approach to the research.
- Strengths of the additional research method can compensate for the weaknesses of the other method.
- Can provide stronger evidence for a conclusion.
- Can reveal insights that would not have been evident with use of only one research method.
- Can increase the generalizability of the results to a larger population.

Limitations of using a mixed method approach to research can include:

- May require a research team.
- Will require the researcher to have a thorough understanding of the intricacies of each method in order to successfully combine them.
- Will require the researcher to accurately interpret conflicting results that are generated.
- Can be more time consuming than use of quantitative research or qualitative research alone, requiring the use of additional personnel, and more expensive, requiring a more expansive budget and potentially additional time spent in fundraising activities (University of South Alabama, n.d.).

DECIDING TO UTILIZE A MIXED METHOD APPROACH

The DNP researcher who is considering the use of a mixed method approach should determine if the purpose of the research is congruent with the potential benefits of combining the research approaches. For example, the desire for triangulation is a frequently used reason for initiating mixed method research. **Triangulation** means the researcher uses the different methods in order to achieve corroboration of results achieved from the different approaches. This can increase the validity of the study. **Complementarity** is another excellent reason for using the mixed method approach. This means the researcher is striving to enhance, illustrate, or clarify the results achieved through use of input from both quantitative and qualitative designs. This can also increase the validity of the research, and can further increase the interpretability of the results generated. Other purposes for choosing a mixed method approach can be the desire to extend the range of the inquiry used in the study as well as the desire to use results achieved so that one method strengthens the other method. This can mean that the researcher is able to include sampling that would not have been possible without using mixed methods (University of South Alabama, n.d.).

MIXED RESEARCH APPROACHES

There are two major types of mixed research—mixed model research and mixed method research. **Mixed model research** is used when quantitative and qualitative approaches are either mixed within the research process or across the various stages of the process. Mixed model research that occurs within the research stages could consist of using a questionnaire for data collection that includes both open-ended and closed-ended questions. Mixed model research that occurs across the research stages could consist of data collection through open-ended interviews, with the results of those interviews then quantified. There are six research designs that are across-stage mixed model designs:

- Qualitative research objectives that lead to collection of qualitative data, which initiate the researcher performing quantitative analysis
- Qualitative research objectives that lead to collection of quantitative data, which initiate the researcher performing qualitative analysis
- Qualitative research objectives that lead to collection of quantitative data, which initiate the researcher performing quantitative analysis
- Quantitative research objectives that lead to collection of qualitative data, which initiate the researcher performing qualitative analysis
- Quantitative research objectives that lead to collection of qualitative data, which initiate the researcher performing quantitative analysis
- Quantitative research objectives that lead to collection of quantitative data, which initiate the researcher performing qualitative analysis

In comparison, **mixed method research** occurs when both a qualitative phase and a quantitative phase are included in the same research study. Mixed method research designs are classified according to time order and paradigm emphasis. This means that the designs are classified according to the researcher's desire to conduct phases concurrently, at roughly the same time, or sequentially so that one occurs before the other. Also, the designs are classified according to the researcher's need to use either a dominant status design, with either a qualitative or quantitative design being the primary focus of the research, or an equal status design that has essentially an equal focus on both quantitative and qualitative aspects of the design. What does knowledge of these research approaches mean to the DNP researcher? It means that unless the researcher is positive that he or she has a fluent understanding of the inner workings of both qualitative and quantitative research, the mixed research approach should not be utilized (University of South Alabama, n.d.).

SPECIFIC MIXED RESEARCH DESIGNS

Once the DNP researcher decides that a mixed approach to the research would best serve the needs of the study and that he or she has sufficient knowledge to implement such an approach, a specific mixed design must be selected. The most common approach to mixing methods is the triangulation design (Creswell & Plano Clark, 2007).

Triangulation Design

In congruence with the definition of triangulation earlier in the chapter, this design is used to obtain different data that are still complementary on the same topic of research. This can be an effective design to use when a researcher wants to compare and contrast quantitative statistical results with qualitative findings or to further validate or clarify quantitative numerical results with qualitative data. Implementation of the design occurs when the researcher implements the quantitative and qualitative methods at the same time and with both methods carrying equal weight in the study. The design involves the collection and analysis of quantitative and qualitative data during the same time frame yet during separate collection procedures for increased understanding of the research problem. The two data sets will then be merged; this can be done by transforming data from qualitative to quantitative and vice versa to facilitate the combining of the data sets during data analysis (Creswell & Plano Clark, 2007).

Because the triangulation design seems to have a "common-sense" appeal, it is frequently a wise choice for novice researchers who are new to mixed research. It is also an excellent design if a team of researchers is available, because quantitative and qualitative data can be collected and analyzed separately. However, the aspects of this design that make it so appealing also make it very challenging. Because all data collection occurs during the same time frame, the design may require a great deal of effort and expertise, necessitating the use of a team of researchers. This translates into a study that will be both lengthy and expensive. This may not be an appropriate design for the researcher who recognizes that a team will not be available. Furthermore, the researcher must decide before implementation of the design how discrepancies in the quantitative and qualitative results will be addressed (Creswell & Plano Clark, 2007).

Embedded Design

The embedded design is used when one data set provides a secondary yet supportive role in a study that is based primarily on the other major research method. It is used when the researcher needs to include qualitative or quantitative data to answer a research question that is included within a study that is primarily quantitative or qualitative. It is particularly useful when there is a need to include a qualitative section within a quantitative design. As mentioned earlier in the chapter, the hallmark of the embedded design is the inclusion of one type of data within a methodology that is framed by the other type of data. Although both types of data are included, one type always plays a secondary role within the design (Creswell & Plano Clark, 2007).

A primary advantage of this design is that it can be used when the researcher does not have enough time or resources to commit to extensively researching both quantitative and qualitative data collection because one data type will be viewed as being supplementary. Also, because the primary focus of the design is traditionally quantitative, agencies tend to be more willing to provide funding for such a design than other types of research. The two research methods will be used to answer different research questions, so the researcher can keep the two sets of results generated separate in the research report and may even opt to report them in separate reports. There is no need to merge the two different data sets in order to answer the same research question, such as is required with the triangulation design (Creswell & Plano Clark, 2007).

Explanatory Design

The explanatory design consists of two phases, with the basic premise being that qualitative data will assist in explaining initial quantitative results. This type of design is well suited for a study in which the researcher needs to explain nonsignificant results, unexpected results, or statistical outliers that did not fall into the mainstream pattern. This design begins with the collection and analysis of quantitative data, followed by collection and analysis of qualitative data. The qualitative phase of the design is formulated to follow from the results of the quantitative phase. Typically, greater emphasis is placed on the quantitative phase (Creswell & Plano Clark, 2007).

The explanatory design has two variations: the follow-up explanations model and the participant selection model. The follow-up explanations model is used when the researcher needs qualitative data to help in explaining quantitative results. The researcher will identify specific quantitative findings that need additional explanation and will then collect qualitative data from research subjects who can most successfully explain these findings. The participant selection model is used when a researcher needs quantitative information to identify research subjects to participate in a follow-up qualitative study. This model will also primarily emphasize the qualitative phase (Creswell & Plano Clark, 2007).

The explanatory design may be a wise choice for the DNP researcher who does not have access to a team to assist in the research process. It is straightforward to implement because the two methods are conducted in separate phases and only one type of data is collected at a time; therefore, one researcher can implement the design. The final report also may be easier for readers to follow because it can be written in two phases. However, the explanatory design requires an extensive amount of time to implement because of its two-phase format, with the qualitative phase being the most lengthy. Another challenge for the researcher can be the need to decide whether the same individuals should be used for both phases of the design, whether subjects from the same sample should be used for both phases, and also whether subjects should be drawn from the same population of potential participants for the phases. A significant drawback can be the difficulty in obtaining approval from an internal review board for this design because the researcher will not be able to specify how subjects will be selected for the second phase of the research until the initial findings are obtained (Creswell & Plano Clark, 2007).

Exploratory Design

The researcher who chooses the exploratory design has the premise that the results of the qualitative method can help develop the quantitative method. Further development or exploration can be needed because measures or instruments are not available, variables are unknown, or no guiding framework is utilized. This design can be particularly effective when the researcher is exploring a phenomenon because it begins qualitatively, and also is well suited to the development and testing of an instrument or the identification of important variables to study quantitatively. The exploratory design has two phases that start with qualitative data to initiate exploration of a phenomenon and then progress to a second phase that uses quantitative data. Researchers build on the results of the qualitative phases by developing an instrument, identifying variables, or stating proposed reasons for testing based on an emergent theory. These developments will forge a connection between the initial qualitative phase and the quantitative component of the research. The qualitative phase usually is given greater emphasis with the exploratory design (Creswell & Plano Clark, 2007).

There are two major variations of the exploratory design: the instrument development model and the taxonomy development model. The instrument development model is used to develop and implement a quantitative instrument based on qualitative findings. The researcher will first explore the research topic qualitatively using only a few participants. The qualitative findings will serve as a guide for the development of a quantitative survey instrument. The researcher will then implement and validate the instrument quantitatively. Researchers who choose this variation of the exploratory design tend to emphasize the quantitative component.

In comparison, the taxonomy development model is used when an initial qualitative phase is conducted to identify important variables, develop a classification system, or develop a theory, and then a second phase is carried out consisting of quantitative tests to study the results in more detail. The initial qualitative phase will produce specific categories that then can be used to direct the research question and data collection in the second quantitative phase (Creswell & Plano Clark, 2007).

Because it uses separate phases, this design is usually straightforward to implement as well as report; however, the researcher should recognize that the use of two phases requires additional time to implement. Also, the researcher may have difficulty specifying the procedures of the quantitative phase when applying for initial institutional review board approval. A decision will be required regarding the use of the same individuals for participation in both the qualitative and quantitative phases of the research (Creswell & Plano Clark, 2007).

SELECTING A TYPE OF MIXED RESEARCH DESIGN

Researchers should consider some key factors when selecting a mixed research design for a research project. These include timing, weighting, and mixing. Timing refers to the order in which the researchers use the data within a study. In a mixed research design, timing is classified as concurrent or sequential. **Concurrent timing** means the researcher implements both quantitative and qualitative methods during a single phase of the research study. **Sequential timing** occurs when the researcher implements the methods in two distinct phases, using one type of data before using the other data type (Creswell & Plano Clark, 2007).

Weighting refers to the emphasis of the two methods used in the study. This means the researcher decides whether the quantitative or qualitative component will have equal priority or if one component will have a greater priority than the other. Weighting is greatly influenced by practical considerations. Because it requires more time, money, and personnel to implement a study that equally weights the two methods, a researcher with limited resources may choose to prioritize one method over the other and dedicate less of his or her budget and time to the secondary method (Creswell & Plano Clark, 2007).

The decision of how to mix the quantitative and qualitative methods will also be a concern when choosing a mixed method design, in addition to timing and weighting. The two data sets can be merged, one set can be embedded within the other, or the two sets can be connected. The data sets can be merged by analyzing them separately in a results section and then merging the two sets of results together during the discussion phase, or by transforming one data type into the other type. Connecting of the data sets can occur when analysis of one type of data leads to the need for the other type of data (Creswell & Plano Clark, 2007).

STAGES OF THE MIXED RESEARCH PROCESS

A specific sequence of steps should be followed to implement a mixed research approach. They can be followed in a different order as the needs of the researcher change or as problems arise that must be addressed. The steps consist of:

1. Determine the appropriateness of the use of a mixed design.
2. Decide if the purpose of the research is congruent with the rationale for using a mixed design.
3. Select the mixed model or mixed method research design.
4. Collect the data. Primary data collection methods consist of tests, questionnaires, interviews, focus groups, observation, and already existing data. Data collection will be discussed in detail in Chapter 9.
5. Analyze the data, bearing in mind that qualitative data can be converted into quantitative data and vice versa. Data analysis in mixed research consists of:

   - **Data reduction**—Reduces the volume of qualitative and quantitative data. This can be accomplished through memoing, for example, for qualitative data, and descriptive statistics such as averages and percentages for quantitative data.
   - **Data display**—Describes quantitative and qualitative data pictorially. This can be done using charts, graphs, and tables.
   - **Data transformation**—Allows quantitative data to be converted into narrative data that can be analyzed qualitatively and qualitative data to be expressed quantitatively using numerical coding and then statistics.

- **Data correlation**—Involves the correlation of quantitative and qualitative data for clarity.
- **Data consolidation**—Combines quantitative and qualitative data to create new sets of data.
- **Data comparison**—Involves the comparison of data from both the qualitative and quantitative sources
- **Data integration**—Allows both quantitative and qualitative data to be integrated into a cohesive data set or to become two separate but equally important parts of an entire data set (Johnson & Onwuegbuzie, 2004).

6. Validate the data. Data validation should occur throughout the research project. The study has internal validity if the design provides a logical basis to show that the independent variable does or does not cause a specific change in the dependent variable. External validity is present if the results can be generalized to the larger population (Manhiem, Rich, & Willnat, 2002).

7. Interpret the data. Data interpretation should begin with the collection of the first piece of datum and should continue throughout the study. Use reflexivity and negative-case sampling throughout data interpretation. **Reflexivity** means the researcher uses self-awareness and critical self-reflection to better understand his or her personal biases and the way these may affect the research process and conclusions. **Negative-case sampling** means the researcher attempts to locate and scrutinize cases that do not confirm his or her expectations and the tentative explanations that have been proposed (University of South Alabama, n.d.).

8. Write the research report. The writing process can actually begin during data collection. The report should reflect that mixing occurred during the research process (University of South Alabama, n.d.).

The researcher who is considering implementing a mixed research study should first gain experience with both quantitative and qualitative research before attempting to implement mixed research. The researcher should be able to craft quantitative hypotheses, select the method of data collection most appropriate for this method, understand how to use statistical analysis, and verify that the instrument used provides both reliability and validity—the results generated can be generalized to the larger population and scores received from participants are consistent over time. In addition, the researcher must be able to develop qualitative research questions, must be familiar with how to use interviews, and must understand how to code text and develop themes based on the codes. The researcher who is considering implementing mixed research should determine if there is adequate time to collect and analyze two different types of data. Furthermore, adequate resources and personnel must be available for the collection and analysis of both quantitative and qualitative data. Once the DNP researcher has decided which type of research design will be most effective for the research project, other issues pertaining to organizing the study must be addressed (Creswell & Plano Clark, 2007). The following chapter will discuss issues pertaining to obtaining a sample of research subjects, while subsequent chapters will address data collection and data analysis.

TABLE 7-1   Comparison of the Major Mixed Methods Designs

Type of Design	Variations	Timing	Weighting of Methods	Mixing
Triangulation	Convergence Data transformation Validation of quantitative data Multilevel	Concurrent, with quantitative and qualitative data collection occurring at the same time	Both methods are usually considered to be equal in importance	Data are merged during the interpretation or analysis phase
Embedded	Embedded/ experimental Embedded/ correlational	Concurrent and sequential	Unequally weighted	Embed one type of data within a larger design using the other type of data
Explanatory	Follow-up explanations Participant selection	Sequential: quantitative, then qualitative	Usually quantitative is weighted more significantly	Connect data between the two phases
Exploratory	Instrument development Taxonomy development	Sequential: qualitative, then quantitative	Usually qualitative is weighted more significantly	Connect data between the two phases

Source: Creswell & Plano Clark, 2007.

■ GLOSSARY

compatibility thesis The idea that the quantitative and qualitative research methods can be compatible and can be used together in a research study.

complementarity The researcher is striving to enhance, illustrate, or clarify the results that are achieved through use of results from both quantitative and qualitative designs.

concurrent timing The researcher implements both quantitative and qualitative methods during a single phase of the research study.

data comparison Involves the comparison of data from both qualitative and quantitative sources.

data consolidation Quantitative and qualitative data are combined to create new sets of data.

data correlation Involves the correlation of quantitative and qualitative data for clarity.

data display Describing quantitative and qualitative data pictorially. This can be done using charts, graphs, and tables.

data integration Allows both quantitative and qualitative data to be integrated into a cohesive data set or to become two separate but equally important parts of an entire data set.

data reduction Reducing the dimensions of qualitative and quantitative data. This can be accomplished through memoing, for example, for qualitative data, and descriptive statistics such as averages and percentages for quantitative data.

data transformation Allows quantitative data to be converted into narrative data that can be analyzed qualitatively and qualitative data to be expressed quantitatively using numerical coding and then statistics.

mixed method research Occurs when both a qualitative phase and a quantitative phase are included in the same research study.

mixed model research Used when quantitative and qualitative approaches are mixed either within the research process or across the various stages of the process.

negative-case sampling The researcher attempts to locate and scrutinize cases that do not confirm his or her expectations and the tentative explanations that have been proposed.

pragmatism A researcher should use any approach or combination of approaches that will function the best in a real-world situation, regardless of assumptions of paradigms or philosophies.

reflexivity The researcher uses self-awareness and critical self-reflection to better understand his or her personal biases and the way these may affect the research process and conclusions.

sequential timing The researcher implements qualitative and quantitative methods in two distinct phases, using one type of data before using the other type of data.

triangulation The researcher uses qualitative and quantitative methods in order to achieve corroboration of results achieved from the different approaches.

■ LEARNING ENHANCEMENT TOOLS

1. You are a DNP researcher who is considering using a mixed method approach to design a research study on addressing the needs of hospice patients who speak English as a second language. How can you most effectively use the principle of complementarity to design a study using a mixed method approach to the research?

2. Describe an original approach to mixed model research that mixes the quantitative and qualitative approaches within the stages of the research process.

3. Describe an original approach to mixed model research that mixes the quantitative and qualitative approaches across the various stages of the research process.

4. Describe a possible research study for an across-stage mixed model research project using one of the following research designs:

   a. Qualitative research objectives, collection of qualitative data, performing quantitative analysis. Describe what should occur in the stages of the mixed research process for such a design, including how data analysis should occur.

   b. Qualitative research objectives, collection of quantitative data, performing qualitative analysis. Describe what should occur in the stages of the mixed research process for such a design, including how data analysis should occur.

   c. Qualitative research objectives, collection of quantitative data, performing quantitative analysis. Describe what should occur in the stages of the mixed research process for such a design, including how data analysis should occur.

   d. Quantitative research objectives, collection of qualitative data, performing qualitative analysis. Describe what should occur in the stages of the mixed research process for such a design, including how data analysis should occur.

   e. Quantitative research objectives, collection of qualitative data, performing quantitative analysis. Describe what should occur in the stages of the mixed research process for such a design, including how data analysis should occur.

   f. Quantitative research objectives, collection of quantitative data, performing qualitative analysis. Describe what should occur in the stages of the mixed research process for such a design, including how data analysis should occur.

5. Describe a possible research study that could be developed using a triangulation mixed research design. Discuss how, as the lead DNP researcher for this project, you will plan to circumnavigate the challenges associated with this design.

6. Describe a possible research study that could be developed using an embedded mixed research design. Discuss how, as the lead DNP researcher for this project, you will plan to circumnavigate the challenges associated with this design.

7. Describe a possible research study that could be developed using an explanatory mixed research design. Discuss how, as the lead DNP researcher for this project, you will plan to circumnavigate the challenges associated with this design.

8. Describe a possible research study that could be developed using the variation of the explanatory mixed research design known as the follow-up explanations model. Discuss how, as the lead DNP researcher for this project, you will plan to circumnavigate the challenges associated with this design.

9. Describe a possible research study that could be developed using the variation of the explanatory mixed research design known as the participant selection model. Discuss how, as the lead DNP researcher for this project, you will plan to circumnavigate the challenges associated with this design.

10. Describe a possible research study that could be developed using an exploratory mixed research design. Discuss how, as the lead DNP researcher for this project, you will plan to circumnavigate the challenges associated with this design.

11. Discuss the various factors that must be considered in opting for a mixed method research design. Draw a decision tree illustrating the researcher's progress through these factors.

12. Compare and contrast the four major types of mixed method research designs.

13. Describe a possible research study that could be developed using the variation of the exploratory mixed research design known as the instrument development model. Discuss how, as the lead DNP researcher for this project, you will plan to circumnavigate the challenges associated with this design.

14. Describe a possible research study that could be developed using the variation of the exploratory mixed research design known as the taxonomy development model. Discuss how, as the lead DNP researcher for this project, you will plan to circumnavigate the challenges associated with this design.

■ RESOURCES

Adcock, R., & Collier, D. (2001). Measurement validity: A shared standard for qualitative and quantitative research. *American Political Science Review, 95*(3), 529–546.

Bartlett, J., Kotrlik, J., & Higgins, C. (2001). Organizational research: Determining appropriate sample size in survey research. *Information Technology, Learning, and Performance Journal, 19*(1), 43–50.

Creswell, J. (2003). *Research design: Qualitative, quantitative, and mixed methods approaches.* Thousand Oaks, CA: Sage.

Manheim, J., Rich, R., & Willnat, L. (2002). *Empirical political analysis: Research methods in political science.* New York: Addison Wesley Longman.

Mason, J. (2006). Mixing methods in a qualitatively driven way. *Qualitative Research, 6*(1), 9–25.

Onwuegbuzie, A., & Johnson, R. (2006). The validity issue in mixed research. *Research in the Schools, 13*(1), 48–63.

Onwuegbuzie, A., & Leech, N. (2007). On becoming a pragmatic researcher: The importance of combining quantitative and qualitative research methodologies. *International Journal of Social Research Methodology: Theory & Practice, 8*(5), 375–387.

Onwuegbuzie, A., & Teddlie, C (2003). *Handbook of mixed methods in social and behavioral research.* Thousand Oaks, CA: Sage.

Sandelowski, M., Volls, C., & Barraso, J. (2006). Defining and designing mixed research synthesis studies. *Research in the Schools, 13*(1), 29–40.

Tashakkori, A., & Teddlie, C. (2003). (Eds.). *The handbook of mixed methods in the social and behavioral sciences.* Thousand Oaks, CA: Sage.

■ REFERENCES

Creswell, J., & Plano Clark, V. (2007). *Designing and conducting mixed methods research.* Thousand Oaks, CA: Sage.

Johnson, R., & Onwuegbuzie, A. (2004). Mixed methods research: A research paradigm whose time has come. *Educational Researcher, 33*, 14–26.

Manheim, J., Rich, R., & Willnat, L. (2002). *Empirical political analysis: Research methods in political science.* New York: Addison Wesley Longman.

Palmer, J. (2009). Nursing research: Understanding the basics. *Plastic Surgical Nursing, 29*(2), 115–121.

University of South Alabama. (n.d.). *Chapter 14: Mixed research: Mixed method and mixed model research.* Accessed December 9, 2009, from www.southalabama.edu/coe/bset/johnson/lectures/lec14.htm

Sampling

8

■ OBJECTIVES

Upon completion of this chapter, the reader should be prepared to:

1 Describe the importance of obtaining a representative sample.

2 Describe the importance of simple random sampling and discuss ways to implement this type of sampling.

3 Describe the importance of stratified random sampling and discuss ways to implement this type of sampling.

4 Discuss the difference between proportional and disproportional stratified sampling.

5 Describe the importance of cluster random sampling and discuss ways to implement this type of sampling.

6 Discuss the difference between one-stage and two-stage cluster sampling.

7 Describe the importance of convenience sampling and discuss the most effective way to implement this type of sampling.

8 Describe the risk of bias and degree of representativeness associated with convenience sampling.

9 Describe the importance of quota sampling and discuss the most effective way to implement this type of sampling.

10 Describe the importance of purposive sampling and discuss the most effective way to implement this type of sampling.

11 Describe the importance of snowball sampling and discuss the most effective way to implement this type of sampling.

12 Discuss the difference between random selection and random assignment.

13 Describe the procedure for determining the sample size when random sampling is utilized.

14 Describe the primary characteristics of maximum variation sampling.

15 Describe the primary characteristics of homogeneous sample selection.

16 Describe the primary characteristics of extreme case sampling.

(continues)

17 Describe the primary characteristics of typical case sampling.

18 Describe the primary characteristics of critical case sampling.

19 Describe the primary characteristics of negative case sampling.

20 Describe the primary characteristics of opportunistic sampling.

21 Describe the primary characteristics of mixed purposeful sampling.

22 Describe sampling strategies for recruiting participants for a sample for qualitative research.

INTRODUCTION TO THE PROCESS OF SAMPLING

The procedure used to obtain the sample of research subjects for participation in a research study is of such vital importance that even a minor error on the part of the researcher can prevent him or her from generating accurate data and a credible report. The researcher's goal in sampling is to obtain a **representative sample**—this means the sample is similar to the **population** from which it was drawn in all areas except that it contains fewer people than the population (University of South Alabama, n.d.).

QUANTITATIVE SAMPLING DESIGNS

Sampling in quantitative research is either random sampling or nonrandom sampling. Random sampling is particularly important because it will generate representative samples, whereas nonrandom sampling will not.

Types of Random Sampling

A researcher who intends to utilize quantitative research should be familiar with several types of random sampling:

■ **Simple random sampling**—This is the most basic type of random sampling. It allows everyone in the group from which the sample is being drawn to have an equal chance of being selected for the final sample. Simple random sampling can be implemented in its most basic form by putting all of the names of potential research participants from the population into a receptacle and then withdrawing the needed number of names at random. A computer program also can be used for simple random sampling. This is known as a random number generator that assigns each person in the population a number. The program will then provide the researcher with a list of randomly selected numbers within a range that the researcher provides. After receiving the random numbers, the researcher identifies the people with those assigned numbers and contacts them to determine their willingness to participate in the research study (University of South Alabama, n.d.).

- **Systematic sampling**—Systematic sampling uses what is known as a **sampling interval**. This is the population size divided by the desired sample size. A number will be randomly selected between 1 and the sampling interval. This will determine which research subjects will be selected for the sample out of the sampling frame. The **sampling frame** is a list of all the potential participants that make up the population. For example, if the sampling interval is 20 and the randomly selected number between 1 and 20 was 7, then the researcher reviews the numbered list of potential participants and selects subjects 7, 14, 21, and 28. A potential problem that can occur with sampling is periodicity, which means a cyclical pattern emerges in the sampling frame, usually because several ordered lists have been attached together. This can be avoided by reorganizing the multiple lists into one general list (University of South Alabama, n.d.).

- **Stratified random sampling**—This type of sampling occurs when the researcher initially selects a stratification variable. This can be anything that is used to classify the sampling frame, such as gender or race. If race is used as the stratification variable, the researcher will then select a random sample from each race in the sampling frame. The various sets of subjects will be put together and the final sample is then generated. There are two types of stratified random sampling:
  - **Proportional stratified sampling**—This occurs when the researcher makes certain that the subsamples that are selected (such as those based on race or gender) are in proportion to their sizes in the population.
  - **Disproportional stratified sampling**—This occurs when the researcher is not concerned with ensuring that the subsamples selected are in proportion to their sizes in the population (University of South Alabama, n.d.).

- **Cluster random sampling**—This type of sampling is utilized when clusters or groups of potential participants, rather than individual subjects, are included only if the clusters are approximately equal in size. If the clusters are known to be unequal in size, probability should be considered to be proportional to the size of the group utilized. This will allow a representative sample to be produced. There are two types of cluster random sampling:

- **One-stage cluster sampling**—To utilize this type of sampling, the researcher initially selects a random sample of the clusters or groups. The researcher then includes in the final sample all of the individual names included in the chosen clusters.
- **Two-stage cluster sampling**—To utilize this type of sampling, the researcher selects a random sample of the clusters or groups, just as would be done in one-stage cluster sampling. The second stage involves taking a random sample of potential subjects from each of the clusters that was selected in the first phase (University of South Alabama, n.d.).

Types of Nonrandom Sampling

In comparison, there are four primary types of nonrandom sampling techniques that can be utilized with quantitative research:

- **Convenience sampling**—This type of sampling is utilized when the researcher selects people who are most easily located or who are most available for participation in the research study. The major advantage for this type of sampling is the ease with which the researcher can locate research subjects; the major disadvantage is the risk of researcher bias is greater than in any other type of sampling. Because the researcher will obtain information only from people who volunteer to participate, the factors motivating people to volunteer should be determined. People who opted to participate may not constitute a representative sample in relation to the overall population. This is considered to be the weakest form of sampling in relation to generalizability to the greater population (LoBiondo-Wood & Haber, 2002).
- **Quota sampling**—This is a variation on convenience sampling. It involves setting quotas and then using convenience sampling to select participants to fill the quotas. This allows the researcher to use the knowledge available about the population to build some representativeness into the sample being selected. However, researcher bias will still be an issue for this type of sampling, as previously discussed with convenience sampling (LoBiondo-Wood & Haber, 2002).
- **Purposive sampling**—With this type of sampling, the researcher specifies the characteristics of the population of interest and then locates individuals who match those characteristics. The researcher typically chooses subjects who are considered to be typical of the population. Purposive sampling is particularly effective when:

- The population being studied is very unusual, such as a group of patients with a rare disease.
- There is a newly developed instrument that requires pretesting.
- There is a scale or test that needs to be validated, when the researcher needs to collect exploratory data regarding a very specific population.
- The researcher wants to describe the lived experience of a phenomenon, such as patients who have been victims of domestic violence.

A significant limitation of this type of sampling is that the researcher must assume that errors of overrepresenting or underrepresenting segments of the population will somehow resolve themselves. However, this is not a valid assumption (LoBiondo-Wood & Haber, 2002).

- **Snowball sampling**—Each subject being used in the research study is asked to identify other potential research subjects who have the characteristics being studied. This technique is particularly effective with a population that is difficult to find and therefore has no sampling frame (University of South Alabama, n.d.). However, it also risks a breach of confidentiality as research subjects identify other individuals with characteristics of interest to the researcher.

Convenience sampling, quota sampling, and purposive sampling would all be wise choices for the DNP researcher who has access to a continuous source of patients.

LoBiondo-Wood and Haber (2002) have developed a summary of the various types of sampling separated according to their respective risk of bias and degree of representativeness. This is included in the chapter table.

RANDOM SELECTION AND RANDOM ASSIGNMENT

In implementing sampling designs, it is important to recognize the difference between random selection and random assignment. Random selection means that the researcher uses an equal probability selection method to select a sample from a population using a random sampling technique. Each element of the population has an equal chance of being included in the sample. The sample that is produced as a result of this procedure will be a mirror image of the overall population (LoBiondo-Wood & Haber, 2002).

In comparison, random assignment occurs when the researcher already has a sample of research subjects that is then randomly divided into two or more groups. Usually the groups will be mirror images of each other and will be roughly equivalent on all variables (University of South Alabama, n.d.). The ultimate purpose of random assignment is the distribution of research participants into either the experimental group or the control group of the research project on a random basis, with each research subject having an equal probability of being assigned to any group. Random assignment is important because it assumes that any important variables will be equally distributed between the groups, and thus variation will be kept to a minimum (LoBiondo-Wood & Haber, 2002).

DETERMINING SAMPLE SIZE

Once the researcher has decided which type of quantitative sampling is most appropriate for the research study, practical issues related to the sampling process must be handled. Such issues include deciding the size sample to collect based on the type of research being implemented. Clearly the researcher should attempt to get as large a sample as possible for the study in order to make it as representative of the overall population as possible. However, if the population is inclusive of 100 individuals or fewer, the researcher should not select a sample, but should instead include the entire population (Manheim, Rich, & Willnat, 2002).

Manheim, Rich, and Willnat (2002) have identified several factors that can help a researcher determine how large a sample will be needed for a research project. One such factor is **homogeneity**. This is the degree to which individuals who compose a population resemble one another in regards to the characteristics being studied in a research project. The more homogeneous the individuals in a population, the smaller the sample required to be representative of that population. In addition, the more variables being studied by the researcher, the larger the sample will need to be. This is a requirement because the more questions asked in the research project, the more likely the researcher will be to find differences among the subjects. Furthermore, the degree of accuracy required by the researcher is also a consideration. Because the sample estimates the characteristics of the population, this estimate is always going to contain a margin of error. The researcher must determine how much sampling error can be tolerated. The greater the degree of accuracy desired, the larger the sample must be. In addition, always plan to utilize a larger sample when:

- The population is heterogeneous, meaning it differs in multiple characteristics.
- The goal is to break down the data into multiple categories.
- The researcher expects that a weak relationship will be shown between variables.

- A less efficient sampling technique is used.
- A low response rate is expected (University of South Alabama, n.d.).

Web-based sample size calculators are available to provide the researcher with a specific sample number. Usually, such a tool will calculate the size sample needed for the project based on the size population utilized and the confidence interval desired. The **confidence interval** is the extent to which the sample mean deviates from the population parameter (Singleton & Straits, 1999). The sample size calculator will tell the researcher that x number of research subjects should be sampled in order to have a 95 percent level of confidence, plus or minus 5 percent. The researcher should bear in mind that in order to ensure a small confidence interval, such as plus or minus 2 percent, a large sample size will be required (Neuendorf, 2002).

QUALITATIVE SAMPLING DESIGNS

As previously mentioned, sampling for qualitative research tends to be purposive in nature so that cases will be selected that will yield relevant data. The sample usually originates from a theory that either is in the process of being tested or is growing progressively. In addition, the sample usually evolves as the study progresses, data are analyzed, and new insight is revealed. The process of sampling will continue until virtually no new information is being revealed. The researcher who will be utilizing sampling for qualitative research should be cognizant of the kinds of research subjects to be included in the sample, the optimum time to contact potential research participants, and the kinds of situations that will be studied. The researcher may encounter difficulty in recruiting participants for a sample when the topic being studied is particularly sensitive, when the potential participants are not offered any type of incentive, or when there are no existing relationships that may be used to assist in recruitment. To circumvent these potential problems, the researcher can:

- Attempt to partner with a group that is already affiliated with the type of people who would be most desirous as participants
- Contact potential participants through informal networks of colleagues
- Recruit participants for sample from existing organizations, using contact people to assist in gaining admittance to agencies
- Recruit from lists of professionals, such as nurse practitioners
- Send follow-up invitations to arrange interviews and set meeting times that do not conflict with the participants' other obligations (MacDougall & Fudge, 2001)

As previously mentioned, sampling in qualitative research is usually purposive in nature. Specific purposive sampling techniques can be used. These include:

- *Maximum variation sampling*—The researcher selects a wide range of cases from which to compose the sample.
- *Homogeneous sample selection*—The researcher selects a small but homogeneous set of cases with the intent of studying them closely.
- *Extreme case sampling*—The researcher chooses cases that represent extremes on a specific variable.
- *Typical-case sampling*—The researcher selects cases that seem to be average for the variable being studied.
- *Critical-case sampling*—The researcher selects cases that are considered to be very important in relation to the variable being studied.
- *Negative-case sampling*—The researcher selects cases that are opposite to the generalizations being made about a variable to confirm that he or she is not selectively finding cases to support his or her personal theory.
- *Opportunistic sampling*—The researcher selects useful cases as the opportunity presents itself.
- *Mixed purposeful sampling*—The researcher combines the sampling strategies previously mentioned into a more complex design that is based on the researcher's specific needs (University of South Alabama, n.d.).

QUALITATIVE SAMPLING STRATEGY

MacDougall and Fudge (2001) have described a multi-stage process for recruiting participants for a sample used in a qualitative research project. The stages consist of:

1. *Prepare*—The researcher should describe the desired sample by preparing a list of geographic locations that will be utilized as well as the characteristics that will be sought in potential participants.

   a. Comprehensive lists of sources of information regarding potential subjects should be obtained. Contact should be made with people who are familiar with communities of potential participants. MacDougall and Fudge (2001) categorize these as key contacts or champions, with **key contacts** being people who can suggest possible groups or participants who might take part in the study, and **champions** being people who are interested in the research and will either assist in recruiting participants or allow the researcher to use the champion's credibility in the community to recruit.

b. The researcher should also contact colleagues to seek out recent related research projects to determine how they involved groups or potential participants in their projects. This is important so that the current recruitment strategies of the project in progress can build on existing relationships. As the researcher begins to build lists of groups, key contacts, and champions that should provide participants with desired characteristics for the sample, alternative possibilities should also be developed, particularly if potential participants will be difficult to reach or if the topic being researched is particularly sensitive.

2. *Contact*—In this stage, the researcher should personally seek endorsement from key contacts with communities who may develop into champions, providing written information about the research project and stressing the valuable insights that potential participants can provide not only for the research project, but also for the community as a whole.

a. If the researcher discovers that the key contact will not develop into a champion but instead has assumed the role of a gatekeeper who is making it difficult to make contact with potential participants, the researcher should begin to tactfully withdraw contact and move on to another key contact. This prevents time wasted in negotiations that will not lead to the desired goal of contact with participants, but will only produce awkward entanglements.

b. The researcher preferably should arrange to meet individual participants in the presence of the key contact or champion. The participants should be given a description of the research, opportunities for questions, and an information sheet written specifically for them. At this point, consent forms should be in place that have been approved by the institutional review board, a time and place for interviews to be conducted should be announced, and the researcher should have arranged a way to effectively yet ethically obtain addresses of potential participants to maintain communication with them as the research project progresses.

c. The researcher should plan to communicate with potential participants after announcing the meeting time and place and then again approximately two weeks before the meeting, asking for a confirmation of plans to attend. At this point, a plan should also be in place to allow for continued communication with key contacts, champions, or participants who show particular enthusiasm regarding the project and would like to be kept abreast of progress being made and actions that have resulted from the research.

3. *Follow-up*—This phase ensures that relationships will be maintained with the research participants even after the research is concluded. A plan should be in place to continue involvement with useful agencies that will be interested in learning about actions that have resulted from the prepare and contact phases.

   a. The researcher should ensure that participants are given feedback on the themes that were discussed in the focus group or the interviews. Also, participants should be given the opportunity to give the researcher feedback on their experience during the research process. If appropriate, the contributions of the key contacts and champions should be acknowledged in some manner.
   b. If there are public events associated with the research, the researcher should ensure that key contacts and champions are invited and their contributions acknowledged.
   c. The researcher should ensure that time has been allotted for participation in actions that are a direct result of the research project (MacDougall & Fudge, 2001).

Once the researcher has developed the research problem, completed the literature review, completed the necessary requirements of an institutional review board, selected a design for the research project, and developed a plan for how sampling will proceed, the researcher is prepared to proceed with data collection. The following chapter will discuss how the researcher can decide on the most appropriate data collection method to utilize based on the type of research study being pursued.

■ GLOSSARY

champion In qualitative research, someone who is interested in the research and will either assist in recruiting participants or allow the researcher to use their credibility in the community to recruit.

cluster random sampling This type of sampling is utilized when clusters or groups of potential participants, rather than individual subjects, are randomly selected.

confidence interval The extent to which the sample statistic deviates from the population parameter; for example, 95 percent confidence that the population mean is between 2.0 and 3.0.

convenience sampling This type of sampling is utilized when the researcher selects people who are most easily located or who are most available for participation in the research study.

TABLE 8-1   Sampling Types Separated According to Risk of Bias and Degree of Representativeness

Type of Sampling Strategy	Risk of Bias	Degree of Representativeness
NONPROBABILITY SAMPLING		
Convenience	Greatest of any sampling strategy	Questionable representativeness because sample is self-selecting
Quota	Can have unknown sources of bias that will affect the external validity of the research study	Representativeness can be built in through knowledge of the population of interest
Purposive	The greater the heterogeneity of the population, the greater the bias; conscious bias on the part of the researcher can be present	Representativeness is limited, as is the ability to generalize to a larger population due to the sample being hand-selected
PROBABILITY SAMPLING		
Simple random	Low risk of bias	Maximum level of representativeness; as sample size increases, possibility of nonrepresentativeness decreases
Stratified random	Low risk of bias	High degree of representativeness
Cluster	Greater risk of sampling errors than simple or stratified random sampling	Less representative than simple random or stratified random sampling
Systematic	Easy to inadvertently introduce bias due to lack of randomization	Because bias can occur as a result of coincidental nonrandomness, tends to be less representative than other types of probability sampling

Source: LoBiondo-Wood & Haber, 2002.

disproportional stratified sampling This occurs when the researcher is not concerned with ensuring that the subsamples selected are in proportion to their sizes in the population.

homogeneity Degree to which the individuals in a population resemble one another in regards to the characteristics being studied in a research project.

key contacts In qualitative research, people who can suggest possible groups or participants who might take part in the study.

one-stage cluster sampling To utilize this type of sampling, the researcher initially selects a random sample of the clusters or groups; the researcher then includes in the final sample all the individual names included in the chosen clusters.

population The full set of people from whom the sample is being drawn.

proportional stratified sampling This occurs when the researcher makes certain that the subsamples that are selected are in proportion to their sizes in the population.

purposive sampling The researcher specifies the characteristics of the population of interest and then locates individuals who match those characteristics.

quota sampling This is a variation on convenience sampling; it involves setting quotas and then using convenience sampling to select participants to fill the quotas.

representative sample The sample is similar to the population from which it was drawn in all areas except that it contains fewer people than the population.

sampling frame A list of all of the potential participants that make up the population.

sampling interval The population size divided by the desired sample size.

simple random sampling This is the most basic type of random sampling; it allows everyone in the group from which the sample is being drawn to have an equal chance of being selected for the final sample.

snowball sampling Each subject being used in the research study is asked to identify other potential research subjects who have the characteristics being studied. This technique is particularly effective with a population that is difficult to find and therefore has no sampling frame.

stratified random sampling Occurs when the researcher initially selects a stratification variable that is used to classify the sampling frame, such as gender or race.

systematic sampling Utilizes a sampling interval to generate a representative sample.

two-stage cluster sampling To utilize this type of sampling, the researcher selects a random sample of the clusters or groups just as would be done in one-stage cluster sampling. The second stage involves taking a random sample of potential subjects from each of the clusters that was selected in the first phase.

■ LEARNING ENHANCEMENT TOOLS

1. You are a DNP researcher who is trying to decide whether to utilize simple random sampling or systematic sampling in your research study. Describe how each type of sampling can be implemented, and the advantages or limitations of each type.

2. Discuss the differences between proportional and disproportional stratified sampling. Describe how each type would be utilized in a research study.

3. Discuss the differences between one-stage and two-stage cluster sampling. Describe how each type would be utilized in a research study.

4. Outline a plan for a research study that would utilize convenience sampling. Describe the advantages and limitations of this type of sampling

5. Outline a plan for a research study that would utilize quota sampling. Describe the advantages and limitations of this type of sampling.

6. Outline a plan for a research study that would utilize purposive sampling. Describe the advantages and limitations of this type of sampling.

7. Outline a plan for a research study that would utilize snowball sampling. Describe the advantages and limitations of this type of sampling.

8. You are a DNP researcher who is preparing to conduct qualitative research using in-depth interviews with nurse managers who have had experience with nurse employees engaging in substance abuse. Describe your plan for recruitment strategies to generate a sample of participants for this study.

9. You are a DNP researcher who is preparing to conduct qualitative research using in-depth interviews with nurse managers who have had experience with nurse employees receiving discipline of their nursing license by the state Board of Nursing. You are interested in using mixed purposeful sampling in this research project. Discuss in detail how you could implement this technique, describing specifically the sampling strategies that you will select to incorporate into the final sampling plan.

10. You are a DNP researcher who is preparing to conduct qualitative research using in-depth interviews with nurse managers who have had experience with nurse employees receiving discipline of their nursing license by the state Board of Nursing. You are developing a plan for recruiting participants for a qualitative sample. Describe in detail the strategies you will use in recruiting subjects during the "prepare" phase of the recruitment process.

11. You are a DNP researcher who is preparing to conduct qualitative research using in-depth interviews with nurse managers who have had experience with nurse employees receiving discipline of their nursing license by the state Board of Nursing. You are developing a plan for recruiting participants for a qualitative sample. Describe in detail the strategies you will use in recruiting subjects during the "contact" phase of the recruitment process.

12. You are a DNP researcher who is preparing to conduct qualitative research using in-depth interviews with nurse managers who have had experience with nurse employees receiving discipline of their nursing license by the state Board of Nursing. You are developing a plan for recruiting participants for a qualitative sample. Describe in detail the strategies you will use in recruiting subjects during the "follow-up" phase of the recruitment process.

13. You are a DNP researcher who is making the final decision regarding a sampling strategy for your research project. Describe how you will decide on a nonprobability sampling strategy based on risk of bias and desired level of representativeness.

14. You are a DNP researcher who is making the final decision regarding a sampling strategy for your research project. Describe how you will decide on a probability sampling strategy based on risk of bias and desired level of representativeness.

■ RESOURCES

Bernardo, J. M. (1997). Statistical inference as a decision problem: The choice of sample size. *The Statistician, 46*, 151–153.

Campbell, M., Thomson, S., Ramsay, C., MacLennan, G., & Grimshaw, J. (2004). Sample size calculator for cluster randomized trials. *Computers in Biology and Medicine, 34*(2), 113–125.

Connelly, L. (2003). Balancing the number and size of sites: An economic approach to the optimal design of cluster samples. *Controlled Clinical Trials, 24*(5), 544–559.

Cosby, R., Howard, M., Kaczorowski, J., Willan, A. R., & Sellor, J. (2003). Randomizing patients by family practice: Sample size estimation, intracluster correlation and data analysis. *Family Practice, 20*(1), 77–82.

Hayes, R., & Bennett, S. (1999). Simple sample size calculation for cluster-randomized trials. *International Journal of Epidemiology, 28*(2), 319–326.

Lake, S., Kammann, E., Klar, N., & Betensky, R. (2002). Sample size re-estimation in cluster randomization trials. *Statistics in Medicine, 21*(10), 1337–1350.

Lee, S., & Zelen, M. (2000). Clinical trials and sample size considerations: Another perspective. *Statistical Science, 15*, 95–103.

Lindley, D. (1997). The choice of sample size. *The Statistician, 46*, 129–138.

Talbot, L. (Ed.). (1995). Populations and samples. *Principles and practice of nursing research*. St Louis, MO: Mosby.

Turner, R., Prevost, A., & Thompson, S. (2004). Allowing for imprecision of the intracluster correlation coefficient in the design of cluster randomized trials. *Statistics in Medicine, 23*(8), 1195–1214.

Wears, R. (2002). Advanced statistics: Statistical methods for analyzing cluster and cluster-randomized data. *Academic Emergency Medicine, 9*(4), 330–341.

■ REFERENCES

LoBiondo-Wood, G., & Haber, J. (2002). *Nursing research: Methods, critical appraisal, and utilization.* St. Louis, MO: Mosby.

MacDougall, C., & Fudge, E. (2001). Planning and recruiting the sample for focus groups and in-depth interviews. *Qualitative Health Research, 11*, 117–126.

Manheim, J., Rich, R., & Willnat, L. (2002). *Empirical political analysis: Research methods in political science.* New York: Addison Wesley Longman.

Neuendorf, K. (2002). *The content analysis guidebook.* Thousand Oaks, CA: Sage Publications.

Singleton, R., & Straits, B. (1999). *Approaches to social research.* New York: Oxford University Press.

University of South Alabama. (n.d.). *Chapter 7: Sampling.* Retrieved December 28, 2009, from www.southalabama.edu/coe/bset/johnson/lectures/lec7.htm

Data Collection

9

■ OBJECTIVES

Upon completion of this chapter, the reader should be prepared to:

1 Describe the steps involved in instrument development.

2 Discuss the advantages and disadvantages of the use of physiological measurements as a data collection method.

3 Discuss the advantages and disadvantages of the use of participant observation as a data collection method.

4 Describe the different types of participant observation.

5 Discuss the advantages and disadvantages of the use of the e-mail interview as a data collection method.

6 Discuss the advantages and disadvantages of the use of existing records as a data collection method.

7 Describe content analysis as a data collection method.

8 Describe the steps in the typical process of content analysis as a research process and data collection technique.

9 Describe the disadvantages of the traditional mail survey and the telephone survey.

10 Discuss how a researcher could utilize the focus group as a data collection method.

11 Describe the differences between structured and unstructured observational methods.

12 Identify special issues that are unique to data collection occurring in mixed method research.

13 Describe how the programmatic research approach will affect data collection.

14 Discuss the different types of questions that can be utilized in most questionnaires.

INTRODUCTION TO THE PROCESS OF DATA COLLECTION

For the DNP researcher, the process of data collection should flow naturally from the progress that has already been made on the project thus far, although selecting the appropriate method and the specific instrument to utilize can be time-consuming. The method of data collection must be appropriate to the problem being researched, the hypothesis that has been formulated, the research setting, and the population of interest. For example, if the researcher is interested in observing the behavioral changes exhibited in patients suffering from Alzheimer's disease, it would be inappropriate to use a lengthy questionnaire that would require the patient to concentrate for long periods to answer questions (LoBiondo-Wood & Haber, 2002).

The process of data collection actually has its origin in the literature review, because it is then that the researcher begins to define variables and determine how they will be **operationalized**, or measured. This provides the germ of an instrument that will be useful in measuring the defined variables. The researcher can even construct his or her own instrument, although this can be a time-consuming process that can overwhelm the novice researcher. Instrument development can be a tedious process because of its multiple steps. It requires:

- Defining the concept to be measured.
- Developing the items to be included on the instrument.
- Assessing the items for **content validity**—this means determining whether the instrument and its items are representative of the content the researcher intends to measure.
- Developing instructions for the research participants.
- Developing a pre-test for the items.
- **Pilot testing** the items—this serves as a pre-test to the major survey.
- Estimating **reliability**—this means determining the instrument is consistent and will give the same results if the research is replicated.
- Ensuring **validity**—this means ensuring the instrument measures what it was intended to measure.

The DNP researcher who is involved in a time-limited capstone project should avoid constructing an original instrument and instead utilize an existing instrument, if one exists with proven validity and reliability (LoBiondo-Wood & Haber, 2002).

TYPES OF DATA COLLECTION METHODS

There are five general types of data collection methods, some of which can be used with both qualitative and quantitative research. These consist of physiological measurements, observational methods, interviews, questionnaires, and records or other types of existing data. The advantages and disadvantages of each type will be discussed, along with the most relevant uses of each as a data collection method.

A brief discussion is required here of programmatic research, an approach to nursing research that is discussed in this chapter because of its profound effect on the data collection process. Programmatic research is usually considered to be research conducted on a large scale by teams of researchers. It is designed to be a lengthy endeavor and is usually research that is considered to be for the public good. Data collection will occur on a team-wide basis with multiple researchers all collecting data simultaneously. Generally, a large amount of funding is required for such a project, and this amount of funding will not be awarded without evidence of prior completion of multiple extensive projects. Because of the multiple researchers involved and the resources required for such an effort, a plan will need to be in place to sustain the research with adequate resources, both financial and personnel-related, and to guide the research so data collection can occur over a lengthy period of time as needed. Collaboration will be required not only among multiple researchers, but also among multiple agencies. Because data collection occurs simultaneously with multiple researchers in the same research project, strict oversight is required to ensure that the same procedures and protocols are being used by all to avoid bias as well as problems with reliability and validity. Although a DNP researcher would certainly function well as a researcher in such a project, it is not recommended that a DNP clinician spearhead such an extensive and lengthy project (University of Ballarat Institute for Regional and Rural Research, 2004).

Physiological Measurements

Physiological measurements can consist of the data nurses collect about their patients on an everyday basis, such as temperature, pulse, respiration, and blood pressure, in addition to body weight, results of laboratory tests, and radiological examinations. Physiological data collection usually is objective, precise, and sensitive. Unless a technical malfunction of the equipment occurs, two readings of the same piece of equipment taken by two different nurses simultaneously will usually generate the same result. The instrument used will usually detect small changes in the variable being studied, such as variations of a tenth of a degree in body temperature. Also, a patient usually cannot distort his or her physiological information to any great degree without actually ingesting a toxifying substance. However, the instruments used in physiological data collection can usually be obtained only in a hospital because of their cost and occasionally due to the training required to utilize them. In addition, some instruments used in physiological data collection are so sensitive that environmental changes can affect them (LoBiondo-Wood & Haber, 2002).

The researcher must bear in mind that physiological measurements in DNP research will be multi-faceted, composed of:

- The true value of what is being measured, such as 140/90 as a blood pressure reading.
- The degree to which the measure varies, such as being lower in the morning and higher in the evening, in the case of blood pressure.
- The accuracy of the instrument with which the variable is being measured, such as a sphygmomanometer.
- The position of the patient, as in blood pressure fluctuating depending on whether the patient is lying or standing.
- The skill of the person obtaining the measurement.

This is another situation in which both reliability and validity will be critical issues. For example, if the patient's pulse is measured every five minutes by the same nurse using the same technique, it is expected that similar results would be obtained. This would be reliability. When multiple readings of a measurement are assessed from the same person, it is known as **intra-rater reliability**. If multiple readings of a measurement are assessed from several nurses, it is known as **inter-rater reliability**. The validity that the researcher must be concerned with in such a case is **criterion-related validity**. This requires the comparison of the measure in question with the best existing measure of the variable (Ciliska, Cullum, & Dicenco, 1999).

Observational Methods

Observational methods include participant observation, which Key (1997) described as the researcher keeping detailed records of what is occurring with the subjects being studied, while occasionally reviewing records as a social scientist and constantly monitoring both the observations and records for any intrusion of personal bias. There are five types of participant observation:

- *External participation*—This is the lowest degree of involvement by the researcher, with the observation being done usually via television or videotape.

- *Passive participation*—The researcher is present at the scene with the subject in the role of spectator but does not attempt to interact with the subject or participate in the scene with him or her.
- *Balanced participation*—The researcher walks a tenuous tightrope between being a participant and a spectator. The researcher is not a full participant in all of the research subject's activities.
- *Active participation*—The researcher generally does what the majority of the participants in the research setting are doing. Active engagement by the researcher will occur as he or she learns the rules of the research setting.
- *Total participation*—This is the highest level of involvement for the researcher and means that the researcher becomes a natural participant. This type of observation generally is used when the researcher chooses to study something in which he or she already functions as a natural participant (Key, 1997).

Participant observation is an effective data collection method when the researcher is interested in gathering information about a research subject's physical symptoms, verbal communication, nonverbal behavior, performance of specific skills, or environment. It is important to note that participant observation is considered to be an unstructured observational method. This means the researcher has a high degree of contact with the research population being studied, tries to collect information within the structures that are meaningful to the research subjects, and tries not to allow his or her own ideas and values to become injected into the situation being studied. The most common forms of record-keeping in this type of data collection are logs and field notes. Logs are considered to be a record of both events and conversations that will be maintained on a daily basis, while field notes can certainly include a log but tend to be more analytical. Field notes will not merely list a record of what has occurred, but will also give the researcher's interpretation of the events (Polit & Hungler, 2000).

In comparison, structured observational methods involve the development of a system for categorizing, recording, and encoding the observations. Also, record-keeping forms will be prepared in advance and will usually be quite elaborate. Because of the in-depth categorizing that is required and the extensive record-keeping forms utilized, it is not recommended that the novice DNP researcher utilize a structured observational method when an unstructured observational method is a viable alternative (Polit & Hungler, 2000).

According to Hoepfl (1997), observation can provide the researcher with a deeper understanding than an interview alone because it provides information about the context in which events occur. Thus, observation can give the researcher knowledge regarding areas that participants are not aware of or that they have chosen not to discuss. It is especially valuable for its ability to allow the researcher a complete understanding of a particularly complex situation. Proponents of this method of data collection believe that more structured methods may be too constricting to provide an accurate account of human behavior and its intricate nature.

Critics of participant observation point out that observer bias and influence from the observer are particular problems with this method. The researcher may have difficulty in maintaining objectivity as observations are recorded, and may record inaccurate events due to memory errors. In addition, the researcher may experience difficulty in entering a group intended for study and being accepted as a fellow member. Emotional involvement on the part of the researcher tends to occur as the researcher begins to participate in the activities of the group. This means that participant observation may be ineffective as a data collection method for the DNP researcher who is studying a research population of employees in a facility where he or she has just been hired, because the researcher will be struggling with the dynamics of organizational behavior in becoming incorporated into the group (Polit & Hungler, 2000).

Interviews and Questionnaires

Interviews used in research studies typically can be structured in several ways:

- *Structured interviews*—These can consist of a fixed series of questions that cannot be altered or a fixed series of questions that contain prompts to the interviewer so he or she can obtain more detailed answers from the subject.
- *Semistructured interviews*—These usually consist of a series of issues the interviewer wants to discuss; they can be addressed in any order.
- *Structured interviews*—These are completely open-ended interviews without a structured set of questions.

As technology has progressed, the e-mail interview has become a frequent data collection tool of researchers. It has several advantages that can make this a recommended tool for the DNP researcher. For example, the e-mail interview is a wise choice for the researcher with a particularly slim budget, because it allows multiple interviews to be conducted simultaneously and requires no travel expenses, no additional equipment to be obtained, and no additional personnel to be hired and trained. In addition, the e-mail interview allows research subjects to be interviewed at an unlimited distance, so participants could literally be obtained globally. Such an interview also provides the research subject with time for reflection, because there is no time constraint and the participant may feel that he or she can formulate an e-mail response more freely than they could verbalize a face-to-face response to questions (Hunt & McHale, 2007).

There are some potential disadvantages to the e-mail interview that the DNP researcher should be prepared to accommodate. For example, it will be difficult to obtain a representative sample, because potential respondents who do not have Internet access will be excluded. Also, the researcher will not be able to be certain that he or she is interviewing the person they think they are interviewing. This can open both validity and ethical issues.

The respondent may lose enthusiasm for the interview if it becomes too lengthy or complicated and may decide either to not complete the interview or to withdraw from the interview. This can leave the researcher with a partially completed interview that may not be usable for data analysis or with the ethical issue of not knowing whether the person has withdrawn or is simply taking a lengthy time for completion. Finally, an e-mail interview eliminates the possibility of the researcher being able to interpret the nonverbal cues of the respondent such as facial expressions or hand movements (Hunt & McHale, 2007).

There are guidelines that can assist the DNP researcher who opts to use the e-mail interview as a data collection tool in circumventing these disadvantages. These suggestions include:

- Alert participants regarding the number of questions they will be asked as part of the entire interview process.
- Encourage the participant to ask questions before the interview begins.
- Have clear-cut procedures that will address informed consent, the right to withdraw from the interview procedure, and how to ensure that the person completing the interview is truly the research participant.
- Set time limits for how long the interview can be reviewed by the participant before a response must be submitted.
- Plan to close the time period when the interview is open for completion with a statement thanking the participant for participating and asking for the participant's comments and feedback (Hunt & McHale, 2007).

While the e-mail interview is increasing greatly in popularity, the use of the traditional mail survey is decreasing in popularity with researchers because of its expense, the extensive amount of time required to prepare the mailouts and accumulate residential addresses, and the frequently low return rate of the surveys. Telephone surveys, however, are still in use. Random digit dialing can be used to generate a sample of all area telephone numbers. The drawback of this type of survey is primarily related to the poor response received from respondents after the first few questions. As respondents begin to tire of answering the questions, they may begin to give unreliable answers or simply hang up on the interviewer. In addition, this type of survey will become more difficult to implement as more people rely on cell phones as their primary telephones and no longer have listings in residential telephone books (O'Sullivan & Rassel, 1999).

As previously mentioned, the design of a new instrument is never recommended when an existing one with proven validity and reliability that has already been pilot tested is available. However, the DNP researcher should be able to discern what type of question will best collect the data he or she is focusing on. There are five main types of questions that will typically be used on most questionnaires:

- *Structured interviews*—This type can easily be used to measure the general attitude of the interviewee, is easy to understand, and is quickly completed. Researchers can also add a text box for respondents to put a response to any of the questions in their own words. Instructions should be included, particularly if the researcher wants respondents to give free text responses to specific questions. The researcher should recognize, however, that free text responses will require additional time and effort on the part of the researcher to code and analyze.
- *Rating scales*—This type of question can describe the interviewee's attitude on either a five- or seven-point scale and also can differentiate between positive and negative. It can be used with interviewees who are capable of understanding linear scales and the meaning of numerical values.
- *Visual analogue scales*—This type of question can precisely measure an interviewee's attitude. The data will need to be transformed to allow for statistical analysis. This question type can be used with interviewees who understand linear scales and who also have no difficulties with their vision.
- *Structured interviews*—This type of question is similar to a numerical rating scale. It is easier to utilize than other question types for interviewees who are visually challenged, those with low literacy levels, and children.
- *Open-ended items*—This type of question requires analysis with qualitative methods. Although it is well suited to creative participants, it may make a negative impression on interviewees who have difficulty putting thoughts and feelings on paper in detail (Boynton & Greenhalgh, 2004).

If the researcher is not vigilant he or she can run into various pitfalls associated with the wording of questionnaires. For example, if the researcher presents a question that uses the word *frequently*, the implication is that there is a frequency involved. A more appropriately worded question would avoid the word *frequently*, and instead would present a rating scale that is frequency-based with options such as hourly, once daily, once every three days, once weekly, and so on. Another example of a potential wording pitfall would be the use of the word *regularly*. This implies that a pattern of activity is present. This can mean different things to different people, with one patient thinking that "regularly" attending cardiac rehabilitation means three times weekly without variation, while another patient might believe that "regularly" means once weekly with an additional time attended if convenient (Boynton & Greenhalgh, 2004).

Focus Groups

The focus group is a form of in-person interviewing that can be used to obtain in-depth information from a group of participants on a specific group of topics. The group interaction is the hallmark of the focus group. Such an interview technique consists of the preparation phase, the formation of the groups, the interviewing of the participants, and finally the analysis and reporting of the results. The researchers should decide on the purpose of the study and what information is needed, and then compose no more than 10 open-ended questions to pose to the focus group participants. It is important to ensure that all of the participants have the opportunity to discuss each question and respond as desired. The focus group can consist of as few as four members but usually no more than 15 people. The participants should be people who have never met prior to arriving at the site for the group interaction; however, the participants should be similar enough to prevent the majority of the group time from being taken up with attempting to find common ground among the group members. The similarity between group members can be that they are all nurses, for example, or all cancer patients (O'Sullivan & Rassel, 1999).

The researcher organizing a focus group will need to arrange for a moderator for the group as well as someone to serve as a transcriber and possibly an additional person to set up recording equipment. Videotaping of the participants will entail distribution of an informed consent form. The moderator is vital to the progression of the group because it is his or her duty to lead the group from question to question and prevent participants from getting stagnated in complicated questions or conversation that has no bearing on the group's topic of discussion. Once the focus group has concluded, the moderator and observers will assemble to discuss the conversational progression of the participants and to record their impression of each of the participants and their individual contributions to the group as well as to the overall interview (O'Sullivan & Rassel, 1999).

A unique feature of the focus group is the topic guide, which is a list of the topics that will be covered. It is most effectively designed as an outline of issues with probing questions listed under each issue, and should be jointly designed with the research team and the moderator. A cue to the degree of detail required in the topic guide will be the degree of experience of the moderator. A less experienced moderator may require a more detailed topic guide with very specific questions written under each issue (Debus, n.d.).

How can an inexperienced researcher know that a focus group might be a more effective means of data collection than an individual interview? According to Debus (n.d.), the researcher should consider using a focus group when:

- Group interaction is likely to produce new thoughts that would not emerge otherwise.
- The subject matter is not so sensitive that participants will hesitate to discuss it in a group.
- The topic is such that participants can voice their thoughts in 10 minutes or less.
- The interviewer is not likely to become fatigued.
- The volume of material is not extensive.
- A single subject matter is being examined.
- It will be helpful for key decision makers to observe first-hand consumer information.
- Target respondents can be easily assembled in one location.
- A quick turnaround is required.
- The researcher has a limited budget.

Records or Existing Data

Records or currently existing data can be used when available data are examined in a new way in order to answer specific research questions. This can be an excellent data collection method for the DNP researcher because of the savings in terms of time. It allows for the examination of trends over the course of time. The researcher also avoids the time involved in approaching potential research subjects to ask for their participation in the research project (LoBiondo-Wood & Haber, 2002).

As might be expected, there are disadvantages attached to the use of existing records as a data collection method. Some facilities may be reluctant to allow researchers access to their records, particularly when there is a concern regarding protected health information. Also, if the researcher is allowed access to records, he or she will be reviewing only those records that have survived over the course of time. If these are not representative of the larger population being studied, then the researcher may face the problem of bias as he or she makes an educated guess regarding the records' accuracy (LoBiondo-Wood & Haber, 2002).

Content Analysis

Content analysis can be a variation on the use of existing data. It is, in its simplest form, the quantitative analysis of message characteristics. It allows the researcher to describe these messages in the media, such as television programs; in documentary data; or in other communications in an objective, systematic, and quantitative manner (LoBiondo-Wood & Haber, 2002). Neuendorf (2002) has described the progression of the typical content analysis research process:

1. *Theory and rationale*—The researcher must decide what content will be described and why it is specifically of interest to the researcher. He or she must develop a literature review to generate either researcher questions or hypotheses.
2. *Conceptualizations*—The researcher decides which variables will be used in the study and how they will be defined.
3. *Operationalizations*—The researcher decides how variables will be measured as well as the unit of data collection. The unit of data collection can be individual words, characters, themes, time periods, or interactions.
4. *Codebook*—The researcher develops a codebook for the coding of variables.
5. *Sampling*—The researcher decides how to randomly sample a subset of the content. This could occur by time period, by issue, by page, by channel, or another similar subset.
6. *Training and pilot reliability*—The researcher should schedule a training session for the personnel serving as coders so that consensus can be developed on the coding of the variables. Reliability of the variables should be determined, so if the study were to be replicated under the same conditions, essentially the same results would be achieved.
7. *Coding*—Intercoder reliability should be established to ensure that all coding is being done consistently.
8. *Tabulation and reporting*—Results can be reported in various ways, with trends over time being a common method of reporting results.

Although content analysis can seem deceptively simple to the novice researcher, it has the disadvantage of requiring the researcher to rely on previously recorded documents or messages. Thus, the accuracy of the existing data can be questionable, and bias may be present.

DATA COLLECTION IN MIXED METHOD RESEARCH

Data collection that occurs in mixed method research has its own particular issues that researchers must be prepared to address. For example, data collection in a research project of this design will occur either concurrently or sequentially. Concurrent data collection occurs when quantitative and qualitative data collection occurs at approximately the same time. Sequential data collection occurs when quantitative or qualitative data are collected first and the results that are achieved are used to provide information for the other form (quantitative or qualitative). Sequential data collection is accomplished with the idea that there will be a connection between the two different forms of the data. Either the first or the second data collection can be considered the greater priority, depending on the research problem and the emphasis the researcher desires (Creswell & Clark,2007).

An additional concern that is unique to mixed method research involves the need to approach institutional review boards. Creswell and Clark (2007) have noted that in an IRB proposal using the concurrent approach, both the quantitative and qualitative forms of data collection can be described at the beginning of the project, whereas in a proposal using the sequential approach, only the initial phase of data collection can be described definitively. This will likely lead to the IRB requiring the researcher to complete an addendum when the second stage data collection procedures have been solidified.

As previously mentioned, the DNP researcher can choose among various approaches to data collection. Although interviews and questionnaires have been discussed in some detail, data collection through survey research has enough unique features to warrant a chapter of its own. The subsequent chapter will discuss data collection through the process of survey research.

■ GLOSSARY

content validity The instrument and its items are representative of the content that the researcher intends to measure.

criterion-related validity Requires the comparison of the measure in question with the best existing measure of the variable.

inter-rater reliability Assessing multiple readings of a measurement from several people for evidence of similarity.

intra-rater reliability Assessing multiple readings of a measurement from the same person for evidence of similarity.

operationalization The process of defining how variables will be measured.

pilot test A small survey that serves as a pre-test to a major survey.

reliability characteristic that allows an instrument to be consistent and give the same results if the research is replicated.

validity Characteristic of an instrument in which it measures what it was intended to measure.

■ LEARNING ENHANCEMENT TOOLS

1. You are a DNP researcher who is conducting research on emotional changes in adolescents who have experienced the death of a sibling. You have decided to develop a new instrument for this study. Describe in detail the process you will go through as you develop the new instrument.

2. Describe a detailed outline for a study you could implement as a DNP researcher that could utilize physiological measurements as a data collection method.

3. Describe a detailed outline for a study you could implement as a DNP researcher that could utilize participant observation as a data collection method.

4. Describe a detailed outline for a study you could implement as a DNP researcher that could utilize the e-mail interview as a data collection method.

5. Describe a detailed outline for a study you could implement as a DNP researcher that could utilize existing records as a data collection method.

6. Describe a detailed outline for a study you could implement as a DNP researcher that could utilize content analysis as a data collection method.

7. As a DNP researcher, you have decided to use content analysis as a data collection method to study current television shows that depict nurses. Describe in detail the various steps you would use to proceed through content analysis for this research project.

8. Describe a detailed outline for a study you could implement as a DNP researcher that could utilize a focus group as a data collection method.

9. You are a DNP researcher and are interested in using an observational data collection method as part of a research project using family members of cancer patients as the research population. Describe how you make the decision of whether to use a structured or unstructured observational method for data collection.

10. Describe a plan that would allow data collection to occur in a research project that has a mixed method design.

11. You are a DNP researcher who is participating in a research project that is using programmatic research as the research design. Describe how use of this type of research will affect data collection for a researcher.

12. You are a DNP researcher who is planning to design a questionnaire on the attitude of nursing staff on a particular floor toward nursing students who were performing clinical rotation on that floor. Describe in detail which types of questions would be best to include in a questionnaire on this topic and also state how many questions of each type you would include.

■ RESOURCES

Buchanan, T., & Schmidt, J. (1999). Using the Internet for psychological research: Personality testing on the World Wide Web. *British Journal of Psychology, 90,* 125–144.

Burke, J., O'Campo, P., Peak, G., Gielen, A., McDonnell, K., & Trochim, W. (2005). An introduction to concept mapping as a participatory public health research method. *Qualitative Health Research, 15,* 1392–1410.

Drewnowski, A. (2001). Diet image: A new perspective on the food-frequency questionnaire. *Nutrition Review, 59,* 370–372.

Emden, C., & Borbasi, S. (2000). Programmatic research: A desirable (or despotic) nursing strategy for the future. *Collegian, 7*(1), 32–37.

Garratt, A., Schmidt, L., Mackintosh, A., & Fitzpatrick, R. (2002). Quality of life measurement: Bibliographic study of patient assessed health outcome measures. *British Medical Journal, 324,* 1417.

Gilbody, S., House, A., & Sheldon, T. (2001). Routinely administered questionnaires for depression and anxiety: Systematic review. *British Medical Journal, 322,* 406–409.

Gosling, S., Vazire, S., Srivastava, S., & John, O. (2004). Should we trust Web-based studies? A comparative analysis of six preconceptions about Internet questionnaires. *American Psychologist, 59*(2), 93–104.

Groger, L., Mayberry, P., & Straker, J. (1999). What we didn't learn because of who would not talk to us. *Qualitative Health Research, 9,* 829–835.

Harris, K., & Graham, S. (1999). Programmatic intervention research: Illustration from the evolution of self-regulated strategy development. *Learning Disability Quarterly, 22*(4), 251–262.

Houtkoop-Steenstra, H. (2000). *Interaction and the standardised survey interview: The living questionnaire.* Cambridge, UK: Cambridge University Press.

Koo, M., & Skinner, H. (2005). Challenges of Internet recruitment: A case study with disappointing results. *Journal of Medical Internet Research, 7*(1). Retrieved January 8, 2010, from www.jmir.org/2005/1/e6

Lohr, K. (2002). Assessing health status and quality of life instruments: Attributes and review criteria. *Quality of Life Research, 11,* 193–205.

Meyen, E., Aust, R., & Gauch, J. (2002). E-Learning: A programmatic research construct for the future. *Journal of Special Education Technology, 17*(3), 37–46.

Minnick, A., & Leipzig, R. (2000). Beyond interviewing skills: Twelve steps for training interviewers. *Outcomes Management for Nursing Practice, 4*(4), 182–186.

Ross, M., Mansson, S., Daneback, K., Cooper, A., & Tikkanen, R. (2005). Biases in Internet sexual health samples: Comparison of an Internet sexuality survey and a national sexual health survey in Sweden. *Social Science and Medicine, 61*(1), 245–252.

Roster, C., Rogers, R., Albaum, G., & Klein, D. (2004). A comparison of response characteristic from Web and telephone surveys. *International Journal of Market Research, 46*(3), 359–373.

Schaeffer, N. (2003). Hardly ever or constantly? Group comparisons using vague quantifiers. *Public Opinion Quarterly, 55*, 395–423.

Trochim, W., Milstein, B., Wood., B., Jackson, S., & Pressler, V. (2004). Setting objectives for community and systems change: An application of concept mapping for planning a statewide health improvement initiative. *Health Promotion Practice, 5*(1), 8–19.

Widerszal-Bazyl, M., & CieSlak, R. (2000). Monitoring psychosocial stress at work: Development of the psychosocial working conditions questionnaire. *International Journal of Occupational Safety Ergonomics*, special issue, 59–70.

Yampolskaya, S., Nesman, T., Hernandex, M., & Koch, D. (2004). Using concept mapping to develop a logic model and articulate a program theory: A case example. *American Journal of Evaluation, 25*, 191–207.

Yuille, J., Marxsen, D., & Cooper, B. (1999). Training investigative interviewers: Adherence to the spirit, as well as the letter. *International Journal of Law and Psychiatry, 22*(3/4), 323–336.

■ REFERENCES

Boynton, P., & Greenhalgh, T. (2004). Hands-on guide to questionnaire research: Selecting, designing, and developing your questionnaire. *British Medical Journal, 328*, 1312–1315.

Ciliska, D., Cullum, N., & Dicenso, A. (1999). The fundamentals of quantitative measurement. *Evidence Based Nursing, 2*, 100–101.

Creswell, J., & Plano Clark, V. (2007). *Designing and conducting mixed methods research*. Thousand Oaks, CA: Sage.

Debus, M. (n.d.). *A handbook for excellence in focus group research*. Washington, DC: Academy for Educational Development Healthcom. Retrieved January 21, 2010, from www.globalhealthcommunication.org/tools/60

Hoepfl, M. (1997). *Choosing qualitative research: A primer for technology education researchers*. Retrieved December 7, 2009, from http://scholar.lib .vt.edu/ejournals/JTE/v9n1/hoepfl.html

Hunt, N., & McHale, S. (2007). A practical guide to the e-mail interview. *Qualitative Health Research, 17*(10), 1415–1421.

Key, J. (1997). *Research design in occupational education*. Retrieved from
  http://www.okstate.edu/ag/agedcm4h/academic/aged5980a/5980/newpage2.htm

LoBiondo-Wood, G., & Haber, J. (2002). *Nursing research: Methods, critical
  appraisal, and utilization*. St. Louis, MO: Mosby.

Neuendorf, K. (2002). *The content analysis guidebook*. Thousand Oaks, CA: Sage
  Publications.

O'Sullivan, E., & Rassel, G. (1999). *Research methods for public administrators*.
  New York: Longman.

Polit, D., & Hungler, B. (2000). *Essentials of nursing research: Methods and
  applications*. Philadelphia: Lippincott.

University of Ballarat Institute for Regional and Rural Research. (2004). *Developing
  a programmatic approach to regional and rural research*. Retrieved January 20,
  2010 from www.ballarat.edu.au/ard/ubresearch/docs/Future_Directions
  _Oct09.pdf

Issues Related to Survey Data Collection

10

■ OBJECTIVES

Upon completion of this chapter, the reader should be prepared to:

1 Describe the different types of information that can be obtained through use of a survey as a data collection method.

2 Describe the various stages of planning the development of a survey for data collection.

3 Discuss the process of recruiting the sample for survey research.

4 Discuss the process of planning the content of a survey instrument.

5 Describe how sampling can occur when survey research is being implemented.

6 Discuss the various cross-sectional survey designs that can be selected for implementation.

7 Discuss the various longitudinal survey designs that can be selected for implementation.

INTRODUCTION TO SURVEY DATA COLLECTION

The DNP researcher who opts to utilize survey research as a method of data collection chooses to do so because he or she wants to make inferences about the larger population. Survey research can produce data that are based on real-world observations. It is more likely than some other research approaches to produce data that are based on a representative sample and that can be generalized to a population. Because surveys can produce a large amount of data in a short period of time at a relatively low cost, a set time span can usually be set for the research project. This can be useful in preparing proposals for institutional review boards (Kelley, Clark, Brown, & Sitzia, 2003). Usually the researcher can obtain five different types of information from the respondents who complete surveys:

- Facts, such as demographics and personal history
- Perceptions, which are statements about what the respondents think they know about the world
- Opinions, which are statements of the respondents' judgments about events that have occurred or specific objects
- Attitudes, which are the respondents' basic orientation toward ideas, objects, or events and can be the basis for respondents' opinions
- Behavioral reports, which are statements of how respondents choose to act in specific situations (Manheim, Rich, & Willnat, 2002)

Once the researcher has decided to utilize survey research as the method of data collection, he or she should begin planning the development of the survey by progressing through specific stages. According to Manheim, Rich, and Willnat (2002), these consist of:

1. *Conceptualizing*—The researcher decides on the purpose of the survey research, develops the hypotheses, specifies the concepts to be utilized, and decides how the concepts will be operationalized (measured) using the survey questions.

2. *Survey design*—The researcher establishes the procedures he or she will utilize in implementing the survey and decides on the nature of the sample that will be used. Kaye and Johnson (1999) recommend that the design of a Web-based survey should allow it to be as short as possible so that respondents can complete it quickly and not have to scroll throughout the survey frequently, use as few graphics as possible so that a Web-based survey can be downloaded rapidly, and use drop-down boxes to save space. In addition, the researcher who is using a Web-based survey should check the survey using a variety of browsers to locate any browser-related design problems.

3. *Instrumentation*—The questions are drafted for the survey and the instrument itself is formatted.

4. *Planning*—The budget is planned, the materials that will be needed are delineated, and personnel that will be needed to assist are either requested, as in the case of graduate teaching assistants, for example, or are recruited from the researcher's company. Kaye and Johnson (1999) recommend that as part of the planning process, the survey should be publicized by listing it with as many major search engines as possible; researchers should offer an incentive for completing the survey, such as continuing education hours; and they should determine the most effective sites for publicizing the survey by asking respondents how they found out about the survey.

5. *Sampling*—The researcher chooses the people to be interviewed. Kaye and Johnson (1999) recommend that respondents can be located by linking the survey to key online sites; announcements should be posted on discussion groups that will be used by the targeted population; and the intended audience should be specified in the introduction to the survey because virtually anyone could potentially complete the survey. Once a sample is selected, the chosen respondents can be e-mailed a request to complete the survey, along with a specific number for identification that will maintain anonymity and a password for accessing the survey on a website.

6. *Training/briefing*—The interviewers or other personnel are prepared so they can administer the survey in a uniform fashion to all participants. The greater the number of interviewers, the longer this will take to complete.

7. *Pre-testing*—The survey instrument is administered to a small group of participants who are similar to the larger sample to be utilized. This ensures that the instructions given to participants can be easily understood and that the survey items will produce the type of response desired by the researcher.

8. *Surveying*—The survey is administered to members of the sample population. Kaye and Johnson (1999) recommend including a verification page with a thank-you response to the respondent so he or she is not left wondering whether the submitted survey was actually transmitted successfully.

9. *Monitoring*—The researcher reviews records of contacts and refusals and discusses administration of instruments with research personnel to verify that the correct people are contacted as potential respondents.

10. *Verifying*—Follow-up contacts are used to make certain interviews are actually performed or surveys are actually returned, whether by e-mail or by actual mail.

11. *Coding*—The data collected at this point are converted into numerical terms to allow for analysis.

12. *Processing*—The data are further organized for analysis.

13. *Analyzing*—The data are analyzed using statistical tools so conclusions can be derived regarding their content and the implications for the greater community.

14. *Reporting*—Findings are summarized into research reports for dissemination into the healthcare community and related stakeholders and possible publication.

As part of the follow-up to the administration, processing, and analysis of survey research, the researcher should closely examine the response rate to the survey. The researcher should determine:

- How many people were sent the survey if it was a mail-out survey?
- What was the method of distribution, and was this a new method of distribution for this type of research? Was this type of research traditionally distributed using a mail-out method but was distributed for the first time using a Web-based survey?
- How many surveys were returned? Of the number returned, how many were completed and therefore usable? Can a reason for the incomplete surveys be determined? Is there a specific question that seemed to confuse respondents?
- If different populations were used, was there a different response rate in various populations? Did certain populations seem to understand the questions differently?
- What specific things were used by the researcher to try to increase the response rate, such as incentives and publicity? Did the incentives seem to be ineffective, or poorly chosen for the target population?
- If the response rate seems to be an extreme case, either extremely high or extremely low, can the aberration be explained? (Baruch & Holtam, 2008)

RECRUITING THE SAMPLE FOR SURVEY RESEARCH

In the process of recruiting the sample for survey research, the researcher frequently has to negotiate access to the potential respondents by going through **purposive sampling**. The gatekeepers are the authority figures who control the researcher's access to the research participants. These can be, for example, nursing school deans if faculty will be surveyed or nurse managers if the survey will involve nurses. The researcher must be prepared to show the gatekeepers that the research is worthwhile and will not negatively affect them or the participants. Also, the researcher must be able to show the gatekeepers that the research has credibility and that he or she has personal credibility (Lindsay, 2005).

Once access to potential participants has been negotiated with the gatekeepers, the researcher must convince the research subjects that the proposed project will benefit them in some way. The subjects will be more likely to agree to participate if they believe the research will provide them with new skills or knowledge they did not have prior to participating. The researcher must be prepared to let the potential participants know the survey will not take long to complete, confidentiality will be maintained, and some type of incentive will be offered for participation. This can be a monetary payment or an hour of continuing education time for nurses (Lindsay, 2005).

An important point in recruiting potential research subjects that is frequently overlooked is timing. When initially negotiating access through the gatekeepers and later recruiting the subjects, the researcher must be flexible enough to present the benefits of completing the survey at a time that is most convenient for the gatekeepers and later for the subjects. This may involve talking with a nurse manager at 4:00 P.M., and with nurses at midnight to speak with the night shift and then at 7:00 A.M. to speak with the day shift (Lindsay, 2005).

PLANNING THE CONTENT OF A SURVEY INSTRUMENT

In planning the format of the questionnaire that will be used in survey research, the researcher should recognize the importance of making the questions clear and easy to read. The use of all capital letters should be avoided. Questions should be numbered and grouped together according to subject. Instructions should be provided at the beginning of the instrument and, if necessary, at the beginning of each new group of questions. In addition, questions that actually consist of two or more subquestions should be avoided. An example of this would be, "How satisfied are you with your current nursing position and with your nurse manager?" Closed-ended questions such as multiple choice questions are answered rapidly by respondents and easy for the researcher to code as well as analyze. Open-ended questions, in which the respondent composes his or her reply rather than choosing one from a selection, can be used in survey instruments as well. Open-ended questions take longer for the research subjects to answer but can provide a rich source of information that would not be available with closed-ended questions. However, they can be very time-consuming for the researcher to code and difficult to analyze, because the researcher will need to decide how to treat partially answered questions and skipped questions, as well as answers that don't seem to be applicable to the question (Kelley et al., 2003). Examples of a survey instrument that uses both open-ended and closed-ended questions may be found in **Figure 10-1**.

When possible, a pilot test of the survey instrument should be conducted. This will allow the researcher to identify questions that are poorly worded or difficult to understand. The researcher should determine whether the majority of respondents seem to understand the questions in the same way. When the researcher uses closed-ended questions, pilot testing should demonstrate whether enough answer options are offered for each question, and whether questions are routinely missed or skipped by respondents. The procedures used in the pilot test should be the same as those that are intended to be used in the administration of the primary survey instrument. This will demonstrate whether procedures used in administration are the source of nonresponses (Kelley et al., 2003).

No matter how the format of the survey instrument is structured, each survey should be accompanied by a cover letter that tells the prospective participant the purpose of the research study, the name and contact information of the researcher, how the information will be used, any potential benefits or harm the research subject can expect, and what will happen to the information he or she provides. An informed consent form should be attached, as well as a

---

FIGURE 10-1   Self-Regulation Questionnaire

The following questions relate to your reasons for participating in nursing classes. Different people have different reasons for participating in such a class, and we want to know how true each of these reasons is for you. There are three groups of items, and those in each group pertain to the sentence that begins that group. Please indicate how true each reason is for you using the following scale:

1	2	3	4	5	6	7
not at all true			somewhat true			very true

A. I actively participate actively in my nursing classes:

_____   1. Because I feel like it's a good way to improve my skills and my understanding of patients.

_____   2. Because others would think badly of me if I didn't.

_____   3. Because learning the content well is an important part of becoming a nurse.

_____   4. Because I would feel bad about myself if I didn't study these concepts.

B. I follow my instructor's suggestions:

_____   5. Because I will get a good grade if I do what he/she suggests.

_____   6. Because I believe my instructor's suggestions will help me nurse effectively.

_____   7. Because I want others to think that I am a good nurse.

_____   8. Because it's easier to do what I'm told than to think about it.

_____   9. Because it's important to me to do well at this.

_____   10. Because I would probably feel guilty if I didn't comply with my instructor's suggestions.

C. The reason that I will continue to broaden my nursing knowledge is:

_____ 11. Because it's exciting to try new ways to work interpersonally with my patients.

_____ 12. Because I would feel proud if I did continue to improve at nursing.

_____ 13. Because it's a challenge to really understand what the patient is experiencing.

_____ 14. Because it's interesting to use the nursing process try to identify what needs the patient has.

DEMOGRAPHIC DATA COLLECTION FORM

Student Classification
☐ Junior   ☐ Senior   ☐ EARN

Sex: _____   **Age:** _____

Ethnicity
☐ Caucasian   ☐ Hispanic   ☐ African-American   ☐ Asian   ☐ Other

Marital Status	**Dependent Children**	**# of Dependent**
☐ Single	☐ 2 parent family	**Children** _____
☐ Married	☐ 1 parent family	
☐ Divorced	☐ no children	
☐ Widowed		

Previous Healthcare Experience   **Current GPA**
☐ Yes   _____ 4.00 to 3.5   _____ 2.99 to 2.50
☐ No   _____ 3.49 to 3.0   _____ 2.49 to 2.00

Number of Hours Spent Independently on School Work Per Week:

_____ <5   _____ 16 to 20   _____ >30
_____ 6 to 10   _____ 21 to 25
_____ 11 to 15   _____ 26 to 30

Number of Hours Spent in Collaboration on School Work Per Week:

_____ <5   _____ 16 to 20   _____ >30
_____ 6 to 10   _____ 21 to 25
_____ 11 to 15   _____ 26 to 30

Hours Employed Per Week:

_____ 0   _____ 11 to 20   _____ 31 to 40
_____ 1 to 10   _____ 21 to 30

Years Since Previous Degree:

_____ 1 to 3 years   _____ 11 to 15 years
_____ 4 to 5 years   _____ > 15 years
_____ 6 to 10 years   _____ No previous degree

Previous Degree GPA:

_____ 4.00 to 3.50   _____ 2.99 to 2.50
_____ 3.49 to 3.00   _____ 2.49 to 2.00

INSTRUMENTATION

The Learning Self-Regulation Questionnaire (LSRQ), originally designed by Williams and Deci (1996) to assess academic self-regulation in a medical school course, was used in this study following minor modification to reflect studies in the field of nursing. This tool has been used in various forms in multiple research studies (Black & Deci, 2000; Ryan & Connell, 1989; Williams & Deci, 1996). Permission to use and modify the LSRQ for this research was obtained from Deci (personal communication, November 10, 2007).

The LSRQ is a 14-item questionnaire which assessed academic self-regulation on two scales, controlled regulation and autonomous regulation. Three primary questions (A, B, & C) were presented with multiple response choices (1–14) to which the respondent indicated the likelihood of that choice using a Likert-type response with answer choices ranging from 1 indicating "not at all true" to 7 indicating "very true." Participant responses were tallied for two subscales: autonomous regulation and controlled regulation. The autonomous regulation subscale score was determined by averaging the answers to the following questions: 1, 3, 6, 9, 11, 13, and 14. The controlled regulation subscale score required to averaging of responses to questions 2, 4, 5, 7, 8, 10, and 12.

Instrument validity refers to the strength of the survey tool to measure what is intended to be measured (Polit & Hungler, 1999). The instrument validity of the LSRQ was ensured through the review of previous published studies which used this research tool and reported good internal consistency and construct validity for this research instrument. The original instrument was used to by Ryan and Connell (1989) to assess learning autonomy in children and was later modified twice by Williams and Deci (1996) to reflect differently curriculum content for use with college students. Williams and Deci reported strong validity for both modified versions of this tool. In addition, Black and Deci (2000) reported construct validity for the LSRQ. This instrument was slightly modified to reflect nursing curriculum similar to the modifications in previous studies.

Reliability refers to the consistency of a measurement tool in measuring a particular attribute (Polit & Beck, 2006). When determining instrument reliability, the instrument should be examined for stability and internal consistency. Stability of an instrument examining a psychosocial construct such as academic self-regulation or learning style preference is questionable. The LSRQ is similar to the VARK Questionnaire which helps students determine their preference for receiving, giving, and processing information as these types of instruments are not designed to be "reliable in terms of consistency of scores of a long period of time" (Fleming, 2006). While test-retest reliability procedures support instrument stability, test-retest methods are not reliable when assessing stability of the instrument due to multiple factors which may impact participant responses such as attitude and mood differences and experience which may have occurred between the two measurements (Polit & Beck).

Internal consistency, the reliability of the LSRQ subscales to measure the expected characteristics, autonomous regulation and controlled regulation, is supported by reviewing the reported Cronbach's alpha reliabilites for the instrument from previous studies. Previous studies report the alpha reliabilities ranging from 0.75 to 0.80 for autonomous regulation subscale and 0.67 to 0.75 for controlled regulation subscale (Black & Deci, 2000; Williams & Deci, 1996).

Since this questionnaire was modified to reflect nursing curricula and questions were generalized to learning efforts related to all nursing courses, not just one specific course, additional factorial analysis was required. The reliability of survey tools utilizing a Likert scale format producing interval and ratio measures can be determined by performing a Cronbach's alpha test of internal consistency (LoBiondo-Wood & Haber, 2006). The desired score of 0.70 or greater on a scale of 0 to 1.0 demonstrates survey tool reliability. The reliability of the modified LSRQ was verified with a reported Cronbach's alpha on the autonomous regulation subscale and the controlled regulation subscale were .768 and .725 respectively.

The DDCT was used to collect the following data: (a) student classification (nominal scale as TBNS or NTBNS); (b) sex (nominal scale); (c) age (interval scale); ethnicity; (d) marital status (single, married, divorced, widowed); (e) family unit (two parent family, single parent family, or no children); (f) number of dependent children; (g) previous healthcare experience; (h) current GPA; (i) number of hours spent independently on school work per week; (j) number of hours spent in collaboration on school work per week; (k) hours employed per week; (l) years since previous degree; and (m) previous degree GPA.

PROCEDURES

Permission to utilize and modify the original LSRQ was obtained. The dean of the Auburn University Montgomery School of Nursing granted the researcher permission to conduct the research. The Auburn University Montgomery Institutional Review Board granted approval of the research study and Auburn University Institutional Review Board also approved the research study as the principal investigator was conducting the research to satisfy degree requirements as a graduate student at Auburn University. The researcher contacted faculty within the School of Nursing to coordinate collection dates.

RECRUITING SCRIPT

Introduction: Hi, my name is Michelle Schutt. I am a doctoral student at Auburn University and I am conducting a study for my dissertation in partial fulfillment for the education doctorate from Auburn University.

Invitation to Participate: You were selected as a potential participant for a research study entitled "Examination of Learning Self-Regulation Variances in Nursing Students" because you are presently enrolled at the Auburn Montgomery School of Nursing. All of you are invited to participate in this study that will evaluate learning self-regulation. I will study the differences in learning self-regulation across different groups of nursing students.

Agreement to Participate: If you agree to participate, I will need you read the information letter. Your completion of the survey conveys consent to participate in this research. The information letter states that participants will anonymously complete a two-sided document with one side being a short demographic tool and the opposite side being a short survey and return the survey in a sealed envelope. There will be no future requirements of the participants.

Anticipated Risks: The risks associated with this study are minimal but could include a breach in confidentiality, social discomforts, or feelings of coercion to participate. Should you need to discuss your feelings about participating in this research, you can speak with me, your advisor or someone at the Auburn Montgomery Counseling Center. Contact information for the Auburn Montgomery Counseling Center is attached to the informed consent form.

Confidentiality of Data: All information obtained about you will remain confidential in a locked filing cabinet in Room 315 Moore Hall. The only other individuals who will review the data will be professors in the Auburn University educational doctoral program assisting with data analysis. No identification will be provided on the forms to link the response to an individual student.

How the study will help: Your participation will greatly benefit future nursing students and will support efforts to improve teaching effectiveness in the Auburn Montgomery School of Nursing, other schools of nursing, and education as a whole.

Decision to Participate or Not and Withdrawal of Consent: Your decision whether or not to participate will not prejudice your future relations with Auburn University, Auburn Montgomery, or the Auburn Montgomery School of Nursing.

If you decide to participate, you are free to withdraw your consent and to discontinue participation at any time without penalty. If you decide to withdraw from the study prior to completing the requested demographic tool and survey, please simply do not return these collection tools. Once these tools are collected, your specific response tool will not be retrievable as it will not have your name or an identifying code on it.

If you have questions concerning the study, presently or in the future, I will be happy to answer/address those concerns. You can contact me by email at mschutt1@aum.edu or by phone at (334) 328-4293.

IRB REQUIRED ALTERNATIVE RECRUITING SCRIPT

NOTE: This script will be used for obtaining informed consent and data collection for two groups of participants: 1) Junior participants during April 2008 and 2) EARN participants during May 2008.

Introduction: Hi, my name is Dr. Debbie Faulk. I am here on behalf of Michelle Schutt, a doctoral student at Auburn University and I am conducting a study for my dissertation in partial fulfillment for the education doctorate from Auburn University.

Invitation to Participate: You were selected as a potential participant for a research study entitled "Examination of Learning Self-Regulation Variances in Nursing Students" because you are presently enrolled at the Auburn Montgomery School of Nursing. All of you are invited to participate in this study that will evaluate learning self-regulation. I will study the differences in learning self-regulation across different groups of nursing students.

Agreement to Participate: If you agree to participate, I will need you to sign an informed consent form. The form states that you agree to the following: Participants will anonymously complete a two-sided document with one side being a short demographic tool and the opposite side being a short survey. There will be no future requirements of the participants.

Anticipated Risks: The risks associated with this study are minimal but could include a breach in confidentiality, social discomforts, or feelings of coercion to participate. Should you need to discuss your feelings about participating in this research, you can speak with me, your advisor or someone at the Auburn Montgomery Counseling Center. Contact information for the Auburn Montgomery Counseling Center is attached to the informed consent form.

Confidentiality of Data: All information obtained about you will remain confidential in a locked filing cabinet in my office in Room 318 Moore Hall until course grades have been entered in Webster in May (August) at which time I will surrender the data collection tools to Mrs. Schutt. The only other individuals who will review the data will be professors in the Auburn University educational doctoral program assisting with data analysis. No identification will be provided on the forms to link the response to an individual student.

How the study will help: Your participation will greatly benefit future nursing students and will support efforts to improve teaching effectiveness in the Auburn Montgomery School of Nursing, other schools of nursing, and education as a whole.

Decision to Participate or Not and Withdrawal of Consent: Your decision whether or not to participate will not prejudice your future relations with Auburn University, Auburn Montgomery, or the Auburn Montgomery School of Nursing.

If you decide to participate, you are free to withdraw your consent and to discontinue participation at any time without penalty. If you decide to withdraw from the study prior to completing the requested demographic tool and survey, please simply do not return these collection tools. Once these tools are collected, your specific response tool will not be retrievable as it will not have your name or an identifying code on it. If you have questions concerning the study, presently or in the future, I will be happy to answer/address those concerns. You can contact me by email at mschutt1@aum.edu or by phone at (334) 328-4293.

Source: Courtesy of Michelle A. Schutt, EdD, RN.

detailed discussion of the safeguards that will be used to guarantee either the anonymity of the research subjects or the confidentiality of the information that they will provide (Kelley et al., 2003). This can be implemented as easily with an electronic version as with a paper version.

SAMPLING DURING SURVEY RESEARCH

Random sampling is usually the type of sampling utilized when questionnaires are being used to collect data. This allows the results to be generalized to a larger population, with the results then being subjected to statistical analysis. There are various types of random sampling, each of which can be utilized in survey research. They include:

- **Simple random sampling**—Each person in the population is chosen by chance and is as likely to be selected as anyone else is.
- **Systematic sampling**—Subjects to be included in the sample are selected at specific intervals within the population; for example, every seventh person.
- **Stratified random sampling**—A specific group is selected from the larger population and a random sample is then chosen from that group. This would be used when the DNP researcher decides to survey nursing students at a college as the greater population, and then selects to random sample only the junior class from the larger population.
- **Cluster sampling**—This technique is frequently used in nationwide research projects, because it randomly assigns research subjects to groups within a much larger population, and then research subjects within the assigned groups are surveyed (Kelley et al., 2003).

Alternatively, nonrandom sampling can be used when the survey instruments are more informal, such as with interviews and focus groups. Just as it sounds, nonrandom sampling targets subjects within a population. There are three main types of nonrandom sampling that can be used in some way with a survey instrument:

- **Purposive sampling**—A specific population is selected and only its members are surveyed; an example would be selecting sophomore nursing students as the population and then surveying only those students who are age 30 or older.
- **Convenience sampling**—The sample is composed of those individuals who are the easiest to recruit; an example would be sending an e-mail to potential subjects in a specific population and asking them to

respond if they would like to be surveyed about a particular topic. Only the respondents would be sent the survey instrument.

- **Snowballing**—The sample actually develops as the survey progresses, because as one person completes the survey, he or she is asked to recommend other potential research subjects who can be asked to participate (Kelley et al., 2003).

The decision of which type of sampling to utilize largely will depend on the degree of sampling error the researcher can tolerate. **Sampling error** is considered to be the possibility that the sample selected is not completely representative of its population of origin. The researcher will never be successful in completely eliminating sampling error, but should recognize that random sampling will always give a better approximation of the population's characteristics than nonrandom sampling (Kelley et al., 2003).

The sample size will depend on the aim of the research project, the statistical analysis the researcher plans, and the resources of the researcher, both personnel and financial. If less formal surveys are planned, such as using focus groups or interviews, the sample size chosen can safely be smaller than the size needed for a more formalized survey. Although the larger the sample size, the more representative it will be of the larger population, for some populations, it will be difficult to obtain a large number of responses. The researcher should ensure that the nonresponse rate is calculated along with all statistics related to the response rate, because there are always implications related to the nonresponse rate. The researcher should determine if a specific section of the population was neglected regarding recruitment, and therefore produced a large number of nonresponders (Kelley et al., 2003).

DESIGNS IN SURVEY RESEARCH

Designs in survey research are usually either cross-sectional or longitudinal in nature. **Cross-sectional designs** gather information about a target population at a specific point in time and essentially produce a "snapshot" about the respondents. **Longitudinal designs** require the researcher to ask the same questions of respondents at two or more points in time. The researcher's choice of survey design is based on the purpose of the research. For example, a cross-sectional survey design can be either a contextual design or a social network design. A **contextual design** would sample cases within specific groups to accurately describe characteristics of the groups' contexts. This could be used, for example, if a researcher is interested in determining whether the increased patient satisfaction with the nursing care provided in the hospitals in a specific area of the state can be explained by the contextual resources available in that area. A **social network design** would be used if the researcher is interested in gaining information on the relationships among individuals and organizations and the processes that link them. Because the researcher will be interested in gaining information on the relationships that are present, this can be a time-consuming technique and will require the surveying of every person in the target population being studied (Singleton & Straits, 1999). This may prove difficult for the DNP researcher to implement because of the time constraints present with a capstone project.

In comparison, a longitudinal design can be a **trend study** if each survey collects data on the same variables with a new sample of the same target population so the researcher is able to observe changes in the population overall. If the researcher decides to study a specific group of individuals over time that typically experience the same significant event within a specific period of time, the research project becomes a **cohort study**. In addition, if the researcher opts to study how specific individuals are changing over time, the design will be that of a **panel study** because the respondents will be surveyed repeatedly (Singleton & Straits, 1999).

After the researcher has decided to use survey research as the method of data collection and has constructed the survey instrument, recruited the sample, and decided on a survey design to utilize in the implementation of the survey itself, the remaining step after implementation is the analysis of the collected data. The subsequent chapter will discuss analysis of the data that are collected, regardless of the type of research project implemented.

■ GLOSSARY

cluster sampling A technique frequently used in nationwide research projects, because it randomly assigns research subjects to groups within a much larger population, and then research subjects within the assigned groups are surveyed.

cohort study The researcher studies a specific group of individuals over time that typically experiences the same significant event within a specific period of time.

contextual design Samples cases within specific groups to accurately describe characteristics of the groups' contexts.

convenience sampling The sample is composed of those individuals who were the easiest to recruit.

cross-sectional design Gathers information about a target population at a specific point in time and essentially produces a "snapshot" about the respondents.

gatekeepers The authority figures who control the researcher's access to the research participants.

longitudinal design Requires the researcher to ask the same questions of respondents at two or more points in time.

panel study The researcher opts to study how specific individuals are changing over time; the respondents will be surveyed repeatedly.

purposive sampling A specific population is selected and only its members are surveyed.

sampling error The possibility that the sample selected is not completely representative of its population of origin. Usually occurs because of an error in the sampling process.

simple random sampling Each person in the population is chosen by chance and is as likely to be selected as anyone else is.

snowballing The sample actually develops as the survey progresses, because as one person completes the survey, he or she is asked to recommend other potential research subjects who can be asked to participate.

social network design Used if the researcher is interested in gaining information on the relationships among individuals and organizations and the processes that link them.

stratified random sampling A specific group is selected from the larger population and a random sample is then chosen from that specific group. This would be used when the DNP researcher decides to survey nursing students at a college as the greater population, and then selects to random sample only the sophomore class from the larger population.

systematic sampling Subjects to be included in the sample are selected at specific intervals within the population; for example, every seventh person.

trend study The survey collects data on the same variables with a new sample of the same target population so the researcher is able to observe changes in the population overall.

■ LEARNING ENHANCEMENT TOOLS

1. You are a DNP researcher who is planning to utilize survey research to collect data on patients' satisfaction with the discharge process from the hospital. You are employed in a 450-bed teaching hospital that is affiliated with a large university that has a nursing school. Describe how you will progress through the process of implementing survey research.

2. You are a DNP researcher who is planning to utilize survey research to collect data on the students' satisfaction with the facilities used for clinical rotation. You are employed by a school of nursing in a large university that is affiliated with a 450-bed teaching hospital. Describe how you will progress through the process of implementing survey research.

3. You are a DNP researcher who is planning to utilize survey research to collect data on the grieving process of siblings of victims of violent crimes. Describe in detail how the planning process of the survey would vary depending on whether a traditional mail-based survey is used or a Web-based survey is used.

4. You are a DNP researcher who utilized a Web-based survey to collect data on the grieving process of siblings of victims of violent crimes. The response rate was extremely low. Describe the process the researcher should use to analyze the response rate to this survey, particularly because it is unusually low.

5. You are a DNP researcher who is interested in using survey research to study nurses' attitudes toward their colleagues who become involved in substance abuse. Describe the process you would use in presenting the idea of the survey research to the hospital Vice President for Nursing, the day shift and night shift house supervisors, and the Neurology floor's nurse manager.

6. You are a DNP researcher who is interested in using survey research to study nurses' attitudes toward their colleagues who become involved in substance abuse. Discuss in detail the process you will use to design the survey instrument for this particular research project.

7. You are a DNP researcher who is interested in using survey research as the primary method of data collection for your research project. Develop a detailed scenario in which you would utilize a survey instrument and the type of sampling selected is:

   a. Simple random sampling

   b. Systematic sampling

   c. Stratified sampling

   d. Cluster sampling

   e. Purposive sampling

   f. Convenience sampling

   g. Snowballing

8. You are a DNP researcher who is interested in using survey research as the primary method of data collection for your research project. Develop a detailed scenario in which you could utilize the following survey designs for your project:

   a. Cohort study

   b. Contextual design

   c. Panel study

   d. Trend study

   e. Social network design

■ RESOURCES

Allen, N., Stanley, D., Williams, H., & Ross, S. (2007). Assessing the impact of nonresponse on work group diversity effects. *Organizational Research Methods, 10*, 262–286.

Badger, F., & Werrett, J. (2005). Room for improvement? Reporting response rates and recruitment in nursing research in the past decade. *Journal of Advanced Nursing, 51*, 502–510.

Bonometti, R., & Jun, T. (2006). A dynamic technique for conducting online survey-based research. *Competitiveness Review, 16*, 97–105.

Burns, K., Kho, M., Meade, M., Adhikari, N., Sinuff, T., & Cook, D. (2008). A guide for the design and conduct of self-administered surveys of clinicians. *Canadian Medical Association Journal, 179*(3), 1–12.

Couper, M., Traugott, M., & Lamias, M. (2001). Web survey design and administration. *Public Opinion Quarterly, 65*, 230–253.

Cycota, C., & Harrison, D. (2002). Enhancing survey response rates at the executive level: Are employee- or consumer-level techniques effective? *Journal of Management, 28*, 151–176.

Cycota C., & Harrison, D. (2006). What (not) to expect when surveying executives. *Organizational Research Methods, 9*, 133–160.

Dillman, D. (2000). *Mail and internet surveys: The tailored design method* (2nd ed.). New York: John Wiley and Sons.

Dillman, D., Phelps, G., Tortora, R., Swift, K., Johrell, J., & Berck, J. (2000). *Response rate measurement differences in mixed mode surveys using mail, telephone, interactive voice response and the Internet.* Paper presentation at Annual Meeting of the American Association for Public Opinion Research, May 2000, Montreal, Canada. Retrieved January 28, 2010, from www.sesrc.wsu.edu/dillman

Dooley, L., & Lindner, J. (2003). The handling of nonresponse error. *Human Resource Development Quarterly, 14*, 99–110.

Groves, R. (2006). Nonresponse rates and nonresponse bias in household surveys. *Public Opinion Quarterly, 70*, 646–675.

Ibeh, K., Brock, J., & Zhou, J. (2004). Drop and pick survey among industrial populations: Conceptualisations and empirical evidence. *Industrial Marketing Management, 33*, 155–165.

Morrel-Samuels, P. (2003). Web surveys' hidden hazards. *Hazard Business Review, 81*, 7, 16–18.

Porter, S. (2004). Raising response rates: What works? *New Directions for Institutional Research, 121*, 5–21.

Porter, S., & Whitcomb, M. (2006). The impact of contact type on web survey response rates. *Public Opinion Quarterly, 67*(4), 579–588.

Rogelberg, S., Conway, J., Sederburg, M., Spitzmuller, C., Aziz, S., & Knight, W. (2003). Profiling active and passive nonrespondents to an organizational survey. *Journal of Applied Psychology, 88,* 1104–1114.

Rogelberg, S., & Stanton, J. (2007). Understanding and dealing with organizational survey nonresponse. *Organizational Research Methods, 10,* 195–209.

Werner, S., Praxedes, M., & Kim, H. (2007). The reporting of nonresponse analyses in survey research. *Organizational Research Methods, 10,* 287–295.

Yoon, S., & Horne, C. (2004). Accruing the sample in survey research. *Southern Online Journal of Nursing Research, 2*(5), 1–17.

▪ REFERENCES

Baruch, Y., & Holtam, B. (2008). Survey response rate levels and trends in organizational research. *Human Relations, 61,* 1139–1160.

Kaye, B., & Johnson, T. (1999). Research methodology: Taming the cyber frontier: Techniques for improving online surveys. *Social Science Computer Review, 17,* 323–337.

Kelley, K., Clark, B., Brown, V., & Sitzia, J. (2003). Good practice in the conduct and reporting of survey research. *International Journal for Quality in Health Care, 15*(3), 261–266.

Lindsay, J. (2005). Getting the numbers: The unacknowledged work in recruiting for survey research. *Field Methods, 17,* 119–128.

Manheim, J., Rich, R., & Willnat, L. (2002). *Empirical political analysis: Research methods in political science.* New York: Addison Wesley Longman.

Singleton, R., & Straits, B. (1999). *Approaches to social research.* New York: Oxford University Press.

Terry, A. (2007). *Annual report of children's health and nursing service in Alabama's public school systems.* Retrieved January 28, 2010, from http://www.abn.state.al.us/main/Research/Document/Annual%20Report%20of %20Health%20Services%20in%20Alabama's%20Public%20Schools-2007.pdf

Data Analysis

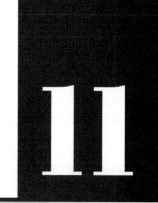

INTRODUCTION TO THE PROCESS OF DATA ANALYSIS

Once the DNP researcher has selected a design for his or her research project, fulfilled all of the requirements of that design such as randomized sampling and instrument design, and collected the data, the next step involves the analysis of the data to determine what the researcher has discovered. The data analysis procedure will vary depending on whether quantitative or qualitative research has been implemented (Trochim, 2006a).

QUANTITATIVE RESEARCH

When quantitative data have been collected, both descriptive and inferential statistics should be generated.

Descriptive Statistics

Descriptive statistics are used to provide summaries about the sample that was used and the measures that were used to describe that sample. Just as the name implies, descriptive statistics merely describe what the data that have been collected show. If the researcher is interested in examining the characteristics of only one variable, this is known as **univariate analysis**. In comparison, **bivariate analysis** examines characteristics of more than one variable. In the interest of simplifying the discussion of statistical methods, only univariate statistics will be reviewed in this chapter. There are several descriptive statistics that would be used in univariate analysis:

- **Distribution**—This is a summary of how often values appear for a variable. This could be as simple as how many students made an *A* as a letter grade on a test, how many made a *B*, and how many made a *C*. A **frequency distribution** can be developed when the values are grouped into ranges and then the frequencies are determined. An example of a frequency distribution is shown in **Table 11-1** (Trochim, 2006a).
- **Central tendency**—This is an estimation of the center point of a distribution of values. There are three major ways to estimate central tendency:
  - **Mean**—The average of a group of values
  - **Median**—The score that is exactly in the middle of a group of values
  - **Mode**—The score that occurs most frequently in a set of values

TABLE 11-1   Example of a Frequency Table

Numerical Grade	Percentage of Students
90–100	40
80–89	30
70–79	10
60–69	10
59 and below	10

Dispersion refers to the spread of the values around the central tendency. Two measures of dispersion are commonly used: the range and the standard deviation. The range is calculated by subtracting the lowest value from the highest value. For example, if the values are dispersed as 10, 20, 30, 40, 50, the range would be 50 − 10 = 40. The other measure of dispersion is the standard deviation. This is calculated by finding the distance between each value and the mean. As would be imagined, the calculations obviously become more complicated at this point. The researcher is by no means advised to attempt hand-calculation of any of the statistics described in this chapter. A DNP researcher in an academic setting will have the advantage of being able to consult a colleague in the Mathematics department for assistance with this area of the project; the researcher in a hospital setting can certainly involve the Information Technology department in the project to receive their input (Trochim, 2006a).

When the question of which descriptive statistical technique is most appropriate for a study arises, the researcher must consider the level of measurement used in the study. Four levels of measurement can be used in a research project:

- **Nominal**—This level is used to classify objects or events into categories. The numbers that are assigned to the categories are only labels and do not indicate more or less of a quantity. The nominal level uses the mode as the appropriate measure of central tendency and the range and frequency distribution as the appropriate measures of variability.
- **Ordinal**—This level ranks objects or events so that an object in a higher category can be considered to have more of a specific attribute than an object in a lower category. The ordinal level uses the mode and median as appropriate measures of central tendency and the range and frequency distribution as appropriate measures of variability.
- **Interval**—This level ranks objects or events on a scale with equal intervals between the numbers on the scale. The interval level uses the mode, median, and mean as the appropriate measures of central tendency and the range and standard deviation as appropriate measures of variability.
- **Ratio**—This level ranks objects or events on a scale with equal intervals between the numbers on the scale and the presence of an absolute zero. This means the numbers represent the actual amount of the condition that an object possesses. Many of the physical characteristics that nurses typically measure in patients can be classified as occurring at the ratio level (LoBiondo-Wood & Haber, 2002).

Inferential Statistics

Inferential statistics are particularly important because they allow the researcher to draw conclusions that reach far beyond a cursory examination of the data. This type of statistics is typically used either to estimate the probability that statistics found in the sample are an accurate reflection of a parameter in the population or to test hypotheses that have been developed about a population. In order for the researcher to make inferences about a population from a sample, the sample must be representative of the larger population. Another requirement for the development of inferences is the interval level of measurement. This is necessary because of the mathematics operations involved in inferential statistics (LoBiondo-Wood & Haber, 2002).

A test known as the **t-test for differences between groups** should be performed when the researcher is interested in comparing the performance of two groups on one measure to determine if a difference exists. This could consist of comparing how long obese male and female patients remained committed to adhering to a weight loss program, for example (Trochim, 2006b).

If the researcher is working with more than two groups or requires measurements to be taken more than once, the **analysis of variance (ANOVA)** can be used. In the same way as the t-test, the ANOVA tests whether group means are different, but also considers the variation that will be present among all of the groups. This statistic takes into account that measures taken at multiple points in time will affect the range of the scores that are generated (LoBiondo-Wood & Haber, 2002).

As previously mentioned, in order for the researcher to be able to make inferences about a population, the data must be at the interval level of measurement or higher. What can a researcher do when the data are not at the interval level? The researcher can use the chi-square statistic to determine if the groups are different. As an inferential statistic, the chi-square will show if the frequency in each category is different from what would be expected to occur by chance. However, chi-square is not usable if samples are very small. Other statistical tests can be used if data are at the ordinal level, including the Kolmogorov-Smirnov test and the Mann-Whitney U test for independent groups (LoBiondo-Wood & Haber, 2002).

Researchers may be interested in examining the relationship that exists between two or more variables, and thus will use statistics such as the Pearson correlation coefficient that will determine the presence of a correlation between the variables. A correlation is literally the degree of association that exists between the variables. In this case, the researcher should use the Pearson correlation coefficient to determine if the value obtained could have been achieved by chance (LoBiondo-Wood & Haber, 2002).

QUALITATIVE RESEARCH

The analytic procedures used for qualitative research will vary considerably from those used with quantitative analysis, primarily because qualitative data incorporates a considerable amount of verbiage. Part of analyzing the data will include determining respondents' motivation for agreeing to participate in a focus group or provide an interview. Peel, Parry, Douglas, and Lawton (2006) found that many research subjects agreed to participate because they felt that it would benefit other people, whereas other subjects reported that interviews in particular actually were therapeutic. Peel and colleagues found that research subjects found it especially beneficial when health professionals showed an interest in hearing the patient's perspective on issues.

Data analysis for a qualitative research project tends to be **interim analysis**, meaning it will be ongoing throughout the project until either the researcher exhausts the time and resources allotted to the project or a complete understanding is achieved of the topic being researched. Qualitative data analysis can be more lengthy than quantitative analysis, because researchers using qualitative data usually engage in **memoing**, meaning they will record notes throughout each field day giving their impression of what is occurring. The memos then are transcribed into a computerized format that can be reviewed more coherently (University of South Alabama, n.d.).

Birks, Chapman, and Francis (2008) explored memoing as a precursor to data analysis and found that the technique can actually serve four important functions. It can be used to:

- *Map research activities*—This allows the researcher to actually create a record of the decision-making process guiding the research, including the circumstances that generated a change in the direction of the research.
- *Establish the meaning of the data*—This allows the researcher to determine what is actually occurring in the data by identifying similarities and differences, exploring relationships, and generating hypotheses.
- *Propel the research project forward*—Because memos document the thought process behind decision making, they eliminate the need to waste valuable research time in second-guessing the logic involved in important decisions. Memos prevent the researcher from over-analyzing decisions and therefore failing to move the research project forward as needed.
- *Maintain open communication among the research team*—Because of the memo's somewhat nonstructured approach, it can be a way to

permit input and comments from all members of the research team without seeming to be judgmental or threatening (Birks, Chapman, & Francis, 2008).

Memoing can be very similar to some researchers' use of a **fieldwork journal**. Considered to be separate from field notes, the fieldwork journal allows the researcher, much as with memoing, to create a precursor to data analysis by recording relevant emotional reactions and self-reflection. The fieldwork journal can assist the researcher with the technique of participant observation, because it will record the capacity in which the researcher was present at the observation and the role he or she assumed (Arber, 2006).

Once all data are collected and transcribed, they must be carefully reviewed and then broken into analytical units. This process is known as **segmenting**. Once segmenting is completed, the researcher then must **code** the data. This means the segments of data are marked with category names. The researcher collects all of the assigned category names in a **codebook**. If multiple coders are used, the researcher must be able to show that a high degree of inter- and intra-coder reliability exists. **Intra-coder reliability** means that each individual coder codes all of the data consistently; **inter-coder reliability** means that among the group of coders the coding process is occurring consistently. If the researcher is able to use a set of codes that already exists, these are known as **a priori codes**; if the researcher opts to develop his or her own codes, these are referred as **inductive codes** (University of South Alabama, n.d.).

Narrative Analysis

Narrative analysis is a qualitative data analysis technique that analyzes a chronological story; it is most effectively used for exploratory purposes. The researcher will primarily be concerned with the sequence of the elements that are included, why some elements are evaluated differently from others, how the past and present are interconnected, and how these shape the events of the future. If the narrative is collected through interviews, the interviewer and the respondent work together to create a narrative framework. The researcher will note **patterns** that actually are recurring speech groupings. Sets of these patterns are considered to be **themes**. Some researchers consider evidence of themes to be sequences of core phrases that recur in multiple interviews. It may be helpful to organize narrative material according to research subjects' chronological accounting of events to encourage the emergence of themes (Garson, n.d.).

Thematic Networks Analysis

Thematic analysis is designed to discover the themes that exist in a narrative. **Thematic networks analysis** involve extracting basic, organizing, and global themes from text and then representing those themes as web-type maps with the relationships between each one illustrated. As previously mentioned, the three classes of themes are:

- **Basic theme**—This is the lowest order theme that can be derived from text. It is a simple idea that is characteristic of the data.
- **Organizing theme**—This organizes the basic theme into clusters of similar ideas.
- **Global theme**—This is a group of organizing themes that together present a position about an issue (Attride-Stirling, 2001).

A thematic network is formulated by starting first with the basic themes and then working inward toward the global theme(s). A collection of basic themes will be classified according to the idea that is characteristic of the data. That characteristic idea will then become the organizing theme when it is used to organize the basic theme into groups of similar ideas. As more than one organization theme develops, the global theme will emerge to represent a position that has developed about an issue. The organizing themes will be brought together to exhibit a single conclusion that will become the global theme (Attride-Stirling, 2001).

The process of creating a thematic networks analysis consists of several steps:

1. *Reduction of the data*—This is accomplished through coding and application of the explicitly defined codes to the text so it is cut into segments.
2. *Identification of themes*—The researcher should reread the text segments within the context of the classified codes so that underlying patterns are revealed. The themes are refined so as to become manageable.
3. *Arrange themes*—The various themes are arranged into similar groupings.
4. *Describe the networks*—Each network is read in sequential order to facilitate understanding of the material.
5. *Summarize*—The researcher presents a summary of the main themes and patterns characterizing the network.
6. *Compile*—This involves compiling the deductions that have been made in the summaries of all the networks along with the relevant theory that will provide more information for the themes, patterns, and structures that emerged in the text.

The process of data analysis can be a cumbersome one, depending on the type of data that have been collected and the number of resources in terms of personnel and expertise that the DNP researcher can call upon to assist. Therefore, for the novice researcher who is working with a minimum of assistance, it is recommended that either qualitative research be implemented in his or her facility of employment and on a small scale, such as pertaining to one department or unit, or quantitative research be performed using a single variable.

Once the researcher has completed data analysis on the project, whether quantitative or qualitative in nature, the next step in the process involves writing the research report in a way compatible with the mission of peer-reviewed journals. The subsequent chapter will discuss how this process can most effectively occur.

■ GLOSSARY

analysis of variance (ANOVA) Tests whether group means are different, but also considers the variation that will be present among all of the groups.

a priori codes Codes that were developed previously and did not require the researcher to develop them as part of the research project.

basic theme The lowest order theme that can be derived from text. It is a simple idea that is characteristic of the data.

bivariate analysis The examination of characteristics of more than one variable.

central tendency An estimation of the center point of a distribution of values.

codebook Contains all of the assigned category names in a master list.

coding The segments of data are marked with category names. to further identify them during the data analysis process.

descriptive statistics Used to provide summaries about the sample that was used and the measures that were used to describe that sample; they describe what the data that has been collected shows.

dispersion The spread of the values around the central tendency.

distribution A summary of how often values appear for a variable.

fieldwork journal Can assist the researcher with the technique of participant observation, because it will record the capacity in which the researcher was present at the observation and the role he or she assumed.

frequency distribution Developed when values are grouped into ranges and then the frequencies are determined.

global theme A group of organizing themes that together present a position about an issue.

inductive codes Developed by the researcher as the data are examined during a research project.

inferential statistics Allow the researcher to draw conclusions that reach far beyond a cursory examination of the data. This type of statistics is typically used either to estimate the probability that statistics found in the sample are an accurate reflection of a parameter in the population or to test hypotheses that have been developed about a population.

inter-coder reliability Among a group of coders, coding of the data is occurring consistently.

interim analysis Data analysis will be ongoing throughout the project until either the researcher exhausts the time and resources allotted to the project or a complete understanding is achieved of the topic being researched.

interval This level of variable ranks objects or events on a scale with equal intervals between the numbers on the scale.

intra-coder reliability Each coder is coding the data consistently.

mean The average of a group of values.

median The score that is exactly in the middle of a group of values.

memoing A researcher records notes throughout each field day giving his or her impression of what is occurring.

mode The score that occurs most frequently in a set of values.

nominal This level of variable is used to classify objects or events into categories. The numbers that are assigned to the categories are only labels and do not indicate more or less of a quantity.

ordinal This level of variable ranks objects or events so that an object in a higher category can be considered to have more of a specific attribute than an object in a lower category.

organizing theme This organizes the basic theme into clusters of similar ideas.

patterns Recurring speech groupings. that are noted as part of narrative analysis.

ratio This level of variable ranks objects or events on a scale with equal intervals between the numbers on the scale and the presence of an absolute zero.

segmenting Data are carefully reviewed and then broken into analytical units.

thematic networks Analysis that involves extracting basic and global themes from text and then representing those themes as web-type maps with the relationships between each one illustrated.

themes Sets of patterns.

t-test for differences between groups Performed when the researcher is interested in comparing the performance of two groups on one measure to determine if a difference exists.

univariate analysis Examines the characteristics of only one variable.

▪ LEARNING ENHANCEMENT TOOLS

1. You are a DNP researcher who is analyzing data gathered from a group of patients. Of the group of 25 patients:

   - 12 were discharged after being hospitalized for 3 days.
   - 7 were discharged after being hospitalized for 4 days.
   - 3 were discharged after being hospitalized for 5 days.
   - 2 were discharged after being hospitalized for 2 days.
   - 1 was discharged after being hospitalized for 6 days.

   Use this information to create a frequency distribution.

2. You are a DNP researcher who is analyzing data gathered from a group of patients. Of the group of 25 patients:

   - 12 were discharged after being hospitalized for 3 days.
   - 7 were discharged after being hospitalized for 4 days.
   - 3 were discharged after being hospitalized for 5 days.
   - 2 were discharged after being hospitalized for 2 days.
   - 1 was discharged after being hospitalized for 6 days.

   Use this information to calculate the mean, median, and mode to estimate central tendency.

3. You have obtained the following values as part of the research project you are implementing: 5, 7.5, 12.4, 15.1, 4.3, 8.3, 12.9, 30.7, 22.7, 25.8. Use this information to calculate the range.

4. You are a DNP researcher who is implementing a research project that involves assigning the various actions that occur during a code situation to specific categories for analysis. Which measure(s) of central tendency and variability will be most appropriate for this project?

5. You are a DNP researcher who is implementing a research project that involves ranking a group of patients according to their acuity levels. Which measure(s) of central tendency and variability will be most appropriate for this project?

6. You are a DNP researcher who is implementing a research project that involves analysis of the oral temperature readings of a group of patients. Which measure(s) of central tendency and variability will be most appropriate for this project?

7. You are a DNP researcher who is implementing a research project that involves analysis of the blood pressure readings of a group of patients. Which measure(s) of central tendency and variability will be most appropriate for this project?

8. You are a DNP researcher who is implementing a research project to study the effectiveness of a student wellness center on a college campus. You observe the students interacting at the wellness center three days a week, and on alternate days, you interview students regarding their impressions of the center and the services available to them. How could you incorporate memoing into your research project as part of your plan for data analysis?

9. You are a DNP researcher who is implementing a research project to study the effectiveness of a student wellness center on a college campus. You observe the students interacting at the wellness center three days a week, and on alternate days, you interview only the female students regarding their impressions of how they feel the exercise programs at the wellness center have affected their body images and self-esteem. How could you incorporate narrative analysis into your research project as part of your plan for data analysis?

10. Select a passage of text from a classic work of literature and document the basic, organizing, and global themes that you can identify.

11. You are a DNP researcher who is conducting a research project on the narratives that cancer patients have written about progressing through the grieving process after their initial diagnosis. Discuss how you could incorporate thematic analysis into your plan for data analysis.

12. You are a DNP researcher who is conducting a research project on the narratives that cancer patients have written about progressing through the grieving process after their initial diagnosis. Discuss how you could develop a thematic network based on this material.

■ RESOURCES

Braun, V., & Clarke, V. (2006). Using thematic analysis in psychology. *Qualitative Research in Psychology, 3*, 77–101.

Burck, C. (2005). Comparing qualitative research methodologies for systemic research: The use of grounded theory, discourse analysis and narrative analysis. *Journal of Family Therapy, 27*(3), 237–262.

Charmaz, K. (2004). Premises, principles, and practices in qualitative research: Revisiting the foundations. *Qualitative Health Research, 14*(7), 976–993.

Eaves, Y. (2001). A synthesis technique for grounded theory data analysis. *Journal of Advanced Nursing, 35*(5), 654–663.

Grinyer, A. (2004). The narrative correspondence method: What a follow-up study can tell us about the longer term effect on participants in emotionally demanding research. *Qualitative Health Research, 14*, 1326–1341.

Guest, G., & McLellan, E. (2003). Distinguishing the trees from the forest: Applying cluster analysis to thematic qualitative data. *Field Methods, 15*, 186–200.

Richards, H., & Emslie, C. (2000). The "doctor" or the "girl from the University"? Considering the influence of professional roles on qualitative interviewing. *Family Practice, 17*(1), 71–75.

Shamai, M. (2003). Therapeutic effects of qualitative research: Reconstructing the experience of treatment as a by-product of qualitative evaluation. *Social Service Review, 77*(3), 455–467.

■ REFERENCES

Arber, A. (2006). Reflexivity: A challenge for the researcher as practitioner? *Journal of Research in Nursing, 11*(2), 147–157.

Attride-Stirling, J. (2001). Thematic networks: An analytic tool for qualitative research. *Qualitative Research, 1,* 385–403.

Birks, M., Chapman, Y., & Francis, K. (2008). Memoing in qualitative research: Probing data and processes. *Journal of Research in Nursing, 13,* 68.

Garson, D. (n.d.). *Narrative analysis.* Retrieved February 2, 2010, from http://faculty.chass.ncsu.edu/garson/PA765/narrativ.htm

LoBiondo-Wood, G., & Haber, J. (2002). *Nursing research: Methods, critical appraisal, and utilization.* St. Louis, MO: Mosby.

Parry, O., Peel, E., Douglas, M., & Lawton, J. (2004). Patients in waiting: a qualitative study of type 2 diabetes patients' perceptions of diagnosis. *Family Practice, 21,* 131–136.

Trochim, W. (2006a). *Descriptive statistics.* Retrieved February 2, 2010, from www.socialresearchmethods.net/kb/statdesc.htm

Trochim, W. (2006b). *Inferential statistics.* Retrieved February 2, 2010, from www.socialresearchmethods.net/kb/statinf.php

University of South Alabama. (n.d.). *Chapter 17: Qualitative data analysis.* Retrieved February 3, 2010, from www.southalabama.edu/coe/bset/johnson/lectures/lec17.pdf

Writing the Research Report for Potential Publication

12

■ OBJECTIVES

Upon completion of this chapter, the reader should be prepared to:

1 Recognize the importance of writing research reports with the intention of ultimate publication in a scholarly journal.

2 Discuss the features of a journal that would be suitable for publication of scholarly research in the DNP researcher's field.

3 Discuss the sections of a manuscript that must be included in order to make it suitable for submission for publication.

4 Analyze a completed manuscript according to the sections that it contains.

INITIATING THE WRITING PROCESS

Once the DNP researcher has completed all of the previously discussed steps in implementing the capstone project, the remaining hurdle is writing the research report, and in particular, writing it with the intention of publication. Submitting research for publication is important because it provides a peer review of the researcher's work; submission of the report also allows networking to occur with individuals who have similar research interests. Publication can certainly be a career boost for the researcher, particularly in academia, and can assist the researcher who is hospital-based in obtaining health-related grants as well as much-needed budgetary resources for additional staff and graduate research assistants (Thompson, 2007).

CHOOSING A JOURNAL FOR MANUSCRIPT SUBMISSION

The researcher must consider several factors when evaluating the merits of journals that may be chosen for manuscript submission. One is the recognition factor of the journal. A journal that is well known and easily recognized by the researcher's peer group will allow his or her research to be seen prominently in the healthcare community. It may be listed in multiple search engines on the Internet and thus be easily accessed by other researchers who may, in turn, cite the research in additional publications (Thompson, 2007).

Another factor for consideration is the scope of the journal. It is important to know whether the journal has a clinical focus that is disease-based, an educational focus that prefers articles pertaining to academia, or an experimental focus that favors research with a strong theoretical basis. The most succinctly written article will be rejected by a publication if it does not fit within the scope of the journal. A researcher who has a clear idea of the specific publication he or she wants to submit a manuscript to should research the journal carefully to determine what types of articles usually achieve acceptance, the length of the articles, their focus, and the writing style that is used (Thompson, 2007). The researcher also should review the journal's "Instructions to Authors" section very carefully. This is the page that delineates every requirement needed for manuscript submission and, hopefully, acceptance. Some journals will not accept a manuscript that is not submitted via an electronic submission process; others still require hard copies sent via U.S. mail. A researcher who favors knowing where the journal reviewers are in the process of analyzing his or her research should select a journal that uses the electronic submission process. The electronic submission process allows the author to find out exactly where the article is in the submission process at that particular time, whether with reviewers or with the main editor. In this day of confidentiality, journals may hesitate to communicate much information by phone when there is no certainty that the publication is actually dealing with the author himself.

The journal instructions will usually state the acceptable font type and size to use, how tables and figures should be formatted, and how photographs can be incorporated into the article. Determine whether the journal states when the author will receive a decision regarding the manuscript. The review process for some journals can take years, requiring one revision after another, before the editors finally decide to accept or reject the article (Thompson, 2007).

As the researcher decides on the journal to use for manuscript submission, he or she should avoid the temptation to submit the article simultaneously to multiple journals in the hope that one of the group will accept the article for publication. This is considered highly unethical, and most journals have stipulations that the author must agree that the manuscript has not been submitted to another journal. The researcher should, however, prepare a list of journals that could be approached regarding publication, because it is common for an article to be rejected upon the initial submission to a journal (Rudner & Schafer, 1999).

FORMATTING THE MANUSCRIPT

The manuscript being formatted for submission to a peer-reviewed journal should consist of several distinct sections that will be discussed in detail. The sections consist of:

- *Title page*—the title should be specific enough to describe the contents of the paper, but not so technical as to overly narrow the scope of your audience. Authors may consist of a primary author, who performed the majority of the research discussed in the article, as well as multiple additional authors who also made a significant contribution (Columbia University, n.d.).
- *Abstract page*—This is a preview of what will be discussed in the article. It allows the reader to determine whether the article meets the needs of their research and should then be reviewed in its entirety. Most journals require that the abstract consist of one paragraph that contains usually no more than 250 words. The abstract should contain the purpose of the research, the research method used, the results achieved, and the conclusions reached by the researcher (Columbia University, n.d.).
- *Introduction*—This should identify the general area of the research. The rationale for the analysis of the problem should be presented, as should the ultimate purpose of the research. The researcher should describe what he or she is trying to achieve by implementing this research (Columbia University, n.d.).
- *Literature review*—This should show how the research is building on prior knowledge in the field by summarizing what is already known about the research problem (Rudner & Schafer, 1999).
- *Method*—This section should include a description of the sample, the materials used in the research, and the procedures utilized. Describe the research subjects, how they were selected, and how they represent the population used. Identify the research design used and the independent and dependent variables. Describe tests that were implemented as well as questionnaires or other instruments that were developed. In the case of a survey or questionnaire, describe how it was scored, validated, and interpreted. Describe the steps included in implementing the study, such as distribution of materials, observation of behaviors, and testing that was implemented. This should be clear enough that another researcher could replicate the study based on the description. Briefly discuss the statistical analysis that was performed (Rudner & Schafer, 1999).

- *Results*—This should include the techniques used in the research as well as the data analysis completed, including both descriptive and inferential statistics. Discuss any complications that were encountered, such as missing data or incomplete survey responses. If tables and graphs are included, they should be self-explanatory (Rudner & Schafer, 1999).
- *Discussion*—At this point, the researcher serves as the expert to interpret the data for the reader, describing the implications of the findings and offering recommendations. Do not overgeneralize the results; rather, allow conclusions to be the natural result of the data presented. Describe the limitations that were noted during the course of the study. Suggest problems that should be researched in order to answer new research questions that have arisen as a result of the original study.
- *References*—References typically are cited according to the American Psychological Association format; however, this may vary depending on the journal. The researcher must ensure that the method of formatting the references and citations in the manuscript are both congruent with the requirements of the journal.

This chapter's appendix contains a manuscript that contains all of these sections.

Appendix
Critique of Clinically Based Research

12A

Enhancing the Ruralization of Alabama's LPN Workforce

Allison J. Terry, PhD, MSN, RN
Assistant Professor of Nursing
Auburn University at Montgomery
Montgomery, Alabama

ABSTRACT

Few studies have focused on nurses in rural counties, and rarely have they centered on the licensed practical nurse. This paper uses the factors that LPNs have reported as enhancing or detracting from their job satisfaction as well as the numbers of LPNs reported to be employed in rural or urban Alabama counties to develop a model that could motivate these workers to remain in rural work environments where they could potentially achieve their maximum potential in the nursing workforce.

Keywords: job satisfaction, nurse, workforce

INTRODUCTION

Although licensed practical nurses (LPNs) have been in the workforce for years, very few studies have focused on the work environments of these nurses. As the nursing shortage continues, some health care facilities are focused on using more LPNs than ever before (1). These nurses are often given increasing amounts of autonomy and accountability in more rural work environments. This paper uses the factors that LPNs have reported as enhancing or detracting from their job satisfaction as well as the numbers of LPNs reported to be employed in rural or urban Alabama counties to develop a model that could motivate these workers to remain in rural work environments where they could potentially achieve their maximum potential in the nursing workforce.

CONCEPTUAL FRAMEWORK

The conceptual framework used for the study was Terry and Lazarus's 2008 (2) work on the state of the licensed practical nurse in Alabama. These authors reported that a statewide survey of LPNs revealed that these nurses indicated the existence of specific factors that either enhanced or detracted from their overall job satisfaction. In descending order, the top five factors that LPNs reported making a positive impact on their current work situations were:

- Reasonable degree of autonomy/good interdependent working relations
- Security in present position
- Good administrative support
- Sufficient support staff for non-nursing duties and
- Reasonable work hours

In comparison, the top five factors that LPNs reported negatively influencing their current work situations were, in descending order:

- Extensive travel commute to work
- Lack of choice in work shift
- Lack of autonomy
- Family responsibilities and
- Inadequate benefits

Terry and Lazarus (2) stated that 52.35% of Alabama's LPNs are employed in urban counties, while 47.65% are employed in work environments located in rural counties. This finding set the stage for the introduction of the second major section of the study's conceptual framework. The Alabama Rural Health Association's (ARHA) definition of "rural" was used to provide a clear-cut distinction between rural and urban counties in the state. The ARHA uses the following criteria to define a "rural" county:

a. the percentage of workers in the county employed by the public school system(s); the more workers employed in school system(s), the more rural a county is considered to be since in many rural counties, the school system is the single largest employer.
b. the dollar value of agricultural production per square mile of land; the greater the value of agricultural production per square acre, the more rural the county.

c. the population per square mile of land; the fewer number of persons per square mile, the more rural the county.
d. a score derived from using the population of the largest city in the county, the populations of other cities in the county, and the population of cities that are in more than one county; counties where the largest incorporated place has a population of under 2,500 are assigned the highest index score of 25, making them the most rural (3).

LITERATURE REVIEW

Ulrich, O'Donnell, Taylor, Farrar, Danis, and Grady (4) surveyed both nurses and social workers regarding job satisfaction and found that being respected, being a valued member of the team, scheduling, and identification with the mission of the institution had the strongest influence on respondents' decision to remain in their current positions. This echoes Terry and Lazarus's 2008 findings regarding factors contributing or detracting from job satisfaction of LPNs.

Further information specific to nurses employed in rural counties was provided by Molinari and Monserud (5), who found that nurses who remained employed in rural areas tended to prefer a rural lifestyle, the incorporation of rural values in the practices of the organization, the role of the nurse generalist along with job variability, and patient variety. The authors expanded on the idea of patient variety by noting that rural nurses typically care for patients whose health issues differ from those in urban populations, since it has been found that rural patients tend to experience more chronic diseases as well as more occupational-related health problems. Rural patient populations have been found be more elderly and obese than urban populations, to have less health insurance, and to require medication that is more expensive. Molinari and Monserud also reported that new graduates who are employed in rural hospitals must exhibit advanced critical thinking skills as well as assessment skills that must cross multiple disciplines.

METHODOLOGY

A model was developed using both LPNs' self-reported factors that either enhanced or detracted from their job satisfaction and the factors that defined a rural Alabama county. A score was generated according to the degree of ruralization of a county, with the counties having the highest scores having the greatest need to fulfill LPNs' job satisfaction areas in order to persuade these workers to remain in practice in rural counties.

Utilization of the model consisted of initially determining the degree of ruralization of the county, using the criteria established by the Alabama Rural Health Association. Ruralization scores could range from 100-400, with a score of 100 generated because the county has:

- 25% of its workers employed by the public school system
- Virtually no agricultural production
- A population of 10,000 people or greater per square mile of land as well as
- A population of 10,000 people or greater in its largest incorporated place.

In comparison, a score of 400 would be generated because the county has:

- 100% of its workers employed by the public school system
- Value of its agricultural production per square acre of land above market value
- A population under 2,500 people per square mile of land as well as
- A population under 2,500 people in its largest incorporated place.

Once the degree of ruralization of the county was determined, the second phase of the model consisted of developing a countywide plan for incorporation of strategies to enhance LPN job satisfaction, with the expansiveness of the plan dependent upon the ruralization score. For example, the county scoring 400 points for maximum ruralization would need to incorporate multiple strategies in all five areas that LPNs have reported can enhance their job satisfaction.

LIMITATIONS

Limitations of the research were identified. A primary limitation of the project was the use of a population specific to Alabama, thus greatly decreasing generalization to other states. A secondary limitation is that the model being proposed is yet untested in a healthcare environment. In addition, it is acknowledged that a more complete picture of the overall nursing workforce and the economic impact of being employed in a rural county could be more thoroughly generated through analysis of both the LPN and RN workforce combined.

IMPLICATIONS

The development and potential use of the model being proposed has implications for nurse administrators, nurse educators, and the nursing profession as a whole. LPNs must initially be recruited by rural hospitals before they can begin to analyze their degree of job satisfaction in their nursing positions. Nurse administrators must recognize that although higher salaries and sign-on bonuses may not be offered by smaller rural hospitals, nurses can be offered incentives such as a slower paced lifestyle, smaller, close-knit schools with teachers who have more personal knowledge of the students, opportunities for middle management career advancement, and great variety in choice of patient assignments (4). Eldridge and Judkins (6) found that rural hospitals tend to have a lower ratio of registered nurses to LPNs and fewer nurses with bachelor's degrees, thus offering additional leadership opportunities for licensed practical nurses.

Keeping an experienced, competent LPN employed in his or her current position could potentially save thousands of dollars annually for a nursing employer who would otherwise need to recruit, orient, and retain a new employee. Recruiting nurses for positions in a medium-sized hospital has been shown to cost as much as three million dollars annually; this amount could increase exponentially in a smaller rural hospital with already limited financial resources and a dwindling, frustrated staff (7). Nurse administrators must recognize that as healthcare continues to be in flux, their challenge will be to avoid unrealistic expectations of new nurses because of the multiple needs of patients in rural hospitals.

It was previously mentioned that new graduate nurses in rural hospitals must possess advanced critical thinking skills (5). For nursing faculty who are educating future licensed practical nurses, fostering the development of critical thinking in this group of practitioners can set the stage for not only their development as an accomplished generalist nurse who can function in a variety of hospital settings, but also for that nurse to further his or her career through additional education. Although the development of critical thinking tends to be mentioned most frequently in connection with registered nurse education, it should be fostered just as diligently in the LPN. This will produce a member of the nursing team who is proficient in his or her role and able to contribute valuable information to the registered nurse's assessment.

Finally, the enhancement of job satisfaction for LPNs localized in rural counties has implications for the overall nursing profession. The nurse who chooses to practice in a rural environment often does so because he or she is familiar with it; perhaps they grew up there and know the people and their daily hardships. The comfort derived from the provision of expert care by a practitioner who is well known to the patient over the course of several years can be immeasurable. Nurses also can receive great fulfillment from the knowledge that they are able to provide expertise to the community where they were born and reared. This may be a very apt solution to the increasing depersonalization of healthcare in general and the nursing profession specifically.

CONCLUSION

This paper used the factors that LPNs have reported as enhancing or detracting from their job satisfaction as well as the numbers of LPNs reported to be employed in rural or urban Alabama counties to develop a model that could be used to motivate these workers to remain in rural work environments. As healthcare costs continue to rise, nurse turnover, whether that of registered nurses or licensed practical nurses, must be curtailed, particularly in financially strapped rural hospitals. Application of the proposed model could potentially decrease that somewhat and ultimately save money through recruitment costs, time spent in lengthy education and training, and the time required to try to develop yet another new nurse into a dedicated employee with a commitment to the patients, the facility, and the profession.

■ REFERENCES

1. Department of Health and Human Services. (2006). Supply, demand, and use of licensed practical nurses. Retrieved September 11, 2007, from http://www.hrsa.gov

2. Terry, A., & Lazarus, J. (2008). Licensed Practical Nurses in Alabama. Retrieved August 31, 2009, from http://www.centerfornursing.alabama.gov

3. Alabama Rural Health Association. (2008). What is rural? Retrieved April 30, 2008, from http://www.arhaonline.org/what_is_rural.htm

4. Ulrich, C., O'Donnell, P., Taylor, C., Farrar, A., Danis, M., & Grady, C. (2007). Ethical climate, ethics stress, and the job satisfaction of nurses and social workers in the United States. *Social Science and Medicine*, *65*(8), 1708–1719.

5. Molinari, D., and Monserud, M. (2008). Rural nurse job satisfaction. *Rural and Remote Health*, *8*, 1055.

6. Eldridge, C., & Judkins, S. (2002). Rural nurse administrators: Essential for practice. *Online Journal of Rural Nursing and Health Care*, *3*(2). Retrieved September 4, 2009, from http://www.rno.org/journal/index.php/online-journal/article/viewFile/116/114

7. O'Malley, J., & Fearnley J. (2007). Can generalist nurses be specialists? How can a rural secondary nursing service be sustained into the future? *Kai Tiaki: Nursing New Zealand*. Retrieved September 4, 2009, from http://findarticles.com/p/articles/mi_hb4839/is_/ai_n29349218?tag=artBody;col1

Model for the Enhancement of Job Satisfaction of LPNs in Rural Alabama Counties

I. Determine the degree of ruralization of the county

a. What percentage of workers in the county are employed by the public school system?

Answer: 25% = Score of 25
50% = Score of 50
75% = Score of 75
100% = Score of 100

b. What is the value of agricultural production per square acre of land?

Answer: virtually no agricultural production = Score of 25
occurs in the county
value is below market value = Score of 50
value is equal to market value = Score of 75
value is above market value = Score of 100

c. What is the population per square mile of land?

Answer: 10,000 people or greater = Score of 25
5,000 people = Score of 50
At least 2,500 people = Score of 75
Under 2,500 people = Score of 100

d. What is the population of the county's largest incorporated place?

Answer: 10,000 people or greater = Score of 25
5,000 people = Score of 50
At least 2,500 people = Score of 75
Under 2,500 people = Score of 100

Score of 400 total = extremely ruralized county
Score of 100 total = least ruralized county

II. Develop county-wide plan in all counties scoring 400 points for incorporation of strategies to enhance LPN job satisfaction (for example):

a. Strategies to encourage reasonable degree of autonomy/good interdependent working relations:

– determine number of LPN charge nurse positions available in long-term care facilities
– determine use of LPNs in home health care agencies
– determine use of LPNs in public schools

b. Strategies to encourage security in present position:
   - organize "town meeting" type groups periodically so that LPNs can voice concerns regarding job security
   - verify that LPNs have a clear-cut job description and concrete criteria for performance review
   - provide opportunities for additional training so that LPNs can enhance their skill
   - level and broaden their range of job experiences

c. Strategies to encourage good administrative support:
   - supervisors should meet with LPNs on a regular basis, apart from other nursing personnel, to allow them to discuss their concerns
   - encourage LPNs to participate in their state and national nursing organizations
   - develop a career ladder specific to LPNs for promotion

d. Strategies to encourage development of sufficient support staff for non-nursing duties:
   - if funding is not sufficient to hire additional support personnel, enhance team-building with specific exercises geared toward this
   - develop volunteer program if none exists
   - develop program to utilize health career students
   - investigate the possibility of providing support staff positions for LPN nursing students

e. Strategies to encourage development of reasonable work hours:
   - have multiple schedule options available
   - develop schedule option that is only for nurses who are in school
   - have part-time, flex-time, job sharing, and prn positions available

▪ Counties found to score 400 points should complete strategies to enhance LPN job satisfaction in all five areas.
▪ Counties found to score 300 points should complete strategies to enhance LPN job satisfaction in four of the five areas.
▪ Counties found to score 200 points should complete strategies to enhance LPN job satisfaction in three of the five areas.
▪ Counties found to score 100 points should complete strategies to enhance LPN job satisfaction in two of the five areas.

Appendix A

Examination of Academic Self-Regulation Variances in Nursing Students

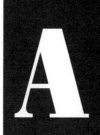

Review the following research project in its entirety. Analyze it to find implementation of each of the steps of the research process.

QUESTIONS TO GUIDE YOUR ANALYSIS

1   What is the research problem? What is the population being studied?

2   Was a hypothesis used or a research question? Was the author's choice appropriate for the type of study implemented? Give your rationale for your answer. Write additional hypotheses or research questions that could have been utilized.

3   Can a theoretical or conceptual framework be identified? If it is not clearly stated, is it implied at some point in the document? Was it an appropriate choice for this project?

4   Was the literature review thorough enough for the topic? Give your rationale for your answer.

5   Was informed consent or an institutional review board utilized in this research project? Was the author's choice to utilize an IRB or not appropriate? Give your rationale for your answer.

6   What type of research design was utilized for this project? How could this project have been implemented differently with a different type of research design?

7   What type of sampling was used in this research project? How could this project have been implemented with a different type of sampling utilized?

8   What type of data collection method was used? Was it the most appropriate one for this study? Give your rationale for your answer.

9   What type of statistical analysis was used with this study? Are there other statistics that could have been utilized but were not selected? Does this study have implications for the population being studied?

10   If you were to replicate this research project, what would you decide to do differently?

Examination of Academic Self-Regulation Variances in Nursing Students[1]

Michelle A. Schutt, EdD, RN
Assistant Professor of Nursing
Auburn University Montgomery
Montgomery, Alabama

ABSTRACT

Multiple workforce demands in healthcare have placed a tremendous amount of pressure on academic nurse educators to increase the number of professional nursing graduates to provide nursing care in both acute and non-acute healthcare settings. Increased enrollment in nursing programs throughout the United States is occurring; however, due to high attrition rates, these increases do not automatically result in more nursing graduates.

The educational focus in nursing education has recently shifted from a student-driven approach wherein learner-centered learning has replaced teacher-centered teaching in an effort to promote student critical thinking ability, autonomy, and professional identity (Billings & Halstead, 2005). Nursing faculty must have an understanding of the theoretical constructs of self-directed learning, academic self-regulation, and learning motivation in order to support student progression toward autonomous learning. The unique needs of individual students as well as possible differences in nursing student groups must be considered when developing educational strategies and methods to promote and enhance student integration of content value and progression toward intrinsic motivation.

The purpose of this research was to determine the existence of statistically significant differences in academic self-regulation behaviors (autonomous vs. controlled) in two distinct groups of nursing students: (a) traditional baccalaureate nursing students, and (b) non-traditional baccalaureate nursing students (licensed nurses returning to nursing school to obtain a baccalaureate degree). In addition, significant differences in the demographic characteristics between the same two groups of baccalaureate nursing students was explored.

Analysis revealed that non-traditional baccalaureate nursing students have statistically significantly higher autonomous regulation subscale (ARS) scores than traditional baccalaureate students. Female participants reported higher

---

[1] Reprinted courtesy of Michelle A. Schutt, EdD, RN.

ARS scores than male participants and participants in a single-parent or two-parent household also reported higher ARS scores. Post-hoc analysis further revealed a statistically significant result for the number of dependent children. Additional findings of interests are explored.

CHAPTER I: INTRODUCTION

This introduction serves as a brief discussion of self-directed learning, academic self-regulation, and the role of learning motivation in student academic success. The statement of the research problem and the purpose of the study will also be discussed. In addition, the research questions, significance of the study, and study limitations will be presented. The terms used in this research will be defined and the organization of the research will be addressed.

Knowles (1980) asserted that self-directed learning is the learning preference of the adult learner. Self-directed learning can be defined as learner ownership and responsibility for the learning process to include the planning, implementation and evaluation of the learning experience (Brockett, 1985; Caffarella, 1993; Merriam & Brockett, 1997). The desire for self-directed learning becomes increasingly prevalent as learners mature over time; however, many learners resist self-directed learning efforts by educators due to increased personal demand and responsibility placed on the student as the student is required to take a more active role in the planning, organization and evaluation of their learning (Brookfield, 2006). Educators must guide and support adult learners as they progress toward learner self-direction.

Pintrich (2000) defines academic self-regulation as the

> active, constructive process whereby learners set goals for their learn-
> ing and then attempt to monitor, regulate, and control their cognition,
> motivation, and behavior, guided and constrained by their goals and the
> contextual features of the environment. These ... activities can mediate
> the relationships between individuals and the context, and their overall
> achievement. (p. 453)

Successful student self-regulation results in increased academic success (Schunk, 1993). Academic self-regulation requires the learner to take ownership and primary responsibility for planning the learning experience, self-motivation, initiative, and persistence (Brookfield, 1994; Caffarella, 1993; Cassazza, 2006).

Academic self-regulation requires learner self-awareness. This awareness, referred to as metacognition, encompasses one's personal knowledge of individual learning needs, learning characteristics and preferred learning strategies, academic motivation, and learner self-efficacy, the knowledge of one's ability to be successful at a learning task (Pintrich, 2000). Academic motivation regulates individual learning outcomes as students who are more highly motivated demonstrate higher academic achievement than those who are not. Learner internalization of the value of the relevance and importance of the current content to future goal attainment is a significant factor which contributes to academic motivation to participate in the learning activity and actively engage in the learning process (Bandura, 1971; Schunk, 2001b).

Learner self-awareness of motivation and individual efforts to control and enhance motivation increase academic success; conversely, anxiety and fear of failure can negatively impact academic motivation, interest and value (Pintrich, 2000).

Motivation can be viewed as a continuum from extrinsic motivation to intrinsic motivation (Zimmerman, 1989); however, academic motivation varies as a result of impacting factors such as learner interest, enthusiasm, learner self-efficacy, and valuation of the relevance of the content to current and future learning and goal attainment (Knowles, Holton, & Swanson, 2005).

Knowles (1989) addressed the adult learner's response to different motivators and recognized the value of both extrinsic motivation and intrinsic motivation. Extrinsic motivation results from the influence of external motivating factors such as the desire for a better job, career progression, or pay improvements. In contrast, intrinsic motivation results from the influence of internal value motivators such as the desire for an increased quality of life, increased job satisfaction, and increased self-esteem.

Intrinsic motivation has been demonstrated to be significantly more beneficial in adult education than extrinsic motivation. While most learners are initially dependent on extrinsic motivation at the beginning of a learning activity (Bruner, 1964), as the learner develops an understanding of the value of the knowledge or content and interest increases, the learner can be expected to shift toward intrinsic motivation (Knowles, Holton, & Swanson, 2005). Most traditional college students are in the process of transitioning from external motivators to internal motivators; however, many mature adults may still be primarily extrinsically motivated. Typically, undergraduate students progress toward intrinsic motivation as they move into their major field of study and begin to study content that they value. External factors in the learning environment, both negative and positive, such as feedback, social support, and the presence of external motivators can contribute to or inhibit academic motivation. These concepts will be further explored in the literature review provided in Chapter II.

Statement of Problem

Occupational employment projections for nurses predict an increase of approximately 587,000 new jobs for registered nurses by the year 2016 (Dohm & Shniper, 2007). This represents an increase of 23 percent. The United States Department of Health and Human Services Health Resources and Services Administration (HRSA) (2004) projects that the current moderate nursing shortage will increase in severity over the next 20 years due to the increased age of the nursing population and attrition due to retirement and retention issues within the workforce. Projections indicate that by 2020, the registered nurse workforce will be twenty percent below the predicted need due to the aging of the nursing workforce and subsequent workforce attrition due to retirements (Buerhaus, Staiger, & Auerbach, 2008).

While these needs are predicted for registered nurses at the bedside, an additional need will exist for advanced practice nurses in outpatient settings such as doctor offices, community health clinics, and home health services as the number of patients served outside the hospital environment increases. This demand will require baccalaureate preparation prior to graduate education. HRSA (2004) further reports that approximately 71,000 registered nurses graduated in 2000 with one-third of these graduates from baccalaureate degree programs. This number reflects a significant decrease in new registered nurses entering into practice, down approximately 12,000 graduates from 1998, just two years prior.

Baccalaureate nursing education is presented with the challenge of successfully educating an increasing number of students to meet the ever growing nursing shortage. The American Association of Colleges of Nursing (AACN) (2006) reported increased enrollment in baccalaureate and graduate nursing programs over the past five years with an 18% increase in enrollment from 2005 to 2006. Unfortunately, while there is increased initial enrollment in baccalaureate nursing programs, this increase does not automatically equate with increased number of graduates and nurses in the work force due to the excessively high attrition rates in nursing academia. Nursing schools in Great Britain, the United States, Israel, and Canada report attrition rates as high as 44% (Pringle & Green, 2005) with academic failure reported as the most common reason for attrition (Ofori & Charlton, 2002).

The primary goal of baccalaureate nursing education is to prepare student nurses for professional practice (AACN, 2001). The National League for Nurses (NLN) (2005) purports that nursing education programs must be "designed to involve students as active participants in the educational enterprise, be flexible to meet constantly changing demands and individual student learning needs, be accessible, and be responsive to diverse student populations" (¶ 1).

The NLN further challenges nurse educators to "focus on student learning and creating environments for students and themselves that are characterized by collaboration, understanding, mutual trust, respect, equality, and acceptance of difference" (¶ 16).

A paradigm shift from teacher-centered teaching to learner-centered learning is presently occurring in higher education, resulting in a change in the learning environment (Barr & Tagg, 1995; Campbell & Smith, 1997; Fink, 2003). The student is now the central component of the learning environment. This shift demands that students develop into self-directed learners. Educators must ensure a supportive learning environment that promotes critical thinking, autonomy, and professional identity (Billings & Halstead, 2005). The shift to student-driven education requires all educators to understand the uniqueness of variances and unique needs of individual students and develop a variety of teaching strategies and learning opportunities which serve to support the variety of learning preferences and learning needs of the student population. Educators must have prerequisite knowledge of the theoretical constructs of adult learning theory and have a firm understanding of the best utilization of teaching methods to support self-directed learning.

The recent paradigm shift in higher education has directly impacted nursing academia. The shift from teacher-centered teaching to learner-centered learning has resulted in a nursing educational environment which is student-driven "where the faculty guides the individual development of students as needed" (Billings & Halstead, 2005, p. xiii). Nurse educators must consider the unique needs of the individual student and the theoretical constructs of self-directed learning, self-regulation, and learning motivation and the use of educational strategies and support methods to promote and enhance student integration of content value and progression toward intrinsic motivation. Academic learning activities focus on the development of critical thinking skills, autonomous decision making, clinical competence, case management skills, and teaching strategies focused on health promotion and disease management (Billings & Halstead, 2005; Cowman, 1998; Keating, 2005; Magena & Chabeli, 2005; Välimäki et al., 1999).

Multiple studies on academic self-regulation have been conducted in nursing education (Bahn, 2007; Birks, Chapman, & Francis, 2006; Cooley, 2008; Delaney & Piscopo, 2004; Hudson, 1992; Mansouri et al., 2006; McEwan & Goldenberg, 1999; Mullen, 2007; Nilsson & Stomberg, 2008; Smedley, 2007; Thompson, 1992; Tutor, 2006; Välimäki et al., 1999; Zuzelo, 2001); however, a review of the literature revealed that no study has been conducted in nursing education to determine the presence or absence of academic motivation differences between groups of nursing students. Nurse educators must understand the unique characteristics of different nursing student subgroups, how to best serve these groups of students, and effective methods to support the academic development of critical thinking and self-directed learning strategies (Billings & Halstead, 2005; Cowman, 1998; Magena & Chabeli, 2005; Välimäki et al., 1999).

Purpose of the Study

The purpose of this study was to determine if there was a difference in self-regulation behaviors (autonomous vs. controlled) in two distinct groups of nursing students: (a) traditional baccalaureate nursing students, and (b) non-traditional baccalaureate nursing students (licensed nurses who have previously completed a diploma or associate degree nursing program and are returning to nursing school to obtain a baccalaureate degree). Research participants were nursing students in a baccalaureate nursing program at one southeastern public Alabama university.

Research Questions

The following research questions were used in this study:

1. Is there a statistically significant difference in academic self-regulation behaviors (autonomous versus controlled) in the following two distinct groups of nursing students: Traditional baccalaureate nursing students and non-traditional baccalaureate nursing students (licensed nurses who have previously completed a diploma or associate degree nursing program and are returning to nursing school to obtain a baccalaureate degree)?
2. Are there significant differences in the following demographic characteristics between the same two groups of baccalaureate nursing students: Age, sex, ethnicity, marital status, family structure, number of dependent children, previous healthcare experience, current GPA, number of hours in independent study per week, number of hours studying collaboratively per week, number of work hours per week, and number of years since previous degree?

Significance of the Study

There are multiple empirical studies from nursing education regarding various aspects of student learning to include teaching strategies such as concept mapping (August-Brady, 2005), coaching (Lemcool, 2007), web-based instruction (Kumrow, 2005), problem-based learning (Alkhasawneh, Mrayyan, Docherty, Alashram, & Yousef, 2008), and reflective audiotape journaling (Kuiper, 2005); factors influencing academic performance such as multiple role demands

(Green, 1987; Lopez, 1992; Thompson, 1992), anxiety (McEwan & Goldenberg, 1999), grade point average (McEwan & Goldenberg; Vincent, 1992), and critical thinking skills (Magena & Chabeli, 2005); self-directed learning strategies (Cowman, 1998; Magena & Chabeli, 2005; Myers, 1999; Välimäki et al., 1999); self-directed learning readiness (Smedley, 2007); achievement motivation (McEwan & Goldenberg), motivational factors (Birks, Chapman, & Francis, 2006; Delaney & Piscopo, 2004; Nilsson & Stomberg, 2008; Thompson, 1992; Tutor, 2006; Zuzelo, 2001), content interest and deep approach to learning (Mansouri et al., 2006), continuing education in professional practice (Bahn, 2007; Cooley, 2008; Välimäki et al., 1999), self-regulation learning strategies in previous degree nursing students in accelerated nursing programs (Mullen, 2007), and graduate education (Hudson, 1992).

This study is significant to nursing education because the findings will provide concrete data on which to base educational decisions regarding content delivery methods, student motivation strategies, and learning activities. Understanding and recognizing possible differences in academic self-regulation across nursing student groups may assist nursing faculty in supporting student learning endeavors and thus increase the number of nursing graduates by limiting the number of students lost to attrition resulting from academic failure.

Nursing faculty in one school of nursing in Alabama can use the resultant data to better serve the two distinct groups of nursing students, traditional and non-traditional baccalaureate nursing students, by recognizing differences in learning motivation resulting from life factor influences and the impact of variances in learning motivation on student academic success. In addition, nursing faculty can provide learning opportunities which promote self-directed learning and offer appropriate supportive feedback in an effort to assist nursing students in the internalization of the value of the content and their individual move toward intrinsic motivation.

Lastly, this research will add to the existing body of knowledge related to self-regulation theory as a whole and promoting self-regulation and the implications of this process within nursing academia and higher education. Educators in higher education, regardless of the discipline, can benefit from these findings by gaining a greater understanding of the complexity of self-regulation.

Assumptions of the Study

For the purpose of this study, the following assumptions were made:

1. Controlled regulation of academic motivation and autonomous regulation of academic motivation were identifiable through participant self-completion of the *Learning Self-Regulation Questionnaire* (LSRQ).

2. Participant demographic data was accurately self-reported on the *Demographic Data Collection Tool* (DDCT).
3. Participants offered honest and accurate responses to both the LSRQ and the DDCT.
4. The LSRQ was assessed for reliability and validity and produced acceptable measurements.

Limitations of the Study

The limitations of this study included the following:

1. The study was limited to 200 participants comprising the two nursing student groups.
2. Only one student sample from one southeastern public Alabama university was sampled, which may have limited the generalizability of the results.
3. Students may not have honestly completed the LSRQ due to concern regarding faculty review.
4. The sample was minimally diverse in regards to ethnicity and gender, which may impact the generalizabilty of the findings.

Definition of Terms

The following operational definitions were used for this study:

Academic self-regulation is "an active, constructive process whereby learners set goals for their learning and then attempt to monitor, regulate, and control their cognition, motivation, and behavior, guided and constrained by their goals and the contextual features of the environment. These ... activities can mediate the relationships between individuals and the context, and their overall achievement" (Pintrich, 2000, p. 453). These processes can be focused on the attainment of a specific educational activity or can be supportive of the attainment of an educational goal, such as course grade or degree achievement (Zimmerman, Bonner & Kovach, 1996).

Andragogy is a central conceptual framework of adult learning and encompasses "any intentional and professionally guided activity that aims at a change in adult persons" (Knowles, Holton, & Swanson, 2005, p. 60).

Autonomous regulation is intrinsic regulation or identified regulation and refers to the learner's tendency toward internal learning motivation on the *Self-Determination Continuum*.

Bachelor of Science in Nursing (BSN) degree is a four-year, 120 semester credit hour program of study resulting in the conferring of the baccalaureate degree in nursing.

Controlled regulation is external regulation or introjected regulation and refers to the learner's tendency toward external learning motivation on the *Self-Determination Continuum.*

Demographic Data Collection Tool (DDCT) is the tool developed to capture demographic data from the participants (see Appendix A-2). This tool captured data on the following variables: (a) student classification (nominal scale as TBNS or NTBNS); (b) sex (nominal scale): 1) female; 2) male; (c) age (interval scale); (d) ethnicity; (e) marital status (single, married, divorced, widowed); (f) family unit (two-parent family, single-parent family, or no children); (g) number of dependent children; (h) previous healthcare experience; (i) current GPA; (j) number of hours spent independently on school work per week; (k) number of hours spent in collaboration on school work per week; (l) hours employed per week; (m) years since previous degree; and (n) previous degree GPA.

Extrinsic motivation refers to an external perceived locus of control. Learners participate in learning projects or activities for the external reward, such as pay improvements, job progression or career enhancement.

Goal proximity refers to the short-term or long-term outcomes associated with goal attainment. Proximal goals are more motivating than distant goals because short-term goal attainment is quicker and movement toward the completion is more noticeable and demonstrates learning progress (Boekaerts, 1995; Cervone, 1993).

Intrinsic motivation (internal motivation) is the innate desire to learn for the pleasure of learning and to satisfy the "itch to learn" (Cross, 1981). Intrinsically motivated learners find sincere pleasure in the learning task (Pintrich & Schunk, 1996), and typically have better learning outcomes than learners who are extrinsically motivated (Deci & Ryan, 1985; Knowles, 1984). Intrinsic motivators include the desire for increased job satisfaction, self-esteem, and increased quality of life.

Junior nursing student is a student in a BSN program who is in their junior year of study, the first year of upper division nursing courses which is comprised of three semesters.

Learning how to learn is an inclusive term referring to student efforts to develop academic skills, learning how to inquire about subjects, and transitioning to self-directed learning. These skills promote future learning and increase the likelihood of significant learning (Myers, 1999).

Learning Self-Regulation Questionnaire (LSRQ) is the survey tool used during this research (see Appendix A-1). This tool was designed for use by

Williams and Deci (1996) with adult learners and assesses learning motivation on two scales, controlled regulation (external regulation or introjected regulation) and autonomous regulation (identified regulation or intrinsic regulation). While these levels of regulation are categorized under external motivation, the differentiation of academic self-regulation between these two categories serves as the transitional point as the learner moves from extrinsic to intrinsic motivation (Ryan & Deci, 2000a). Responses to the two subscale scores were totaled and averaged.

Non-traditional baccalaureate nursing student (NTBNS) is a nursing student who is a licensed registered nurse who has previously completed a diploma or associate degree nursing program. This student is completing three semesters of nursing study to earn a BSN degree.

Self-directed learning is learner ownership and responsibility for the learning process, which includes the planning, implementation, and evaluation of a learning experience (Brockett, 1985; Caffarella, 1993; Merriam & Brockett, 1997).

Self-efficacy is a student's belief in his or her capability to succeed at a given task (Bandura, 1997) and involves regulating one's environment, affective and cognitive processes, patterns of behavior and motivation (Bandura, 2000).

Senior nursing student is a student in a BSN program who is in their senior year of study, the second year of upper division nursing courses which is comprised of two semesters.

Traditional baccalaureate nursing student (TBNS) is a student who has not yet obtained a degree in nursing but may have a degree in another discipline. This student would be completing the curricular requirements of 120 credit hours for completion of the BSN degree in nursing.

Organization of the Study

The understanding of the differences in student achievement motivation across nursing educational environments provides insight to nursing faculty as curricular outcomes and learning outcomes are developed. This study investigated the existence of differences in self-regulation behaviors between two distinct groups of baccalaureate nursing students as measured by scores on the Learning Self-Regulated Questionnaire (LSRQ). Based on the initial findings of variance, further analysis of contributing life factors (age, marital status, number of children in the home, prior work history, etc.) was conducted to determine the possible correlation of independent variables to variances in academic self-regulation.

Chapter II provides a comprehensive review of the literature concerning adult learning theory, social cognitive theory, self-directed learning theory, academic self-regulation theory, and motivation theory. In addition, empirical studies regarding self-directed learning theory, academic self-regulation theory, and motivation theory in both adult education and nursing education will be discussed. Chapter IV will offer a discussion of the results of the research study. Chapter V will conclude with a summary and discussion, implications of the findings, recommendations for use of the findings, and a conclusion based on the study findings.

CHAPTER II: LITERATURE REVIEW

The purpose of this study was to determine if there was a difference in self-regulation behaviors (autonomous vs. controlled) in two distinct groups of nursing students: (a) traditional baccalaureate nursing students, and (b) non-traditional baccalaureate nursing students (licensed nurses who have previously completed a diploma or associate degree nursing program and are returning to nursing school to obtain a baccalaureate degree). Research participants were nursing students in a baccalaureate nursing program at one southeastern public Alabama university.

The research questions addressed in this study are as follows: (a) Is there a statistically significant difference in academic self-regulation behaviors (autonomous versus controlled) in the following two distinct groups of nursing students: Traditional baccalaureate nursing students and non-traditional baccalaureate nursing students (licensed nurses who have previously completed a diploma or associate degree nursing program and are returning to nursing school to obtain a baccalaureate degree)? (b) Are there significant differences in the following demographic characteristics between the same two groups of baccalaureate nursing students: Age, sex, ethnicity, marital status, family structure, number of dependent children, previous healthcare experience, current GPA, number of hours in independent study per week, number of hours studying collaboratively per week, number of work hours per week, and number of years since previous degree?

This study is significant to nursing education because the findings will provide concrete data on which to base educational decisions regarding content delivery methods, student motivation strategies, and learning activities. Nursing faculty in one school of nursing in Alabama can use the resultant data to better serve the two distinct groups of baccalaureate nursing students, traditional and non-traditional, by recognizing differences in learning motivation resulting from life factor influences and the impact of variances in learning motivation on student academic success. In addition, nursing faculty can provide learning opportunities which promote self-directed learning and offer appropriate supportive feedback in an effort to assist nursing students in the internalization of the value of the content and their individual move toward intrinsic motivation.

This chapter provides theoretical foundations related to adult learning theory and presents the concept of self-directed learning theory and the characteristics of the adult self-directed learner. Social learning theory and developmental theory will be discussed. This chapter examines the literature in an effort to explore the theoretical foundations of self-regulation as a component of self-directed learning in the successful achievement of academic pursuits and the significance of motivation in the process of self-regulation. This chapter also discusses the development, implementation, and use of the Self-Regulated Learning Questionnaire. A review of nursing education literature will be integrated into the discussion of self-directed learning, self-regulation, and motivation. The need for further research as identified in the review of the literature will be briefly discussed and a brief summary of the chapter will be provided.

Conceptual Frameworks of Adult Learning Theory

Andragogy is defined as the "concept of an integrated framework of adult learning" and encompasses "any intentional and professionally guided activity that aims at a change in adult persons" (Knowles, Holton, & Swanson, 2005, p. 60). The process of learning throughout life is supported by a continuum of learning opportunities, which begins with pedagogy in childhood, slowly transitions to andragogy in late adolescence and early adulthood, and may at times swing back and forth from pedagogy to andragogy throughout the remainder of the lifespan (Cross, 1981). This continuum of learning is impacted by several factors specific to individual learners including learner experience, readiness to learn, orientation to learning and maturity level.

Variances in the following six learner-focused categories form the theoretical core differences in pedagogy and andragogy (Knowles, Holton & Swanson, 2005). These variances include the learner's need to know, the learner's self-concept, the role of the learner's experience, the learner's readiness to learn, the learner's motivation to learn, and the learner's orientation to learning. At the time of instruction, the child learner only needs to know the content and has a limited need to know how the information being learned will be utilized in later life situations. The child learner's self-concept is that of a dependent personality due to the fact that the learner brings little, if any, experience to the learning situation. The learner gains experiential knowledge in a passive manner through teacher-driven instructional methods (Knowles, 1980). Experience obviously plays a limited role in pedagogy simply due to the fact that the participants in pedagogy, children, do not have sufficient life experiences to relate to the newly learned content. As a result, pedagogical transmittal techniques tend to be limited to lecture presentations, textbook readings and reviews, and audiovisual aids (Knowles, Holton, & Swanson, 2005).

Readiness to learn is determined by the group's developmental ability to learn the information as a group and individual fear of failure at a sufficient level to compel the learner to maintain their learning at the same level of the group. This fear of failure may be prompted by a desire to not disappoint the teacher or parents by earning poor grades or not progressing to the next class (Knowles, 1980). Motivation is directly tied to readiness to learn as children are motivated to learn by negative or positive external motivators such as grades, rewards, and parental and/or teacher response. Orientation to learning is subject-centered and organized in a lock-step logical sequence based on subject-matter content; however, the content learned may not be readily applicable to everyday life situations.

In contrast, the six assumptions of andragogy reveal that life experience plays a major role in the differences between pedagogy and andragogy. Adults need to know the relevance of new knowledge prior to undertaking the effort to learn new content; thus, one of the first acts of facilitation of adult learning is assisting the learner in identifying the benefits of learning new content and the consequences of not learning the given content (Knowles, Holton, & Swanson, 2005). These benefits and consequences can be linked to personal goals, career goals, learner performance or quality of life.

As young adults mature, there is a shift from dependency to self-directed learning. The rate of this shift in self-concept varies among individuals. Most adult learners are typically self-directed in multiple areas of their lives; however, these same adults may need assistance transitioning to self-directed learning due to educational conditioning resulting from traditional pedagogical methodologies in childhood (Knowles, 1980). This shift in self-concept may be directly impacted by the learner's life experiences which serve as a learning resource for future learning encounters, not only for the learner but for fellow learners as well. As a result of these life experiences, the adult learner has a different learning context than the child and can more effectively participate in active learning activities such as lab experiences, discussions, case studies, etc., that draw on the learning groups' various experiences (Knowles, Holton, & Swanson, 2005).

Readiness to learn and motivation are directly linked to the need to know. Adult learners must identify a gap in their learning and thus, the "need to know" specific information is a prerequisite for readiness to learn. The adult learner must value the information presented for the learning to be effective. This process can be facilitated by assisting students in self-identifying gaps in their knowledge and recognizing the personal benefits gained from actively engaging in learning activities. Once identified, these internal benefits, such as increased job satisfaction, self-esteem, pride, etc., serve as motivators for the adult learners (Knowles, Holton, & Swanson, 2005).

Orientation to learning in andragogy shifts from subject-centered learning to life-centered, task-centered or problem-centered learning (Knowles, 1980). Adult learners are motivated to learn information and concepts that will help them be successful in their daily lives. "Issues of motivation, preference for learning style and interest all enter into the attitudes of learners which may either encourage and stimulate self-directed learning, or present obstacles and constraints to learning" (Keirns, 1999, p. 132). In addition, adult learners learn more effectively when information is connected to real-life situations and events (Knowles, Holton, & Swanson, 2005).

Lindeman (1926) presented the following key characteristics of adult learners, which constitute the foundation of adult learning theory: (a) Adults are motivated to learn as they experience needs and interests that learning will satisfy; (b) Adults' orientation to learning is life-centered; (c) Experience is the richest source of adult learning; (d) Adults have a deep need to be self-directing; and (e) Individual differences among people increase with age. Most adult learners pursue additional educational opportunities primarily on a voluntary basis in an effort to increase their work skills and thereby advance their career; however, a considerable number of adult learners engage in learning activities simply for the enjoyment and pleasure of learning new information (Tough, 1979). Adult learners desire active learning activities and expect their life experiences to be respected and drawn on during learning activities.

The Characteristics of Adults as Learners (CAL) framework differentiates adult learners from children learners and suggests teaching strategies to facilitate adult learning (Cross, 1981). The CAL model is composed of both personal characteristics, which describe the learner, and situational characteristics, which describe the learning conditions. Situational characteristics are typically easily distinguished characteristics such as full-time students versus part-time students or voluntary learning versus compulsory learning.

Personal characteristics follow the growth and development of the individual learner across the lifespan and the CAL model suggests three specific growth and development continuums: Physical characteristics related to aging, sociocultural characteristics related to life phases, and psychological characteristics related to developmental stages (Cross, 1981). The individual learner will be at a different point of growth in each area and the precise point of growth and development in each category will contribute to the learner's unique learning characteristics including physical ability, readiness to learn, ego maturity, and self-directedness. Understanding the multiple characteristics of the adult learners and the process of self-directed learning allows adult educators to "gain a more holistic view of the learner" (Merriam & Brockett, 1997, p. 140).

Smith (1982) identified the following four distinctly unique contributing factors which impact adult learning experiences: Life experiences incurred over time; progression through distinct physical, psychological and social developmental phases; multiple role demands and responsibilities; and anxiety and uncertainty about their learning. Additional contributing factors include the maturity level of the learner, the learner's self-confidence, and the learner's perceived self-competence. The adult educator must consider these contributing factors and be ever mindful of the adult learner's individual self-directed learning needs, life responsibilities and multiple role requirements.

Undergraduate education in the United States has undergone a paradigm shift as academic institutions restructure in an effort to transition from a teaching paradigm to a learning paradigm (Barr & Tagg, 1995; Campbell & Smith, 1997; Fink, 2003), resulting in a learning environment focused on producing learning, not providing instruction (Fink). This paradigm shift is supportive of a learning environment that is student-focused, as opposed to educator-focused, and provides learning opportunities for students to develop into self-directed learners (Barr & Tagg). Campbell and Smith differentiated the changes that exist between the old teaching paradigm and the new learning paradigm. Table A-1 provides these changes.

This new learning paradigm requires students to jointly participate with faculty in the development of knowledge construction to become actively engaged in constructing, discovering, and ultimately transforming the knowledge for their own independent purpose (Campbell & Smith, 1997). The adult educator must assume the role of a facilitator, a guide who assists the learner in identifying their personal learning needs and determining effective learning strategies (Hiemstra, 1985). In addition, the educator must serve as a coach, providing timely and effective feedback to support the learner during periods of stress and unease. These actions assist students to develop self-directed learning skills and become self-regulated learners. Svinicki (2004) argues that while novice learners have difficulty understanding the relevance of the current learning content to future academic, professional, and life goals, educators can assist learners in connecting what is being learned today to the knowledge the learner will need in the future.

Nursing education must embrace the paradigm shift to a learner-centered educational approach in an effort to facilitate student nurses who can critically think and take ownership of their life long learning (Billings & Halstead, 2005; Cowman, 1998; Magena & Chabeli, 2005; Välimäki et al., 1999). Greveson and Spencer (2005) further asserted that medical educators should incorporate self-directed learning principals so as to produce individuals who manage learning throughout lifelong careers.

TABLE A-1 Old and New Paradigms for College Teaching

	Old Paradigm	New Paradigm
Knowledge	Transferred from faculty to students	Jointly constructed by students and faculty
Student	Passive vessel to be filled by faculty's knowledge	Active constructor, discoverer, transformer of knowledge
Mode of learning	Memorizing	Relating
Faculty purpose	Classify and sort students	Develop students' competencies and talents
Student growth, goals	Students strive to complete requirements, achieve certification within a discipline	Students strive to focus on continual lifelong learning within a broader system
Relationships	Impersonal relationship among students and between faculty and students	Personal relationship among students and between faculty and students
Context	Competitive, individualistic	Cooperative learning in classroom and cooperative teams among faculty
Climate	Conformity, cultural uniformity	Diversity and personal esteem; cultural diversity and commonality
Power	Faculty holds and exercises power, authority, and control	Students are empowered; power is shared among students and between students and faculty
Assessment	Norm-referenced (that is, grading on the curve); typically use multiple-choice items; student rating of instruction at end of course	Criterion-referenced (that is, grading to predefined standards); typically use performances and portfolios; continual assessment of instruction
Ways of knowing	Logical-scientific	Narrative
Epistemology	Reductionist; facts and memorization	Constructivist; inquiry and invention
Technology	Drill and practice; textbook substitute; chalk-and-talk substitute	Problem-solving, communication, collaboration, information access, expression
Teaching assumption	Any expert can teach	Teaching is complex and requires considerable training

Source: Campbell and Smith, 1997, p. 275.

Development of Self-Directed Learning Principles

To fully understand academic self-directed learning, a comprehensive review of self-directed learning principles is required. Houle (1988) set the stage for today's interest in participation and self-directed learning. Houle identified three interrelated groups of learners and presented the typology of learning orientation. All learners can be categorized as goal-oriented, activity-oriented, or learning-oriented learners. Goal-oriented learners engage in learning activities to meet a specific a specific goal such as degree. Activity-oriented learners participate in the learning activity for the sake of the activity or the social interaction of the learning environment. Learning-oriented learners are life long learners and pursue knowledge for pleasure, not for external accomplishment. Adult learners may engage in different forms of learning for different content areas and individuals have overlapping learning orientations throughout their lifespan and can shift from one orientation to another based on their interest and motivation (Houle, 1988).

Houle's typology led others to investigate to determine adult reasons for participating in learning activities. Boshier (1971) argued that educators need to know what motivates adult learners in an effort to increase the quality of education, to increase the quantity of adult learning experiences, and to decrease the occurrence of attrition. The development and later revision of the Education Participation Scale (EPS) resulted in the determination of five to eight factors which contribute to adult desire to participate in learning activities (Boshier & Collins, 1985; Cross, 1981). Morstain & Smart (1974) replicated Boshier's study to determine group variances in motivational factors resulting from age and gender differences. Factor analysis on EPS was performed to determine the utility of the instrument and a resultant six factors for participation were identified: social relationships, external expectations, social welfare, professional advancement, escape/stimulation, and cognitive interest.

Phillip Candy (1991) focused on explaining the theory of self-directed learning and provided useable strategies for adult educators. Candy differentiated between the goal of self-directed learning and process of self-directed learning and offered a comprehensive review of the literature outlining the research and expository efforts of educators in both venues published from the late 1960's to the late 1970's and explored multiple scholastic works from this time period. Candy offered the term autodidaxy to encompass self-directed learning which occurs outside of a formal learning environment.

Various studies report successful self-directed learning to be contingent on the presence of multiple characteristics and qualities (Bruner, 1964; Caffarella, 1983; Candy, 1991; Guglielmino, 1977; Hiemstra & Judd, 1978; Knowles, 1984; Mezirow, 1981; Smith, 1982; Tough, 1979). The self-directed learner demonstrates the multiple attributes including a methodical and disciplined approach to learning, logic and analytical skills, willingness to self-reflect and self-evaluate, flexibility, persistence, responsibility, creativity, confidence and a positive self-concept (Candy, 1991; Guglielmino, 1977). In addition, a successful self-directed learner, regardless of the learning mode, whether self-directed, collaborative, or formal, must be independent and self-sufficient, have basic knowledge related to learning methods, be motivated and be able sustain their motivation (Smith, 1982).

Tough's (1979) report *The Adult's Learning Project* focused on independent scholarship and presented Tough's theory that self-directed learning is a learning process with specific phases. Tough indicated that two-thirds of all adult learning activities were planned, implemented and evaluated solely by the learner outside of a formal learning environment. Knowles (1980) asserted that future adult educational efforts should focus on the promotion of self-directed learning by promoting learning opportunities that require learners to self-determine their learning needs, develop their own learning objectives, share responsibility for planning and completing learning activities, and actively self-evaluate progress toward the learning objective. This process is challenging for both the educator and the learner as both parties become more comfortable with their roles in the process as growth occurs over time.

Goleman (1995) explored the multiple realms of emotional intelligence as an adjunctive component of individual performance and goal achievement and purported that emotional intelligence is comprised of "self-control, zeal and persistence, and the ability to motivate oneself" (p. xii). Goleman focused on the psychological role that personal emotional competence plays in one's ability to achieve personal goals. Goleman divided the skills of emotional intelligence into two categories, personal competence and social competence. Personal competence comprises self-awareness, self-regulation, and motivation, while social competence consists of empathy and social skills. The subcomponents of the personal competence directly correlate with self-directed learning skills. Learners must be self aware of "one's internal states, preferences, resources, and intuitions" (Goleman, p. 26); thus, Goleman provides the three distinct tasks of self-awareness, emotional awareness, accurate self-assessment and self-confidence. Self-regulation is central to personal competence and encompasses self-control, trustworthiness, conscientiousness, adaptability and innovation. Motivation includes achievement drive, commitment, initiative and optimism (Goleman, 1998).

Fink (2003) presented the Taxonomy of Significant Learning wherein the following six significant areas of learning are categorized: Foundational knowledge, application, integration, human dimension, caring, and learning how to learn (see Figure A-1). While all categories are important to offering successful

FIGURE A-1 Positive factors impacting current work situation of hospital-based RNs.

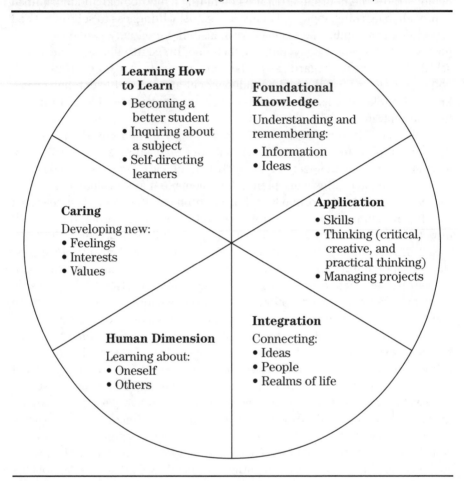

learning opportunities, areas of interest for this discussion include Human Dimensions and Learning How to Learn.

Fink integrates Goleman's concepts of personal competence and social competence under the category of Human Dimension. This category includes the sub-processes of learning about others and one's self, understanding one's self, and how one reacts to others as well recognizing one's personal competence, which includes self-awareness, self regulation and motivation.

The category of learning how to learn includes student efforts to develop academic skills, learning how to inquire about subjects, and transitioning to self-directed learning. These skills promote future learning and increase the likelihood of significant learning (Myers, 1999). Figure A-2 provides a visualization of Fink's

FIGURE A-2 The interactive nature of significant learning.

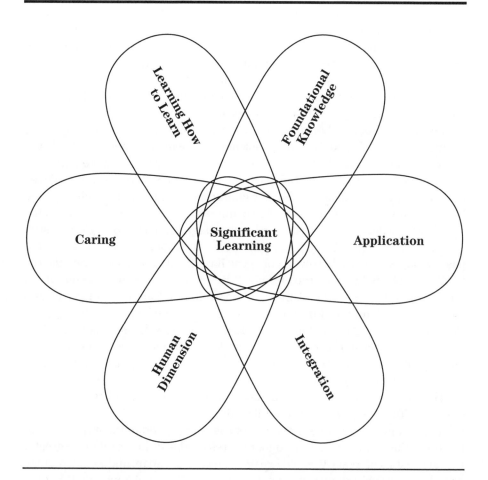

model of the interactive nature of significant learning, which demonstrates how the six constructs work to provide a significant learning opportunity for students.

Brockett and Hiemstra (1991) developed the Personal Responsibility Orientation (PRO) model, a theoretical model which places self-direction in learning as an overriding theme with two related sub-dimensions: (a) self-directed learning based on the elements of the teaching-learning process similar to Knowles' prior definition, and (b) learner self-direction, which focuses on internal individual characteristics which predispose that individual to take primary responsibility for their learning (Brockett & Hiemstra, 1991).

Thomas and Rohwer (1993) offered the Effort Management Hierarchy model based on the four hierarchical levels of study activities, which include monitoring, self-regulation, planning and evaluation and argued that learner self-direction occurs in a continuum of activities, which range from awareness of need to individual control of one's study efforts to include concentration, time and learning effectiveness. Garrison's (1997) model of self-directed learning is quite similar in theory. This model offers the input of initial motivation at the beginning of a task and combines this motivation with self-monitoring and self-management with self-directed learning as the end result. Regulation and reflection are key to self-directed learning.

The Self-Directed Learning Readiness Scale (SDLRS) developed by Guglielmino (1977) and the Oddi Continuing Learning Inventory (OCLI) are two quantitative measurement tools which have contributed to the extensive research regarding self-directed learning. The SDLRS instrument was developed in an effort to measure learner characteristics related to self-directed learning and to assess the learner's readiness to participate in self-directed learning in an academic environment such as high school or college (Hiemstra, 1985). The SDRLS has been used by multiple educational researchers over the past twenty-six years; however, concerns have been expressed regarding the SDRLS accuracy in measurement of self-directed learning due to stability of the factor solutions of the SDLRS and possible resultant inaccurate assessments (Hoban, Lawson, Mazmanian, Best, & Seibel, 2005; Straka & Hinz, 1996). Concerns regarding Guglielmino's SDLRS led Fisher, King and Tague (2001) to develop a 40-item self-directed readiness learning readiness scale for use in nursing education and reported homogeneity and validity; however, further research is necessary to determine content validity.

The OCLI is a 24-item 7-point Likert scale measurement tool which reports on three domains of self-directed learning: (a) proactive/reactive learning drive, (b) cognitive openness/defensiveness, and (c) commitment/aversion to learning (Chou & Chen, 2008). Higher scores on the OCLI correlate to greater characteristics of a self-directed learner. Harvey, Rothman, and Frecker (2006) completed an additional factor analysis on the OCLI and concluded that the original three domains should, in fact, be four domains and offered the following four overlapping dimensions: Learning With Others, Learner Motivation/Self-Efficacy/Autonomy, Ability to be Self-Regulating, and Reading Avidity.

Self-Directed Learning Principles

Self-directed learning is simply defined as learner ownership and responsibility for the learning process, which includes the planning, implementation, and evaluation of a learning experience (Brockett, 1985; Caffarella, 1993; Merriam & Brockett, 1997). Self-directed learning is the learning preference of the true adult learner (Knowles, 1980) and is the central theme in andragogy because adult learners have a "deep psychological need to be generally self-directing" (p. 43). This need becomes more prevalent as the learner matures; however, this process is individualized and many learners may alternate degrees of self-directedness in different environments and as learning situations vary.

Self-directed learning encompasses both external and internal factors which force the learner to engage in more responsibility regarding the learning process (Brockett & Hiemstra, 1991). External factors focus on instructional processes, learning environment, and facilitation methods to assist the learner in self-evaluation, planning, implementing, and evaluating learning. Internal factors include the multitude of personality characteristics that impact a learner's movement toward self-directed learning.

A strong inherent connection exists between self-directed learning and self-concept and multiple social characteristics and personality traits contribute to successful self-directed learning (Merriam & Brockett, 1997). Guglielmino (1977) suggested that self-directed learning is promoted by a mix of learner attitudes, values and abilities and identified fifty-six characteristics and psychological qualities that impact learner readiness to transition to self-directed learning. While the list of characteristics is exhaustive, Guglielmino recognized that self-directed learners tend to be goal-oriented and accept responsibility for their own learning; demonstrate initiative and independence; be persistent and self-disciplined; possess a high degree of curiosity; enjoy learning; have a strong ability to learn independently; and, tend to see problems as challenges, not obstacles.

Four major factors contribute to the learner's degree of self-directedness: (a) the learner's technical skill related to the learning process; (b) the learner's familiarity with the content; (c) the learner's sense of ability to learn the material, or competence; and (d) the learner's commitment to learning (Merriam & Caffarella, 1999). The self-directed learner implements creative and adaptive ways to attain the learning goals by reviewing the learning task, selecting appropriate learning strategies, planning out the learning and studying process, evaluating the learning progress, seeking out feedback from others, and regulating thought processes (Brookfield, 1994; Pintrich & Schunk, 1996; Schunk & Zimmerman, 1994; Thomas & Rohwer, 1986; Warkentin & Bol, 1997; Zimmerman, 1990).

Self-directed learning properties should be viewed as a continuum, not an absolute condition. While learners may demonstrate self-directedness in other areas of life management, frequently students in formal educational environments revert to pedagogical expectations for the learning environment out of habit and familiarity (Knowles, 1980). Self-directed learning is greatly individualized and is impacted by learner maturity and experience; however, the older student may not demonstrate stronger self-directed learning readiness

than a younger student. In addition, the learner's experience in previous learning encounters may have encouraged the use of self-directedness to achieve
the learning outcomes, thus providing a starting point for the learner in the
next encounter (Knowles). Pekrun, Frenzel, Goetz, and Perry (2007) asserted
that self-regulation of learning behavior allows the student to adapt behavior
according to the goal demands and the demand of the learning environment.

A unique set of skills is required for self-directed learning to be successful.
The learner must be curious about the content, recognize the need for the information, be willing to ask questions, and recognize the availability of multiple
resources (Smith, 1982). Adult educators must promote self-directed learning
by providing learning opportunities that require learners to self-determine
their learning needs, develop their own learning objectives, share responsibility for planning and completing learning activities, and actively self-evaluate
progress toward the learning objective (Knowles, 1980); however, this process can be challenging due the number of factors which impact self-directed
learner readiness and faculty willingness to change their instructional style.
Black and Deci (2000) argued the following:

> Instructional style low in autonomy support is likely to be related to stu-
> dents' feeling bad, and possibly to performing badly thus shifts in teaching
> approaches toward providing more support for students' autonomy and
> active learning may hold promise for enhancing students' achievement and
> psychological development. To some extent, this can be accomplished by
> having professors become more student-oriented, more accessible to stu-
> dents, and responsive to their needs and concerns. That, of course, would
> require willingness on the part of faculty to change their orientations, and
> promoting such willingness may be very difficult. (p. 754)

While student learning may be self-directed, the facilitator must be cau-
tious not to isolate the student and leave the student stranded and without
guidance. The educator must assist the learner with assimilation to the role of
a self-directed learner role by helping the learner establish learning goals and
by serving as a consultant by offering their own experience and knowledge as
a source of information (Brockett & Hiemstra, 1991).

Adult educators in the formal and informal learning environment must
assist students in engaging in the process of self-directed learning and serve
as facilitators in the process, not merely teachers of content. Collaborative discussion and exploration to expose the learner to the benefits of learning new
content, assist the learner in determining the learner's desired outcomes, and
help the learner complete a needs assessment to identify "gaps between their
aspirations and their present level of performance" (Knowles, 1980, p. 57). This

process can be unsettling for the learner as self-reflection may reveal needs or subject knowledge deficits not previously recognized or subject knowledge deficits. Self-directed learning can by promoted by exploring multiple learning strategies and available resources and by supporting the learner in determining the best learning partnership (independent study pair work, group work) and learning environment.

The process of evaluation is critical to successful self-directed learning. The adult educator should assist the learner in developing an evaluation tool to promote critical reflection to determine if the learning outcomes were met (Knowles, 1980). These requirements necessitate a greater sense of commitment to the process of self-directed learning than the traditional teaching methods of rote lecture and evaluation as this method of student-driven instruction can be time intensive and demanding. Knowles (1980) further argues the following:

> The truly artistic teachers of adults perceive the locus of responsibility for learning to be in the learner; they conscientiously suppress their own compulsion to teach what they know students ought to learn in favor of helping students learn for themselves what they want to learn. (p. 56)

A resultant period of dissonance may occur during which the learner experiences an uncomfortable state due to the contrast of previous learning experiences wherein the learner was given all the information they need to know and merely had to memorize the content.

Thoughtfully planned learning opportunities are necessary to guide the student and provide social contact with other learners who are also manipulating the learning content to determine relevance and meet the learning outcomes. Adult educators in both formal and informal settings must recognize the attributes of the adult learner and strive to develop appropriate learning opportunities that strengthen the skills required for future successful self-directed learning efforts. Adult educators must value the adult learner on a personal level and respect the learner's unique learning preferences and needs in order to ensure a positive learning outcome.

Not all voices in education heartily support the concepts of self-directed learning. Brookfield (1990) cautioned that the development of self-direction is unsatisfactory in college learning in that it leads to working in isolation instead of promoting collaborative learning. Fifty percent of all learning activities are completed in isolation (Winne, 1995); consequently, educators must diligently work to support self-regulated learning and further their understanding of how learners use self-regulated learning strategies when working alone. Brookfield further encourages the integration of cooperation and self-direction reinforcements, internalized perceived benefits of the skill or knowledge, and self-reinforcements, evaluations of learning behavior (Schunk, 2001a).

While all four components vary with the individual, the fourth component of reinforcement and motivation comprise the subparts of self-regulated learning. These variables give the individual control of the social learning experience (Cross, 1991).

Through self-regulation, the learner can process the reasons for participating in the learning activities and the consequences related to their level of participation (non-participation, poor participation, or active participation), and subsequent learning outcomes. Bandura (1976) argued that "persons can regulate their own behavior to some extent by visualizing self-generated consequences" (p. 392). Bandura further identified three distinct, yet interrelated, subprocesses of self-regulation: self-observation, self-judgment and self-reaction. The concept of self-efficacy, the self-knowledge that an individual can successfully accomplish a given task, is also imperative to the learning process (Bandura, 1997).

Self-regulation can viewed as a continuum in which individuals may demonstrate higher or lower self-regulatory behaviors based on their value of the learning, interest in the content, self-efficacy, and motivation (Pintrich, 2000). Schunk (2001a) argues that self-regulation is situational and context specific; consequently, learner self-regulation varies greatly from person to person and activity to activity. The Social Cognitive Model of the Development of Self-Regulation Competence demonstrates the shift from external to internal sources of self-regulation (Schunk). The first two levels of the model, observational and emulative, are primarily influenced by social factors. During the observational level, learners observe models and process verbal descriptions of appropriate actions during lectures, demonstrations, discussions and through encouragement. At the emulative level, learners demonstrate performance capability but remain dependent on modeling and external feedback. During the self-control phase, level three, learners internalize the self-regulation strategy off of the modeled behavior. At level four, full self-regulation, learners have not only integrated the modeled behavior but have begun to modify strategies and make situational adjustments. In addition, learners who have achieved full self-regulation independently maintain their motivation and self-efficacy (Schunk).

In contrast to social learning theory, Piaget's stages of cognition help explain the way individual learners process, organize and recall information (James & Maher, 2004). Piaget viewed cognitive learning in relation to chronological age and proposed that humans progress through four distinct stages of cognitive development: Sensory-motor (birth to 2 years of age), pre-operational (2 to 6 years), operational (7 to 11 years) and formal or abstract (12 to 20 years)

(Hockenberry & Wilson, 2007). Piaget purported that adults performing at formal or abstract level of cognition can think abstractly and work with hypothetical situations; however, age alone cannot indicate an adult's level of cognitive performance as many adults do not ever truly transition to abstract thinking.

Keefe's taxonomy integrated cognitive, physiological, and affective dimensions of learning in an effort to explain the individual variances which impact the learning process (James & Maher, 2004). Affective dimensions include personality variances such as motivation, emotion, interest and value. These aspects of personality contribute to variances in individual self-regulation of learning. Keefe's taxonomy was foundational to the emergence of learning styles research. Kolb's *Learning Styles Inventory, Myers-Briggs Type Indicator,* the *Keirsey Temperament Sorter,* the *VARK Learning Preference Survey,* and the *Learning Combination Inventory* all provide learner's with information regarding their individual learning style and preferences. Individual understanding of one's personal learning style supports the learner's understanding of one's cognitive function and approach to learning. This knowledge is imperative for the self-regulated learner as this information is foundational to self-monitoring and self-regulation of the learning process (Keirns, 1999; Smedley, 2007). Garrison (1997) argued that self-regulation is a metacognitive process "which requires students to explore their own thought processes so as to evaluate the results of their actions and plan alternative pathways to success" (p. 18); thus, self-regulation is a primary construct of self-directed learning. Zimmerman (1995) further stressed that "it is one thing to possess metacognitive knowledge and skill but another thing to be able to self-regulate its use in the face of fatigue, stressors, or competing attractions" (p. 217).

Empirical studies exploring nursing student learning styles include Lapeyre's (1991) investigation comparing degree and non-degree student learning approaches in which Lapeyre reported that the goal attainment of a degree did not result in a difference in approach to learning in the two groups. Alkhasawneh, Mrayyan, Docherty, Alashram, and Yousef (2008) explored the use of problem-based learning techniques and student learning preferences as reported by the VARK Learning Styles Preference survey, which identified student learning preference in four distinct areas: visual, aural, read/write, kinesthetic. While most nursing students demonstrate a read/write preference, most reported a multimodal learning preference, meaning that they demonstrated a combined aptitude for learning in more than one modality. Alkhasawneh et al. (2008) concluded that nursing students had successful academic outcomes as long as the nurse educator provided various learning activities which supported the four preference areas.

In 1956 Benjamin Bloom and associates proposed the taxonomy of educational objectives in the cognitive domain wherein learning objectives were in an effort to foster the student ability to work together and contribute to a collective effort. While many educators view self-directed learning from the cognitive perspective, that of individual private learning, Greveson and Spencer (2005) caution that learner success is enhanced by social interaction with other learners and the learning environment. Dornan, Hadfield, Borwn, Boshuizen, and Scherpbier (2005) caution educators to ensure that the learner is not isolated and to be aware of the multiple learner support needs that must be met to enable learners to successfully transition to a more self-directed learning style.

Brookfield (2006) discussed student resistance to self-directed learning and cautioned that many educators demand students take responsibility for planning and organizing their learning prematurely. This can place students in the position of designing their learning activities prior to developing a full understanding of the content and can jeopardize student learning outcomes. Guidance provided by educators through evaluations of learning approaches and strategies is imperative to support students as they develop deeper understanding, improve their learning skills, and can help them become aware of new learning needs. In addition, positive feedback and encouragement can deepen student motivation to learn and commitment to the learning process (Brookfield, 2006).

Social Cognitive Perspectives of Learning Self-Regulation

Social cognitive theory is based on the central theme of learning through observation of real and representational models or symbols (Svinicki, 2004). While social cognitive theory will be discussed in detail, a synopsis of theoretical views from other learning theories as set forth by Zimmerman (2001) is replicated in Table A-2. Bandura (1976) argued that social cognitive processes are directly associated with observational learning and recognized four components of observational learning: 1) attentional processes, 2) retention processes, 3) motor reproduction processes and 4) reinforcement and motivational processes. These four internal subprocesses are foundational to the learning experience. Attentional processes refer to the learner's interest in the model, whether it be a teacher modeling behavior, or a television show or book (Schunk, 2001a). Retention processes include the cognitive methods used to commit the actions of a model to memory and recall the information for future use. These methods may be thoughtful or may occur subconsciously. Motor reproduction processes include the learner's physical ability to perform the demonstrated task. Reinforcement and motivational processes vary based on the consequence of learning or not learning given the content or task and include vicarious

TABLE A-2 A Comparison of Theoretical Views Regarding Common Issues in Self-Regulation of Learning Common Issues in Self-Regulation of Learning

Theories	Motivation	Self-Awareness	Key Processes	Social & Physical Environment	Acquiring Capacity
Operant	Reinforcing stimuli are emphasized	Not recognized except for self-reactivity	Self-monitoring, self-instruction, and self-evaluation	Modeling and reinforcement	Shaping behavior and fading adjunctive stimuli
Phenomeno-logical	Self-actualization is emphasized	Emphasize role of self-concept	Self-worth and self-identity	Emphasize subjective perceptions of it	Development of the self-system
Information processing	Motivation is not emphasized historically	Cognitive self-monitoring	Storage and transformation of information	Not emphasized except when transformed to information	Increases in capacity of system to transform information
Social cognitive	Self-efficacy, out-come expectations, and goals are em-phasized	Self-observation and self-recording	Self-observation, self-judgment and self-reactions	Modeling and enactive mastery experiences	Increases through social learning at for successive levels
Volitional	It is a precondition to volition based on one's expectancy/ values	Action controlled rather than state controlled	Strategies to control cognition, motivation, and emotions	Volitional strategies to control distracting environments	As acquired ability to use volitional control strategies
Vygotskian	Not emphasized historically except for social context effects	Consciousness of learning in the Zone of Proximal Development	Egocentric and inner speech	Adult dialogue mediates interna-tionalization of chil-dren's speech	Children acquire inner use of speech in a series of devel-opmental levels
Constructivist	Resolution of cognitive conflict or a curiosity drive is emphasized	Metacognitive monitoring	Constructing schemas, strategies, or personal theories	Historically social conflict or discovery learning are stressed	Development con-strains children's acquisition of self-regulatory processes

Source: Zimmerman, 2001, p. 9.

ranked from the lowest level to the highest level as follows: knowledge, comprehension, application, analysis, synthesis, and evaluation (Bloom, 1971). Anderson and Krathwohl (2001) offered a revision of Bloom's original taxonomy and included metacognitive knowledge, student knowledge of their own cognition and how they approach learning, as a type of knowledge; however, Anderson and Krathwohl posited that the act of self-regulation is a component of the cognitive process dimension. Justice and Dornan (2001) investigated the differences in metacognitive awareness between traditional age and non-traditional age college students and reported that while there was increased metacognition in mature students this did not translate to higher academic performance.

Academic Self-Regulation

Pintrich (2000) offers the following working definition of self-regulation learning:

> Self-regulated learning is an active, constructive process whereby learners set goals for their learning and then attempt to monitor, regulate, and control their cognition, motivation, and behavior, guided and constrained by their goals and the contextual features of the environment. These self-regulatory activities can mediate the relationships between individuals and the context, and their overall achievement. (p. 453)

> These processes can be focused on the attainment of a specific educational activity or can be supportive of the attainment of an educational goal, such as course grade or degree achievement (Zimmerman, Bonner & Kovach, 1996). Students who can self-regulate their learning behaviors are more likely to perform successfully than students with low self-regulation (Schunk, 1993).

While many educators view self-regulation as a set of skills, Zimmerman (1998) argues that "academic self-regulation is not a mental ability, such as intelligence, or an academic skill, such as reading proficiency; rather it is the self-directive process through which learners transfer their mental abilities into academic skills" (p. 1). Academic self-regulation requires learners to be "metacognitively, motivationally, and behaviorally" self-active in the entire learning process (Zimmerman, 2001; Zimmerman, Bandura, & Martinez-Pons, 1992). While the self-regulated learner does not learn in isolation, the individual takes primary responsibility for planning the learning experience, self-motivation, initiative, and persistence and is willing to modify learning strategies and develop new approaches as is necessitated by the learning challenge (Brookfield, 1994; Caffarella, 1993; Cassazza, 2006).

Zimmerman (1989) offered a triadic model demonstrating self-regulated functioning in three specific influence processes: personal, environmental, and behavioral (see Figure A-3). This model reflects social cognitive theory and supports the concept that self-regulated learning is a dynamic process which can be influenced by cognitive, emotional and environmental factors. Fluctuations between processes and variances in reciprocality exist within each self-directed learner. The personal processes includes self-efficacy, motivation, affect and interest in the content area or learning task while the environmental processes include managing the learning environment such that environment is conducive to learning. Behavior processes include the cognitive strategies to organize, learn and recall the information. The triadic model further demonstrates the feedback loop resulting from self-reflection. Effective self-management of the learner's environmental, behavioral, and personal processes is the most visible indicator of a learner's degree of self-regulation (Zimmerman, 1989).

Zimmerman (1989) further proposed multiple self-regulated learning strategies which support the triadic model (see Figure A-3). These strategies include self-evaluating, organizing and transforming learning resources and content to be learned, goal setting and planning, seeking information, keeping records and monitoring performance and progression, environmental structuring, self-consequating and rewarding, rehearsing and memorizing content, seeking social assistance, and reviewing the records.

Kanfer and Heggestad (1999) identified academic self-regulation as one of the four areas of individual variance which impact student success. The remaining areas include the student's preferred learning strategies, the way the student processes information, and the student's self-efficacy. Self-efficacy can be defined as a student's belief in his or her capability to succeed at a given task (Bandura, 1997) and involves regulating one's environment, affective and cognitive processes, patterns of behavior and motivation (Bandura, 2000). A student who is self-efficacious is more open to try new things, less worried about making mistakes, and more willing to exert additional effort to succeed at a specific task. As a result, these students are more "persistent, experiment with learning strategies and have more initiative" (Svinicki, 2004, p. 207). With influence, effective learning strategies, and internalization of values, student self-efficacy can change over time.

There are four common general components of self-regulation theories: (a) self-regulated learners strive for improvement in academic learning and use specific strategies to support this improvement; (b) effective use of a feedback loop of evaluation; (c) motivational differences exist between those who utilize self-regulation behaviors and those who don't; and (d) the regular use of self-regulation requires extra time and effort (Zimmerman & Schunk, 2001). Variances

FIGURE A-3 Triadic analysis of self-regulated functioning (Zimmerman, 1989, p. 330).

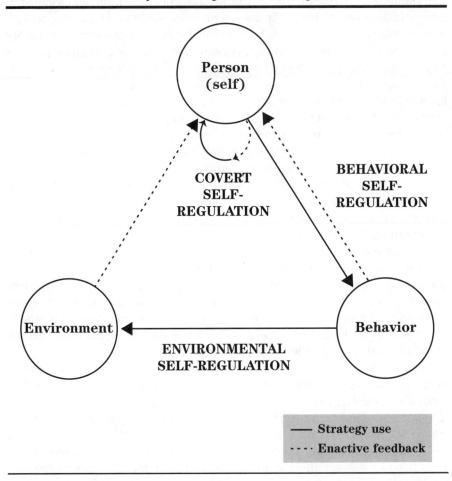

in these four distinct areas of self-regulation can be impacted by an individual's age, maturity level, and internal valuation of the content being learned.

Cassazza's (2006) review of the literature determined the following three principles exist in the construct of self-regulation: (a) Learners who utilize self-regulated learning proactively manage learning by utilizing various adaptive strategies; (b) learning is improved when there is a connection between learning outcomes and learning strategies; and (c) the act of setting learning goals leads to enhanced academic achievement. Schunk (1993) argued that students who successfully transition to college programs have adequate self-regulatory behaviors which include three components: goals, self-efficacy and learning strategies.

Multiple models of self-regulated learning exist. While it would be exhaustive to explain each model in detail, four common assumptions regarding learning and regulation in all models will be discussed. The first assumption, active constructive assumption, assumes all learners are "active, constructive participants in the learning process" (Pintrich, 2000, p. 452). Learners take information offered in the learning environment and link this information to previously internalized information to form personalized meaning, goals, and strategies. Second, potential for control, is the assumption that learners have the ability to self-monitor their thought processes, motivation and behavior and the environment; however, it is not assumed that all learners utilize this self-monitoring ability. Third, goal assumption, assumes that learners set goals and self-regulate their efforts by monitoring thought processes, behavior, and motivation in effort to obtain the goal. The fourth assumption, mediation, recognizes the role of self-regulation of learner cognition, behavior and motivation in the facilitation of the dynamics of the individual, the learning context and the achievement of the goal (Pintrich, 2000).

A framework of the four specific phases of self-regulation serves to assist learners and educators in conceptualizing the process and the distinct steps (Pintrich, 2000). Phase 1 focuses on obtaining knowledge about the learning task and context, planning and goal setting. Phase 2 includes the self-monitoring and metacognitive awareness of the integration of self with the requirements of the task and context. Phase 3, the controlling phase, consists of efforts to self-regulate and manage the different aspects of the task or context. Phase 4 includes self-reflection and self-reaction. Phases 2 and 3 can meld into one another as self-monitoring, metacognition, and self-regulation all concern self-awareness and direction. Pintrich further breaks down these phases into each step and includes appropriate expected action in the realms of cognition, motivation, behavior and context (see Table A-3). These steps do not occur in linear fashion for all learners and some steps may occur synchronously. Self-efficacy, learner belief that they can successfully complete the task, operates during all four phases of self-regulation (Schunk & Ermter, 2000).

Regulation of motivation and affect are important aspects of self-regulation and include regulation of motivational beliefs, self-efficacy, personal interest and value in the task (Pintrich, 2000). Learners' awareness of their motivation and their efforts to control their motivation directly impact learning outcomes. Learners make learning judgments concerning the degree of difficulty of an assignment or content area through metacognition, knowledge of their learning needs and preferred learning strategies in combination with self-efficacy. In addition, learner appreciation of the relevancy of the task and the value to future goals impacts academic motivation to participate and strive for successful learning outcomes. Learner desirability or interest in the content is

TABLE A-3 Phases and Areas for Self-Regulated Learning

Phases	Areas of Regulation			
	Cognition	Motivation/affect	Behavior	Context
1. Forethought, planning & activation	Target goal setting	Goal orientation adoption	[Time and effort planning]	[Perceptions of task]
	Prior content knowledge activation	Efficacy judgments	[Planning for self-observations of behaviors]	[Perceptions of context]
	Metacognitive knowledge activation	Ease of learning judgments; perceptions of task difficulty		
		Task value activation		
		Interest activation		
2. Monitoring	Metacognitive awareness and monitoring of cognition	Awareness and monitoring of motivation and affect	Awareness and monitoring of effort, time use, need of help Self-observation of behavior	Monitoring changing task and context conditions
3. Control	Selection and adaptation of cognitive strategies for learning, thinking	Selection and adaptation of strategies for managing motivation and affect	Increase/decrease effort Persist, give up Help-seeking behavior	Change or renegotiate task Change or leave context
4. Reaction and reflection	Cognitive judgments	Affective reactions	Choice behavior	Evaluation of task
	Attributions	Attributions		Evaluation of context

Source: Pintrich, 2000, p. 454.

also imperative. Conversely, learner anxiety and fear of failure can negatively impact learner interest and value (Pintrich).

Educators can enhance and promote learner self-efficacy, personal interest and value through the effective introduction of new content, linking current learning to future needs, and demonstrating personal value of the content presented and the tasks that students are asked to master (Svinicki, 2004). Educators can provide a pleasant, safe non-threatening learning environment which encourages social interaction among learners thus promoting learner belonging and self-worth; inversely, educators can disrupt the learning environment in an effort to cause dissonance, which can result in cognitive growth (Svinicki). Positive emotions, including pleasure and enjoyment of learning, enhance self-regulation, while negative emotions such as fear and anxiety require extrinsic support (Pekrun, Frenzel, Goetz, & Perry, 2007). Educators have the ability to increase academic motivation by modeling the value of a goal and can influence student goal orientation and value integration during every student-faculty interaction (Svinkcki).

Successful goal attainment does not automatically ensure the use of self-regulation strategies; however, internalization of the value of a goal enhances and sustains motivation (Bandura, 1997; Schunk, 2001b). Learner reflection and self-feedback during the learning process revealing positive learning outcomes can affirm student self-regulation strategies and thus increase motivation and self-efficacy; however, unexpected difficulty or task failure can negatively impact self-efficacy and motivation. Goal properties that support effective self-regulation include goal specificity, goal proximity and difficulty level (Bandura, 1986; Locke & Latham, 1990). Specific goals are easier to measure than non-specific goals and thus, can be more beneficial to motivation. Goal proximity refers to the short-term or long-term outcomes associated with goal attainment. Proximal goals are more motivating than distant goals because short-term goal attainment is quicker and movement toward the completion is more noticeable and demonstrates learning progress (Boekaerts,1995; Cervone, 1993). This concept supports breaking long-term tasks into smaller, more manageable segments.

The difficulty level or attainability of the goal should be appropriate to the learner's ability as a goal that is too easy or too hard does not motivate the learner. Goals should be challenging, but reachable, in order to enhance academic motivation. Locke and Latham (1990) reported that providing feedback increases goal commitment when the feedback focuses on self-improvement, challenge and mastery, and promotes self-efficacy. Challenging the learner by increasing the difficulty level of the learning while maintaining achievability typically results in higher learner performance. Warkentin and Bol (1997) reported significant differences in self-regulatory variances in high achieving and low achieving students and determined that while most students experience difficulty monitoring their personal efforts, lower achieving students tend to memorize content for immediate recall, not long-term future needs.

Locke and Latham (1990) purport that when goals are set by the learner, the learner is more committed to the task and performance is enhanced. If learner performance does not appear to be satisfactory in relation to goal achievement, dissatisfaction can occur, which can lead to increased effort or failure resignation. Learners typically will continue at the learning activity if it is believed that success is possible. Once the goal is successfully reached and the learner has the positive reinforcement associated with success, the learner sets new goals and continues the process (Schunk, 2001b).

Multiple models of self-regulation exist. The Personal Responsibility Orientation model set forth by Brockett and Hiemstra (1991) places self-direction in learning as a overriding theme with two related sub-dimensions. Under the umbrella of self-direction exist the following two constructs: (a) self-directed learning, which incorporates the concepts of the adult learner and teaching-learning process set forth by Knowles, and (b) learner self-direction which focuses on characteristics internal to the individual that "predisposes one toward taking primary responsibility" (p. 29).

The Effort Management Hierarchy model (Thomas & Rohwer, 1993) is based on four hierarchical levels of study activity. These activities include monitoring, self-regulation, planning and evaluating. Thomas and Rohwer purport that learner self-direction occurs in a continuum of activities, which range from awareness of need to individual control of one's study efforts to include concentration, time and learning effectiveness. Regulation and remediation are key to self-directed learning.

Zimmerman's three-phase self-regulation model presents self-regulation as a cyclical process involving learner assessment and feedback of personal, behavioral, and environmental factors during three phases of the learning process: (a) the forethought phase during which goal setting and social modeling occur; (b) performance control during which the learner compares their performance to that of other learners and provides self-instruction regarding learning strategy; and (c) self-reflection, the stage of self-evaluation, resultant feedback, and self-reward for performance success (Schunk, 2001a).

Further discussion regarding self-regulated learning has focused on student interest in the subject matter and the impact of affect on self-regulation and resultant end learning outcomes (Alexander, 1995; Boekaerts, 1995). Bruner (1964) advocated the collaboration of teacher, subject-matter specialist, and psychologist in the development of a curriculum, the learning pace, appropriate points of feedback, and types of feedback. Bruner further argued for the inclusion of multiple teaching strategies and learning activities to facilitate individual learning differences resulting from variations in interest, skills, ease of learning, and cognitive levels.

Additional empirical studies on adult academic self-regulation have focused on specific content areas such as computer skills (Schunk & Ertmer, 1999), reading (Barnett, 2000), writing (Hammann, 2005; Zimmerman, Bandura, & Martinez-Pons, 1992), medical training (Evensen, Salisbury-Glennon, & Glenn, 2001), and vocabulary acquisition (Tseng, Dornyei, & Schmitt, 2006); teaching methods such as the use of hypermedia (Azevedo & Cromley, 2004), case study-based instruction (Ertmer, Newby & MacDougall, 1996), problem-based learning (Evensen, Salisbury-Glennon, & Glenn); and specific cohorts of students such as developmental students (Young & Ley, 2000), students with disabilities (Rubin, McCoach, McGuire, & Reis, 2003), first-year college students, and graduate students. Much effort has focused on adult self-regulated learning related to distance education including Williams and Hellman (2004), Schmidt and Werner (2007), and Artino (2007).

The Role of Motivation in Academic Self-Regulation

While learning may take place in formal educational environments or in an individual's home, individuals participate in learning for different reasons. The reason individuals participate in learning is the core of academic motivational theory. Motivation is a major construct in the personal realm of self-regulation (Zimmerman, 1989). Most often, adults learn because they want to, not because some else wants them to learn (Slotnick, Pelton, Fuller, & Tabor, 1993); however, extrinsic and intrinsic motivators significantly impact adult learner outcomes. The literature is abundant regarding motivation in relation to self-regulation as it pertains to social behavior, healthcare management, workplace performance; however, this discussion will focus solely on academic self-regulation.

Extrinsic and intrinsic motivation can be viewed as the ends of a spectrum or continuum. All learners can be motivated to learn. Knowles (1980) addressed the adult learner's response to different motivators and recognized the value of extrinsic motivator (the desire for a better job, career progression, pay improvements, etc.); however, intrinsic motivators (increased quality of life, increased job satisfaction, increased self-esteem, etc.) are much more beneficial. Young adults are transitioning from external motivators to internal motivators; however, many mature adults may still be primarily extrinsically motivated. Most learners are initially dependent on extrinsic motivation at the beginning of a learning activity (Bruner, 1964). As the learner develops an understanding of the value of the knowledge or content and interest increases, there may be a shift toward intrinsic motivation. In addition, as undergraduate students move into their major field of study, they progress on the continuum of motivation toward intrinsic motivation.

Miller explained the interrelatedness of socioeconomic status and participation in adult education by using Mazlow's theory of hierarchy of needs—basic needs (safety, survival, belonging, shelter, food) must be met before higher needs (recognition, achievement, self-realization) can be considered (Cross, 1981). Miller combined Mazlow's theory with Lewin's force field analysis theory to explain variances in education motivation in different socioeconomic groups. This theory explains why young adults in early independence seek out learning that will increase their stability and income and allow them to support a spouse and family. As these same learners age and the basic needs have been met, focus can shift to achieving status, enjoying learning, and working toward self-realization. This theory also demonstrates why parental obligations and job requirements override learner obligations (Long, 2004).

Tough, Abbey, and Orton (1982) suggested that the learner's conscious expectation of reward for learning exceeds the force of either subconscious or environmental factors and developed a learning model comprised of five stages: (a) engagement, (b) retention, (c) application, (d) gain of material reward (job promotion), and (e) gaining an symbolic reward (degree or certification) (Cross, 1981).

Wlodkowski (1985) reported that six major factors affect motivation to learn and argued that the motivational factors strongly affect how learners learn and what they learn. These factors include attitudes, needs, stimulation, emotion, competence, and reinforcement. Wlodkowski also summarized motivation to be based on the following four desires of adult learners: Success, volition, value, and enjoyment.

Multiple theories attempt to explain reasons why adults are motivated to participate in learning. These theories include the Expectancy-Valence Paradigm developed by Rubenson, the Congruence Model presented by Boshier, and Tough's Anticipated Benefits (Cross, 1981). All models recognize the existence of variances in learner self-regulation motivation specific to the level of extrinsic motivation or intrinsic motivation.

Intrinsic motivation can be defined as the innate desire to learn for the pleasure of learning (Cross, 1981). Intrinsically motivated learners find sincere pleasure in the learning task (Pintrich & Schunk, 1996), and typically have better learning outcomes than learners who are extrinsically motivated (Deci & Ryan, 1985; Knowles, 1984). Intrinsic motivators include the desire for increased job satisfaction, self-esteem, and increased quality of life. While learning occurs in the presence of both intrinsic and extrinsic motivation, tasks that are engaged with high levels of intrinsic motivation are more enjoyable and pleasurable for the learner. In addition, successful learning outcomes provide positive feedback into the motivation loop and increase intrinsic motivation, which then results in increased interest and increased learning (Bandura, 1986).

Superficial or surface learning at the knowledge and comprehension levels is much more indicative of students who possess an extrinsic level of motivation, while deeper learning processes are demonstrated by learners who demonstrate an intrinsic level of motivation (Mansouri et al., 2006; Pintrich, 2000). Walker, Greene and Mansell (2005) investigated the relationship of motivational characteristics of students and reported positive correlations between academics, self-efficacy, and intrinsic motivation related to meaningful cognitive engagement. Their study demonstrated that extrinsic motivation tends to predict superficial cognitive engagement. In addition, multiple quantitative research studies concerning intrinsic and extrinsic factors have been conducted with the majority reporting positive correlations between intrinsic motivation and academic success (Azevedo & Cromley, 2004; Black & Deci, 2000; Grolnick & Ryan, 1987; Ryan & Connell, 1989; Wissmann, 2002). Burton, Lydon, D'Alessandro and Koestner (2006) reported that presenting a learning activity as fun or pleasurable can increase student positive affect and can result in improved learning outcomes.

Self-determination theory is based on the distinct differences between intrinsic and extrinsic motivation and the spectrum of motivation that exists between these two constructs (Burton, Lydon, D'Alessandro, & Koestner, 2006; Ryan & Deci, 2000b).

Internality and externality exist between these two extremes. Four levels or categories of motivation exist and can be conceptualized as a continuum (Svinicki, 2004). Movement from the lowest level to the highest level requires internalization of motivation. At the lowest level of motivation, controlled (external or total extrinsic motivation), the perceived locus of control is external. Learners participate in learning projects or activities for the external reward, such as pay. The learner moves into the next level, introjected motivation, as the motivation to perform the job well for approval of others exceeds the reward of payment. Introjected motivation is more internalized than total extrinsic motivation because the learner's motivation has become the approval of others as opposed to the reward associated with a grade. As the learner moves into the next level, identification, the learner recognizes the value of the learning to his or her future success. Autonomous (complete intrinsic motivation) exists when the learner integrates the values of the society into his or her value structure (Svinicki, 2004).

Deci and Ryan (1985) proposed a continuum of learning motivation which ranges from totally intrinsic motivation where motivation to learn is based on the enjoyment of knowing and the inherent satisfaction of gaining new knowledge to amotivation, a complete lack of any motivation. Deci and Ryan further offered three categories of external events that impact student motivation: (a) informational, regulation events, which support learner autonomy and competence; (b) controlling events, which force control of the learner, restrict creativity and, thus, undermine intrinsic motivation; and (c) amotivation events, which convey inability to achieve mastery of the content which further undermines internal motivation.

Williams and Deci (1996) presented the Self-Determination Model as is applies to medical education (see Figure A-4). They studied the impact of instructor orientation on medical student learning outcomes and approaches to delivery of medical care and partnership with patients; specifically, their research indicated that instructors who have a humanistic orientation, recognize learner differences, and allow individualization in support of adult learner autonomy contribute to greater conceptualization of the content and better psychological adjustment during the learning experience. This in turn contributes to the medical student integration of a humanistic, collaborative approach to patient management.

Ryan and Deci (2000b) further developed the Self-Determination Continuum and provided an updated model which includes the related regulatory styles, loci of causality and corresponding processes (see Figure A-5). This continuum further categorizes extrinsic motivation into four levels: external regulation, introjected regulation, identified regulation, and integrated regulation. Within this model identified regulation is considered somewhat internalized where the learner recognizes the personal importance of the content and consciously values the learning and integrated regulation is viewed as internalized with the learner demonstrating awareness, congruence, and synthesis with self.

Learners who are autonomously regulated report psychological benefits such as enjoyment of learning, better task performance, increased self-efficacy, increased mood, positive coping strategies, better learning outcomes, and better behavioral performance (Black & Deci, 2000; Grolnick & Ryan, 1987; Ryan & Connell, 1989; Zimmerman, 1990). Burton, Lydon, D'Alessandro, and Koestner (2006) suggested that intrinsic motivation and the accompanying interest and enthusiasm predict academic performance.

Bye, Pushkar and Conway (2007) investigated differences in motivation, interest and positive affect in two distinctly different student populations, traditional and non-traditional students, and reported that interest and age were significant predictors of intrinsic motivation to learn. Justice and Dornan (2001) found that while variances in metacognition exist between traditional age and non-traditional age college students, "higher education will need to respond to differences in motivation and learning processes of nontraditional-age students" (p. 248).

FIGURE A-4 Self-determination model applied to medical education (Williams & Deci, 1998, p. 304).

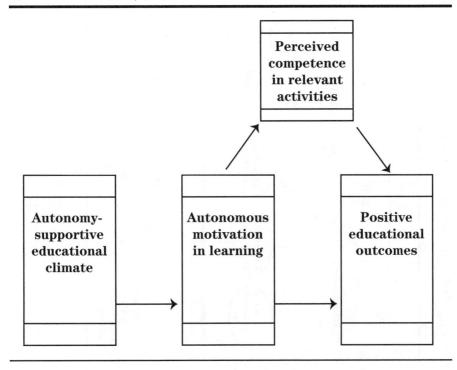

The variable of age as a predictor of self-regulatory behaviors such as cognitive maturity, use of learning strategies, metacognition, and motivation have revealed that older undergraduate students are more self-aware, demonstrate greater self-regulation, and report both intrinsic and extrinsic motivation (Alexander, Murphy, Woods, Duhon & Parker, 1997; Gadzella, Stephens, & Baloglu, 2002; Justice & Dornan, 2001; Kasworm, 2003). Gender differences have been found to relate to variances in motivation as a result of variation in enjoyment of the learning task and variations in response to reward contingencies; however, these variations are common across all individuals and have not been directly linked.

Dornan, Hadfield, Brown, Boshuizen, and Scherpbier (2005) also conducted research on self-directed learning of medical students in the clinical environment and report that academic motivation is increased when the learner has academic support from the educator (Dornan, Hadfield, Brown, Boshuizen, & Scherpbier, 2005). This support can be provided in the following ways in multiple venues: (a) organizational support, (b) pedagogic support, and (c) affective support. Organizational support is comprised of providing opportunities

FIGURE A-5 The self-determination continuum showing types of motivation with their regulatory styles, loci of causality, and corresponding processes (Ryan & Deci, 2000b, p. 72).

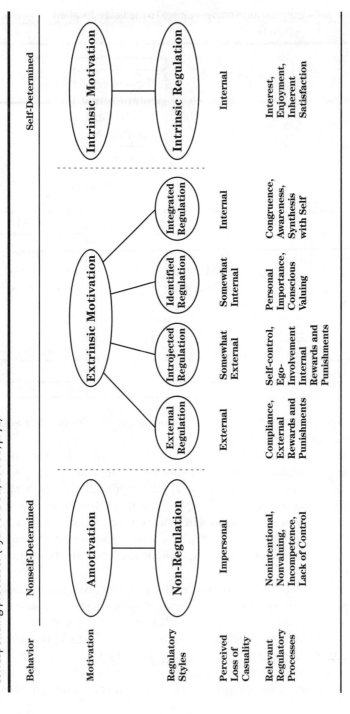

for student learning in an optimal learning environment. Pedagogic support includes guiding the learning in the self-determination of learning objectives, learning strategies, scholastic feedback, and instructional guidance and explanation of content. Affective support consists of supporting students as they transition to a more independent and self-directed learning style, nurturing the student through the process and providing appropriate feedback.

Svinicki (2004) reports multiple opportunities for educators to support academic motivational progression from controlled to autonomous as proposed in self-determination theory. Educators can ensure that learners are provided opportunities to participate in the decision-making process concerning learning approaches and strategies and learners should be granted some control of their work. Collaborating with students to develop course assignments and allowing individualization of course activities support learner autonomy. Educators should strive to model the values that they wish their students to exhibit and base course policies on these values. In addition, timely feedback and encouragement are foundational to the promotion of learner autonomy.

Multiple empirical studies exist regarding educational self-regulation and include extensive exploration and investigation of multiple concepts related to motivation to include the impact of rewards, sharing of knowledge, goal orientation, the importance of parental support, and the role of faculty (Black & Deci, 2000; Cameron & Pierce, 1994; Deci, 1971; Deci & Ryan, 1985; Harder, 2008; Levesque, Zuehlke, Stanek, & Ryan, 2004; Niemiec et al., 2006; Ryan & Deci, 2006; Ryan, Koestner, & Deci, 1991; Ryan, Mims, & Koestner, 1983; Vansteenkiste, Lens, & Deci, 2006; Vansteenkiste, Simons, Lens, Sheldon, & Deci, 2004; Wild, Enzle, Nix, & Deci, 1997). In addition, Cameron (2001) and Deci, Koestner, and Ryan (2001) both provide extensive comprehensive meta-analyses concerning the role of extrinsic rewards in cognitive evaluation theory.

A review of the literature regarding the role of motivation in self-regulation related to self-determination regarding the management of behavioral constructs, psychological health, social development, and physical health management revealed an extensive amount of theoretical offerings (Cameron, 2001; Deci & Ryan, 2000a; Deci & Ryan, 2000b; Deci, Schwartz, Sheinman, & Ryan, 1981; Levesque & Pelletier, 2003; Ryan & Deci, 2000a). In addition, a multitude of empirical investigations have been conducted exploring self-determination as it relates to the previously mentioned topics. These studies are not discussed here since this research is focused on academic self-regulation.

Review of Nursing Education Literature

The literature revealed a minimal number of studies focused on motivation in nursing education and practice with two studies focusing on nurse motivation to persist with continuing education requirements after degree attainment (Bahn, 2007; Cooley, 2008). Both investigations found that nurses pursue continuing education in an effort to stay current, compete with higher educated nurses, and provide safe client care. An additional benefit was the enhancement of their professional self-worth by participating in the continuing education offerings. Välimäki et al. (1999) reported that while nursing students valued self-determination and were willing to exercise self-determination in nursing studies, these same students did not demonstrate self-directed learning behaviors and reported that nurse educators did not support the use of these behaviors.

McEwan and Goldenberg (1999) explored achievement motivation, anxiety, and academic success in first-year graduate nursing students and reported that younger students were more achievement motivated than older students. Research findings suggested that students who were in school to secure employment had a greater anxiety level and more fear of failure with a lower achievement motivation than older students who were currently employed but in school to increase their economic status.

Green (1987) found that most graduate nursing students are female, between 30 and 40 years of age, and have multiple role demands which can result in increased stress and poor academic performance. Thompson (1992) reported that multiple role requirements of older students to include that of parent, spouse and student, increased the stress of the academic experience. Lopez (1992) explored the impact of demographic, academic, and personal variables on nursing student attrition and reported that nursing grades, family support and academic support are supporting factors which limit nursing student attrition. Vincent (1992) also reported that a grade point average of 3.0 or more in the nursing major courses was predictive of degree attainment. Further research by Smedley (2007) reported self-directed learner readiness increases with life experience; consequently, older students typically demonstrate more tendencies toward self-directed learning than younger students. Smedley asserts that nursing curricula must include both teacher-directed and student-directed learning activities.

Lee (2007) discussed nursing student use of academic help-seeking behaviors and explored theory related to self-efficacy, motivation and self-regulation interspersed with anecdotal comments and provided suggestions for nurse educators and academic administrators to promote nursing student help-seeking behaviors in three specific areas—culture, communication, and commitment. Ofori and Charlton (2002) reported that help-seeking behaviors prove to be more predictive of academic success than entry qualifications; in addition, older students tend to demonstrate more willingness to seek out support, which results in overall higher academic success. Additional empirical research suggests that nursing students with a greater self-reported interest in the content utilize a deep approach to learning, which results in increased academic success (Mansouri et al., 2006).

Tutor (2006) explored associate degree nursing student motivational factors and reported that academic self-efficacy, achievement goal orientation, and self-regulation of learning were significant predictors of academic success. This finding supports the need for faculty support of both self-efficacy and self-regulation learning strategies as ways to support positive student learning outcomes and limit attrition. Nilsson and Stomberg (2008) surveyed Swedish nursing student learning motivation throughout three years of nursing study and reported that extrinsic motivators such as teacher involvement, curricular design, social relationships, and successful nursing certification were more common than the intrinsic motivation of the pleasure of learning. Nilsson and Stomberg urge further investigation utilizing a more specific measurement tool.

Myers (1999) compared the learning strategies of associate degree nursing students and baccalaureate degree nursing students to determine variances in the use of metacognition, metamotivation, metamemory, critical thinking, and resource management and considered multiple variables to include age, gender, previous degree, previous healthcare experience, previous work experience, martial status, residence conditions and location, and grade point average. While the sample size was small (34 associate degree students and 19 baccalaureate students), the findings support the conclusion that associate degree students utilized metamotivation learning strategies more frequently than baccalaureate students. Myers asserts that associate degree nurses may have demonstrated higher intrinsic motivation because the pursuit of a nursing degree would help to solve an acute problem such as the need for financial gain or single parenting demands. In addition, Myers offers the explanation that baccalaureate students are typically younger and most sought degrees in nursing due to the "extrinsic value of employment pursuits and monetary rewards" (1999, p. 92).

Myers (1999) recommended that future efforts focus on the intrinsic reasons for choosing a career in nursing, such as caring for others and contributing to society and argued that the modification of "internal values must be changed before outward motivation can be exhibited" (p. 94). Myers further suggests that kindergarten children be introduced to hospitals and visit the sick and infirmed in an effort to promote this intrinsic valuation of caring for the ill. While this is a novel idea, intrinsic motivation is much more than seeking nursing as a career to satisfy altruistic desires to serve the sick. Nursing is a demanding scientific educational discipline and students should be encouraged to recognize that altruistic desires serve to promote motivation, but this motivation can waiver during periods of stress and fear, as reported by McEwan and Goldenberg (1999).

Walker et al. (2007) explored the differences in student motivation for learning between second-degree and traditional nursing students and reported that second-degree students, regardless of age, had higher intrinsic motivation; however, these same students reported a greater desire for faculty guidance and organized classroom activities and placed a higher importance on the final course grade than traditional nursing students. Hudson (1992) investigated why individuals pursue graduate nursing degrees in relation to the expectancy–valence theory, cognitive motivation theory, and multiple independent variables including age, incentive, enrollment statues, and grade point average and determined that no correlation existed. The study found that the independent variables were not predictors of incentive for graduate nursing students. Hudson recommends improving the measurement tool and further investigation to determine whether incentives can be found to be significant predictors of academic success or attrition.

Delaney and Piscopo (2004) investigated associate degree nurses' motivation to obtain a baccalaureate nursing degree and determined that multiple factors serve as motivation for further degree attainment including the desire to compete in the work environment, experience professional advancement, and personal growth. Barriers to continuing academic pursuit included family and work demands, role conflict, financial concerns, and the lack a strong support system (Birks, Chapman, & Francis, 2006; Campaniello, 1988; Lengacher, 1993; Thompson, 1992; Zuzelo, 2001).

Research has been conducted concerning the use of hybrid learning environments, those which integrate web-based support with traditional classroom management approaches, in nursing education. Kumrow (2005) examined the predictability of five self-regulatory resource management strategies in determining nursing student academic success within a hybrid learning environment. The management strategies explored included time management, study environment, effort regulation, help seeking, and peer learning. While the sample size was limited to 31, Kumrow asserts the importance of help-seeking behaviors in the successful completion of a web-based hybrid course and encourages nurse educators of current and future web-based courses to provide sufficient help-seeking pathways to ensure that the student does not learn in isolation and suggests that further research efforts focus on the cognitive, metacognitive, and motivational aspects of self-regulation theory and how these other elements predict academic success in web-based hybrid courses.

Lemcool (2007) investigated the impact of coaching on the use of self-regulated learning strategies on nursing student academic performance and attitudes toward self-regulated learning strategies. Again, the sample size was rather small (26 with 13 participants in the experimental group and 13 participants in the control group), which Lemcool contributes to the resultant lack of significance; however, Lemcool argues that high-academic achieving students utilize self-regulated learning strategies and that the study should be replicated with an increased sample size to determine if coaching does in fact promote increased use of self-regulation learning strategies.

Academic Motivation Measurement Tools

Additional learning motivation measurement tools are available. The Motivated Strategies for Learning Questionnaire (MLSQ) consists of an 81-item self-reported survey which provides information concerning student goal and value beliefs, skill requirements, assessment anxiety and cognitive and metacognitive learning strategies specific to a single course (Artino, 2007; Pintrich, Smith, Garcia, & McKeachie, 1993). Pintrich, Smith, Garcia, and McKeachie (1991) reported research conducted with the MSLQ indicates that traditional students demonstrate higher extrinsic goal orientation than non-traditional students. Vallerand et al. (1992) proposed the Echelle de Motivation in Education, the French precursor to the English version named the Academic Motivation Scale, in an effort to further explore three proposed subcategories of intrinsic motivation: (a) intrinsic motivation to know, (b) intrinsic motivation to accomplish tasks, and (c) intrinsic motivation to experience stimulation. Additional literature focuses on the validity of this instrument and possible future uses of the Academic Motivation Scale to further the understanding of the impacting factors and the peculiarities of intrinsic motivation (Vallerand et al., 1993).

Ryan and Connell (1989) developed the Academic Self-Regulation Scale, which has been used for assessing the level of autonomous regulation in children and has been modified for students with learning disabilities. This measurement tool is comprised of four questions regarding student reasons for completing various learning behaviors including homework, classwork, asking questions in class, and general overall school performance. Each question is followed by multiple responses which can be classified into one of the four self-regulation categories: external regulation, introjected regulation, identified regulation, and intrinsic motivation.

The Learning Self-Regulation Questionnaire (LSRQ), designed for use with adult learners, assesses learning motivation on two scales, controlled regulation (external regulation or introjected regulation) and autonomous regulation (identified regulation or intrinsic regulation). While these levels of regulation are categorized under external motivation, the differentiation of academic self-regulation between these two categories serves as the transitional point as the learner moves from extrinsic to intrinsic motivation (Ryan & Deci, 2000a). This measurement tool has been used to assess academic self-regulation in particular college courses such as organic chemistry (Williams & Deci, 1996) and organ systems (Black & Deci, 2000). Scoring can be based on the two scales, autonomous regulation and controlled regulation, or a Relative Autonomy Index can be calculated by subtracting the controlled subscale z-score from the autonomous subscale z-score. Previous studies report the following alpha reliabilities for the two subscales: approximately 0.75 for controlled regulation and 0.80 for autonomous regulation (Black & Deci; Williams & Deci). This measurement tool will be used for this research project.

Multiple research studies have investigated the variable of age as a predictor of self-regulatory behaviors such as cognitive maturity, use of learning strategies, metacognition, and motivation and reported that older undergraduate students demonstrate more self-awareness, greater self-regulation, and both intrinsic and extrinsic motivation (Alexander, Murphy, Woods, Duhon & Parker, 1997; Gadzella, Stephens, & Baloglu, 2002; Justice & Dornan, 2001; Kasworm, 2003); however, none of these studies have investigated the differences of academic self-regulation between different groups of nursing students, specifically previous degree nurses seeking a baccalaureate degree and traditional baccalaureate nursing students. The different reasons individuals have for participating in learning form the basis of motivation variances in adult learners (Cross, 1981).

August-Brady (2005) investigated the effect of metacognitive intervention on baccalaureate nursing student academic self-regulation and reported educators must understand student approaches to learning and self-regulation of learning. In addition, educators must understand the effectiveness of teaching practices on self-regulated learning development. August-Brady encouraged further nursing education research in this specific area. Wissmann (2002) explored nursing student metacognition and recognized a strong relationship between nursing student learning effort and interest and motivation; furthermore, Wissmann reported that motivation was directly impacted by nursing students' personal goals for adequate performance and the importance of current content to future nursing practice.

Alexander and Murphy (1999) recognize the need for further multidimensional research on individual adult learner variances and the impact of motivational factors on student success in the formal learning environment. Bye, Pushkar, and Conway (2007) argued that further study is warranted to determine if there is a correlation between age, degree persistence, and intrinsic motivation. Understanding the impact of life factors on variances in academic motivation can facilitate educators in the development of more effective instructional environments and learning activities.

Summary

The paradigm shift from a teacher-centered teaching to learner-centered learning requires educators to understand the uniqueness of different nursing student subgroups and how to best serve these groups of students during the academic development of critical thinking and self-directed learning strategies (Billings & Halstead, 2005; Cowman, 1998; Magena & Chabeli, 2005; Välimäki et al., 1999). Nurse educators must consider the unique needs of the individual student and the theoretical constructs of self-directed learning, self-regulation, and learning motivation and the use of educational strategies and support methods to promote and enhance student integration of content value and progression toward intrinsic motivation.

The specific problem investigated in this study is the variance of academic self-regulation and the possible impact of various independent factors on the individual motivation. Chapter III will present the research design and data analysis. The results of the research study will be discussed in Chapter IV. Chapter V will conclude with a summary and discussion, implications of the findings, recommendations for use of the findings, and a conclusion based on the study findings.

CHAPTER III: METHODS

The purpose of this study was to determine if there was a difference in self-regulation behaviors (autonomous vs. controlled) in two distinct groups of nursing students: (a) traditional baccalaureate nursing students, and (b) non-traditional baccalaureate nursing students (licensed nurses who have previously completed a diploma or associate degree nursing program and are returning to nursing school to obtain a baccalaureate degree). Research participants were nursing students in a baccalaureate nursing program at one southeastern public Alabama university.

This chapter presents the methods used in this research study to include the purpose and design of the study, population and sample selection, instrument validity and reliability, and data collection strategies. The chapter will conclude with a discussion of the data analysis process.

Design of the Study

This was a cross-sectional study focused on the identification of academic self-regulation differences in two distinct groups of nursing students wherein the data was collected during a single encounter with each participant in an effort to describe the differences among groups of participants (Houser, 2008). This type of research design is beneficial when attempting to solicit data on attitudes, behaviors, and demographic data from a large number of participants as it is relatively inexpensive, does not involve an intervention or treatment, and has limited loss of subjects from attrition. Disadvantages to this type of research include the inability to measure change over time due to the single collection of data and difficulty determining causal association. Cross-sectional studies are often used as a pilot study prior to conducting longitudinal research (Houser).

The primary independent variable of this study was student designation as either a TBSN student or NTBSN student. Additional independent variables of interest included demographic data collected by participant completion of the Demographic Data Collection Tool (DDCT). The dependent variable was nursing students' academic self-regulation as operationalized by the autonomous regulation subscale (ARS) score and the controlled regulation subscale (CRS) score as determined from the LSRQ questionnaire.

Research Questions

The research questions for this study were:

1. Is there a statistically significant difference in academic self-regulation behaviors (autonomous versus controlled) in the following two distinct groups of nursing students: Traditional baccalaureate nursing students and non-traditional baccalaureate nursing students (licensed nurses who have previously completed a diploma or associate degree nursing program and are returning to nursing school to obtain a baccalaureate degree)?
2. Are there significant differences in the following demographic characteristics between the same two groups of baccalaureate nursing students: Age, sex, ethnicity, marital status, family structure, number of dependent children, previous healthcare experience, current GPA, number of hours in independent study per week, number of hours studying collaboratively per week, number of work hours per week, and number of years since previous degree?

Sampling

The sample studied consisted of all nursing students enrolled in a baccalaureate nursing program and included two groups: (a) traditional BSN students, and (b) non-traditional baccalaureate nursing students (students who are licensed nurses, have previously completed a diploma or associate degree nursing program, and are returning to academia to obtain a baccalaureate degree). The university selected for this study was a small southeastern university established in 1967 with an enrollment of 5,124 undergraduate and graduate students. This university offers degrees in Business, Education, Liberal Arts,

Nursing and Science. The average student age is 25 with over one-third of the student body comprised of students 24 years or older. Approximately 80% of the students are employed part time or full time and many commute to campus (Auburn University Montgomery, 2008).

The sample was a non-probability convenience sample of available students enrolled in the nursing program. Criteria for participant selection included enrollment in upper division nursing courses. All enrolled nursing students were invited to participate in the study on a voluntary basis. Power analysis was not conducted prior to the study; however, the use of 100 or more subjects supports the generalizability of the findings (Houser, 2008). The minimum number of participants was set at 100. The initial sample consisted of a total of 215 participants; however, fifteen participants did not complete all aspects of the DDCT and these subjects' contributions were not included in the sample.

The final sample comprised 200 participants with 149 traditional baccalaureate nursing students (74.5%) and 51 non-traditional baccalaureate students (25.5%). The age range of the participants was from 19 to 55 years with a mean age of 27.79 years, mode of 21 years, median of 24 years, and a standard deviation of 8.44. The sample included 154 Caucasians (77%), 37 African-Americans (18.5%), three Hispanics (1.5%), two Asians (1%), and four participants indicated "other" (2%). The 168 participants (84%) were female and 32 participants (16%) were male.

Study Variables

The primary independent variable of this study was student type which consisted of TBSN and NTBNSD students. The dependent variable was nursing student academic self-regulation as operationalized by the total scores of the responses on the LSRQ survey. Additional independent variables of interest were collected through use of the DDCT.

Instrumentation

The Learning Self-Regulation Questionnaire (LSRQ), originally designed by Williams and Deci (1996) to assess academic self-regulation in a medical school course, was used in this study following minor modification to reflect studies in the field of nursing. This tool has been used in various forms in multiple research studies (Black & Deci, 2000; Ryan & Connell, 1989; Williams & Deci, 1996). Permission to use and modify the LSRQ for this research was obtained from Deci (personal communication, November 10, 2007).

The LSRQ is a 14-item questionnaire (see Appendix A-1) which assessed academic self-regulation on two scales, controlled regulation and autonomous regulation. Three primary questions (A, B, & C) were presented with multiple response choices (1–14) to which the respondent indicated the likelihood of that choice using a Likert-type response with answer choices ranging from 1 indicating "not at all true" to 7 indicating "very true." Participant responses were tallied for two subscales: autonomous regulation and controlled regulation. The autonomous regulation subscale score was determined by averaging the answers to the following questions: 1, 3, 6, 9, 11, 13, and 14. The controlled regulation subscale score required the averaging of responses to questions 2, 4, 5, 7, 8, 10, and 12.

Instrument validity refers to the strength of the survey tool to measure what is intended to be measured (Polit & Hungler, 1999). The instrument validity of the LSRQ was ensured through the review of previous published studies which used this research tool and reported good internal consistency and construct validity for this research instrument. The original instrument was used to by Ryan and Connell (1989) to assess learning autonomy in children and was later modified twice by Williams and Deci (1996) to reflect different curriculum content for use with college students. Williams and Deci reported strong validity for both modified versions of this tool. In addition, Black and Deci (2000) reported construct validity for the LSRQ. This instrument was slightly modified to reflect nursing curriculum similar to the modifications in previous studies.

Reliability refers to the consistency of a measurement tool in measuring a particular attribute (Polit & Beck, 2006). When determining instrument reliability, the instrument should be examined for stability and internal consistency. Stability of an instrument examining a psychosocial construct such as academic self-regulation or learning style preference is questionable. The LSRQ is similar to the VARK Questionnaire, which helps students determine their preference for receiving, giving, and processing information as these types of instruments are not designed to be "reliable in terms of consistency of scores of a long period of time" (Fleming, 2006). While test-retest reliability procedures support instrument stability, test-retest methods are not reliable when assessing stability of the instrument due to multiple factors which may impact participant responses such as attitude and mood differences and experiences which may have occurred between the two measurements (Polit & Beck).

Internal consistency, the reliability of the LSRQ subscales to measure the expected characteristics, autonomous regulation and controlled regulation, is supported by reviewing the reported Cronbach's alpha reliabilites for the instrument from previous studies. Previous studies report the alpha reliabilities ranging from 0.75 to 0.80 for autonomous regulation subscale and 0.67 to 0.75 for controlled regulation subscale (Black & Deci, 2000; Williams & Deci, 1996).

Since this questionnaire was modified to reflect nursing curricula and questions were generalized to learning efforts related to all nursing courses, not just one specific course, additional factorial analysis was required. The reliability of survey tools utilizing a Likert scale format producing interval and ratio measures can be determined by performing a Cronbach's alpha test of internal consistency (LoBiondo-Wood & Haber, 2006). The desired score of 0.70 or greater on a scale of 0 to 1.0 demonstrates survey tool reliability. The reliability of the modified LSRQ was verified with a reported Cronbach's alpha on the autonomous regulation subscale and the controlled regulation subscale were .768 and .725 respectively.

The DDCT (see Appendix A-2) was used to collect the following data: (a) student classification (nominal scale as TBNS or NTBNS); (b) sex (nominal scale); (c) age (interval scale); (d) ethnicity; (e) marital status (single, married, divorced, widowed); (f) family unit (two-parent family, single-parent family, or no children); (g) number of dependent children; (h) previous healthcare experience; (i) current GPA; (j) number of hours spent independently on school work per week; (k) number of hours spent in collaboration on school work per week; (l) hours employed per week; (m) years since previous degree; and (n) previous degree GPA. The study demographic variable results of the DDCT are presented in Tables A-4 to A-7.

Procedures

Permission to utilize and modify the original LSRQ was obtained from Deci. The dean of the Auburn University Montgomery School of Nursing granted the researcher permission to conduct the research. The Auburn University Montgomery Institutional Review Board granted approval of the research study and Auburn University Institutional Review Board (IRB) also approved the research study as the principal investigator was conducting the research to satisfy degree requirements as a graduate student at Auburn University. The researcher contacted faculty within the School of Nursing to coordinate collection dates.

Students were approached at the end of class time. The Recruitment Script (see Appendix A-3) was read to each student group by the principal investigator; it provided an overview of the research study and invited students to participate in the study on a voluntary basis. The researcher was course faculty for two groups of participating students; consequently, in an effort to limit risk and discomfort related to coercion, a colleague agreed to support this research effort by conducting the data collection portion of the research for these two groups. This required the use of an alternative recruitment script (see Appendix A-4). In addition to the Recruitment Script, each potential participant was provided an Information Letter which reiterated the information provided in the recruitment script.

TABLE A-4 Study Variables Including Sex, Ethnicity, Marital Status, and Family Structure

Variable	TBNS		NTBNS	
	n	%	n	%
Sex				
Female	129	86.6	39	76.5
Male	20	13.4	12	23.5
Ethnicity				
Caucasian	118	79.2	36	70.6
African-American	22	14.8	15	29.4
Hispanic	3	2.0	0	0.0
Asian	2	1.3	0	0.0
Other	4	2.7	0	0.0
Marital Status				
Single	108	72.5	11	21.6
Married	31	21.0	33	64.7
Divorced	10	6.5	7	13.7
Widowed	0	0.0	0	0.0
Family Structure				
No children	111	74.5	12	23.5
Two-parent family	26	17.5	33	64.7
One-parent family	12	8.0	6	11.8

N = 200

There was no direct compensation for participants involved in this research study. Participation was strictly voluntary with participants being fully aware that refusal to participate was acceptable. Participants were advised to withdraw from the study prior to completing the requested LSRQ and DDCT by simply not returning the two surveys. Participants were further informed that once these tools were collected, the participant's specific response tool would not be retrievable as it would not have identifiable information on it. The average time to complete the data tool was five minutes.

There were minimal risks associated with study participation. The primary identified risk was that of a breach of confidentiality. This was addressed by the use of anonymous, uncoded data and limited access to the data by only the researcher and faculty sponsor. Another possible risk was psychological or

TABLE A-5 Study Variables Including Number of Dependent Children, Previous Healthcare Experience, and Current GPA

Variable	TBNS		NTBNS	
	n	%	*n*	%
Number of Dependent Children				
None	110	73.8	14	27.5
One	20	13.4	16	31.3
Two	11	7.4	19	37.2
Three	6	4.1	1	2.0
Four	1	0.6	1	2.0
Five	1	0.6	0	0.0
Previous Healthcare Experience				
Yes	56	37.6	51	100
No	93	62.4	0	0.0
Current GPA				
2.0 – 2.49	1	0.6	0	0.0
2.5 – 2.99	31	21.0	8	15.7
3.0 – 3.49	74	49.7	21	41.2
3.5 – 4.0	43	28.7	22	43.1

$N = 200$

social discomfort resulting from the social pressure to participate to please the researcher or to be part of the social group. The research tools were returned to the research in a sealed envelope in an effort to limit this risk. Lastly, participants may have felt coerced to participate because of the progression requirements in the school of nursing or due to the fact the researcher was faculty of record for two participant groups. Participants were encouraged to discuss concerns regarding feelings about participating in this research with the researcher, the participant's advisor, or the university counseling center. Contact information for the counseling center was provided on the information letter. Additionally, to help decrease the risk of students' feeling coerced to participate and to protect confidentiality, the following measures were taken:

- No faculty member teaching the participant was involved in recruitment or data collection.
- Participants were counseled not to complete any question which made the participant uncomfortable.

TABLE A-6 Study Variables Including Number of Independent Study Hours and Collaborative Study Hours per Week

Variable	TBNS		NTBNS	
	n	%	*n*	%
# of Hours Spent Independently on School Work per Week				
< 5	2	1.3	2	3.9
6 to 10	14	9.4	7	13.7
11 to 15	30	20.1	8	15.7
16 to 20	46	30.8	13	25.5
21 to 25	22	14.8	7	13.7
26 to 30	17	11.4	6	11.8
> 30	18	12.1	8	15.7
# of Hours Spent in Collaboration on School Work per Week				
< 5	46	30.1	15	29.4
6 to 10	32	21.4	11	21.6
11 to 15	18	12.1	10	19.6
16 to 20	14	9.4	5	9.8
21 to 25	11	7.4	4	7.8
26 to 30	10	6.7	4	7.8
> 30	18	12.1	2	3.9

N = 200

- Data was collected anonymously in a sealed envelope.
- Sealed envelopes were not opened until grades were submitted for the courses.
- Only the researcher and faculty sponsor had access to the individual data collection tools.

The researcher entered the collected data into an Excel spreadsheet after which the data collection tools were then stored in a locked cabinet in the researcher's office. Only the researcher and the faculty sponsor had access to the data for analysis.

Two anticipated benefits of participation in this study were identified. First, participants might gain a greater sense of appreciation for research related to adult education and nursing education. Specifically, the participants were required to successfully complete a course on research in nursing. Participation in this research effort may have provided an opportunity to witness the actual research process thus enforcing the importance of research

TABLE A-7 Study Variables Including Number of Hours Employed per Week and Years Since Previous Degree

	TBNS		NTBNS	
Variable	n	%	n	%
# of Hours Employed per Week				
0	80	53.7	2	3.9
1 to 10	15	10.1	0	0.0
11 to 20	40	26.8	4	7.8
21 to 30	11	7.4	2	3.9
31 to 40	3	2.0	42	82.4
> 40	0	0.0	1	2.0
Years Since Previous Degree				
1 to 3 years	17	11.5	15	29.4
4 to 5 years	20	13.4	16	31.3
6 to 10 years	8	5.3	17	33.4
11 to 15 years	0	0.0	3	5.9
> 15 years	0	0.0	0	0.0
No previous degree	104	69.8	0	0.0

$N = 200$

procedures such as IRB approval, informed consent, consideration of methods to ensure confidentiality and proper data storage, and data collection tools. In addition, students may have gained a sense of self-contribution to the larger field of knowledge regarding adult education and academic self-regulation.

Statistical Analysis

Data was originally entered into an Excel spreadsheet and then imported into Statistical Package for the Social Sciences (SPSS) Version 15 for further analysis. For this study, descriptive statistics were used to analyze the demographic data and scores on the LSRQ. A one-way Analysis of Variance (ANOVA) was completed to determine the differences between self-regulated learning in the two distinct groups of nursing students. The student group was the independent variable and the differences in student academic self-regulation between groups was the dependent variable. The one-way ANOVA is used to test the difference among the independent groups and analyzes categorical or nominal independent variables and continuous (interval or ratio data) variables (Polit & Beck, 2006).

The data collected was analyzed in the following manner:

1. A one-way ANOVA was conducted on both autonomous regulation sub-scale (ARS) scores and the controlled regulation subscale (CRS) scores to determine if statistically significant differences existed between to two groups. Statistical significance was set at $p < 0.05$.
2. The demographic variables were further analyzed with follow-up ANOVAs and subsequent post-hoc analysis was performed, as appropriate, to further isolate any reported differences between groups.
3. Simple linear regression analyses of the demographic data of participant age and the number of dependent children in relation to the ARS was also conducted. Results from the study will be further discussed in Chapter IV.

Summary

While nursing academia has long assumed academic self-regulation differences in nursing students in different educational settings, limited research exists which has focused on the academic self-regulation in nursing students. The understanding of the differences in student achievement motivation across nursing educational environments would provide insight to nursing faculty as coursework outcomes and learning outcomes are developed. In addition, academic self-regulation theory may provide an impetus for faculty decision making regarding teaching methods such as hybrid or online course offerings. This research explores the existence of differences in academic self-regulation across distinct nursing student populations and provides insight into the impact of additional variables such as age, gender, race, socioeconomic status, family size, and fiscal responsibility on academic self-regulation.

This chapter presented the methods used in this research study to include the purpose and design of the study, population and sample selection, instrument validity and reliability, data collection strategies, and the data analysis process. The results of the data analysis will be discussed in detail in Chapter IV.

CHAPTER IV: RESULTS

The purpose of this study was to determine if there was a difference in self-regulation behaviors (autonomous vs. controlled) in two distinct groups of nursing students: (a) traditional baccalaureate nursing students, and (b) non-traditional baccalaureate nursing students (licensed nurses who have previously completed a diploma or associate degree nursing program and are returning to nursing school to obtain a baccalaureate degree). Research participants were nursing students in a baccalaureate nursing program at one southeastern public Alabama university.

Research Questions

The following research questions were used in this study:

1. Is there a statistically significant difference in academic self-regulation behaviors (autonomous versus controlled) in the following two distinct groups of nursing students: Traditional baccalaureate nursing students and non-traditional baccalaureate nursing students (licensed nurses who have previously completed a diploma or associate degree nursing program and are returning to nursing school to obtain a baccalaureate degree)?
2. Are there significant differences in the following demographic characteristics between the same two groups of baccalaureate nursing students: Age, sex, ethnicity, marital status, family structure, number of dependent children, previous healthcare experience, current GPA, number of hours in independent study per week, number of hours studying collaboratively per week, number of work hours per week, and number of years since previous degree?

The data collected was analyzed in the following manner:

1. A one-way Analysis of Variance (ANOVA) was conducted on both ARS scores and the CRS scores to determine if statistically significant differences existed between to two groups. Statistical significance was set at $p < 0.05$.
2. The demographic variables were further analyzed with follow-up ANOVAs and subsequent post-hoc analysis was performed, as appropriate, to further isolate any reported differences between groups.
3. Simple linear regression analyses of the demographic data of participant age and the number of dependent children in relation to the ARS was also conducted.

The final sample consisted of 200 participants, 149 traditional baccalaureate nursing students (TBNS) and 51 non-traditional baccalaureate nursing students (NTBNS). The researcher initially entered the data into a Microsoft Excel spreadsheet and then imported the data into Statistical Package for the Social Sciences (SPSS) Version 15 for analysis. Further analysis was completed using R-Project software. For this study, descriptive statistics were used to analyze the demographic data and scores on the LSRQ. A one-way ANOVA was completed to determine the differences between self-regulated learning in two distinct groups of nursing students. The student group was the independent variable and the student academic self-regulation as operationalized by the participants' scores on the LSRQ acted as the dependent variable.

Study Design

This is a cross-sectional study which focused on the identification of academic self-regulation differences in two distinct groups of nursing students in an effort to assist nurse educators in understanding the varying self-regulation of nursing students. As an exploratory method, descriptive studies garner a large amount of data which can then be explored in a cross-sectional manner to determine possible relationships between suspected variables (LoBiondo-Wood & Haber, 2006) and additional variables can be readily examined to determine new information about a phenomena (Merriam & Simpson, 1995). This study design compared student learning self-regulation as measured by scores on the Learning Self-Regulation Questionnaire (LSRQ) for two distinct groups of nursing students, TBNS and NTBNS, through the use of a one-way ANOVA. The differentiation in student classification served as the independent variable and the dependent variable was the three resultant LSRQ scores. The assumptions associated with the ANOVA test were met. The scores were normally distributed in the population. Random and independent sampling took place. Levene's Test of Equality of Error Variances ($p = .710$) indicated the group variance was not statistically significantly different; therefore, the assumption of equal variances was not violated.

Sample size with a minimum of 100 participants was desired by the researcher in an effort to ensure power and generalizability of the findings. The initial sample consisted of a total of 215 participants. Fifteen of 215 participants did not complete all aspects of the Demographic Data Collection Tool (DDCT); consequently, those participants' responses were not included in the analyzed sample. The final sample was comprised of 200 participants. The TBNS group consisted of 149 participants, 74.5% of the overall sample, and the NTBNS group consisted of 51 participants, 25.5% of the overall sample.

Descriptive Statistics

The age range of the participants was from 19 to 55 years with a mean age of 27.79 years, mode of 21 years, median of 24 years, and a standard deviation of 8.44. The sample included 154 Caucasians (77%), 37 African-Americans (18.5%), three Hispanics (1.5%), and two Asians (1%). Four participants indicated "other" ethnicity (2%). The sample consisted of 168 female participants (84%) and 32 male participants (16%). A breakdown of the additional independent variables obtained from the DDCT is provided in Tables A-8 to A-11.

TABLE A-8 Review of Study Variables Including Sex, Ethnicity, Marital Status, and Family Structure

	TBNS		NTBNS	
Variable	*n*	%	*n*	%
Sex				
Female	129	86.6	39	76.5
Male	20	13.4	12	23.5
Ethnicity				
Caucasian	118	79.2	36	70.6
African-American	22	14.8	15	29.4
Hispanic	3	2.0	0	0.0
Asian	2	1.3	0	0.0
Other	4	2.7	0	0.0
Marital Status				
Single	108	72.5	11	21.6
Married	31	21.0	33	64.7
Divorced	10	6.5	7	13.7
Widowed	0	0.0	0	0.0
Family Structure				
No children	111	74.5	12	23.5
Two-parent family	26	17.5	33	64.7
One-parent family	12	8.0	6	11.8

N = 200

Instrumentation

Prior to analyzing the data, instrument reliability of the LSRQ was ensured by performing a Cronbach's alpha test of internal consistency on the instrument. Cronbach's alpha tests were computed for both the ARS and the CRS subscales. The reported Cronbach's alpha on the items used to calculate the ARS and the CRS were .77 and .73 respectively. These scores fall within the desired score of 0.70 or greater on a scale of 0 to 1.0 (LoBiondo-Wood & Haber, 2006), which indicates that the LSRQ provided a consistent measure. "As a rough rule of thumb, a measure is considered reliable for most research and practical purposes if its reliability coefficient is .80 or higher. (In the case of one type of reliability coefficient, Cronbach's Alpha, a value of .70 or higher is usually sufficient)" (Gall, Gall & Borg, 2005, p. 140). Assurance of survey tool

TABLE A-9 Review of Study Variables Including Number of Dependent Children, Previous Healthcare Experience, and Current GPA

Variable	TBNS		NTBNS	
	n	%	*n*	%
Number of Dependent Children				
None	110	73.8	14	27.5
One	20	13.4	16	31.3
Two	11	7.4	19	37.2
Three	6	4.1	1	2.0
Four	1	0.6	1	2.0
Five	1	0.6	0	0.0
Previous Healthcare Experience				
Yes	56	37.6	51	100
No	93	62.4	0	0.0
Current GPA				
2.0 – 2.49	1	0.6	0	0.0
2.5 – 2.99	31	21.0	8	15.7
3.0 – 3.49	74	49.7	21	41.2
3.5 – 4.0	43	28.7	22	43.1

N = 200

reliability was imperative as the tool was slightly modified to reflect nursing curricula and questions were generalized to learning efforts related to all nursing curriculum courses. In previous studies, the LSRQ was designed to focus solely on one particular course (Black & Deci, 2000: Williams & Deci, 1996).

Data Analysis

The LSRQ provides a total of three scores for each participant: (a) the ARS score; (b) the CRS score; and (c) the Relative Autonomy Index score. Since the Relative Autonomy Index score is comprised of further calculation of the two subscales, analysis of the Relative Autonomy Index score was not performed. The ARS score was determined by averaging participant answers to the following questions: 1, 3, 6, 9, 11, 13, and 14. The CRS score required averaging of participant responses to questions 2, 4, 5, 7, 8, 10, and 12. Table A-12 provides the means and standard deviations for participant responses on the LSRQ for

TABLE A-10 Review of Study Variables Including Number of Independent Study Hours and Collaborative Study Hours per Week

Variable	TBNS		NTBNS	
	n	%	*n*	%
# of Hours Spent Independently on School Work per Week				
< 5	2	1.3	2	3.9
6 to 10	14	9.4	7	13.7
11 to 15	30	20.1	8	15.7
16 to 20	46	30.8	13	25.5
21 to 25	22	14.8	7	13.7
26 to 30	17	11.4	6	11.8
> 30	18	12.1	8	15.7
# of Hours Spent in Collaboration on School Work per Week				
< 5	46	30.1	15	29.4
6 to 10	32	21.4	11	21.6
11 to 15	18	12.1	10	19.6
16 to 20	14	9.4	5	9.8
21 to 25	11	7.4	4	7.8
26 to 30	10	6.7	4	7.8
> 30	18	12.1	2	3.9

N = 200

all 14 questions. The means for the questions utilized to calculate the ARS scale (1, 3, 6, 9, 11, 13, and 14) are significantly higher than the means for the questions specific to the CRS scale (2, 4, 5, 7, 8, 10, & 12) as a direct result of the use of a Likert-type responses to which the participants indicated the likelihood of that choice using a Likert-type response with answer choices ranging from 1 indicating "not at all true" to 7 indicating "very true."

Table A-13 presents the means and standard deviations by group for the ARS score and the CRS score. A one-way ANOVA was computed comparing the ARS scores and the CRS cores for the two participant groups. An ANOVA is used to analyze the relationship of one categorical independent variable and one continuous variable (Cronk, 2008). Although the TBNS group consisted of approximately three times the number of participants than the NTBNS group (n = 149, n = 51 respectively), a statistically significant difference between groups was found for the ARS scores (F (1,198) = 5.336, p = 0.022). This analysis revealed that participants in the NTBNS group had higher ARS scores

TABLE A-11 Review of Study Variables Including Number of Hours Employed per Week and Years Since Previous Degree

	TBNS		NTBNS	
Variable	n	%	n	%
# of Hours Employed per Week				
0	80	53.7	2	3.9
1 to 10	15	10.1	0	0.0
11 to 20	40	26.8	4	7.8
21 to 30	11	7.4	2	3.9
31 to 40	3	2.0	42	82.4
> 40	0	0.0	1	2.0
Years Since Previous Degree				
1 to 3 years	17	11.5	15	29.4
4 to 5 years	20	13.4	16	31.3
6 to 10 years	8	5.3	17	33.4
11 to 15 years	0	0.0	3	5.9
> 15 years	0	0.0	0	0.0
No previous degree	104	69.8	0	0.0

$N = 200$

($m = 6.45$, $sd = 0.63$) than participants in the TBNS group ($m = 6.19$, $sd = 0.68$). No statistically significant difference was determined for the CRS score ($F(1,198) = 0.162$, $p = 0.687$).

The initial results prompted follow-up analysis. The data collected from the DDCT was further analyzed with a one-way ANOVA for each demographic variable to determine if any additional statistically significant differences existed between ARS scores and CRS scores and participant demographics variables. While a multiple t-test could be conducted to determine group differences, this analysis is subject to the risk of inflating the Type I error and inappropriate interpretation of the results (Cronk, 2008). The ANOVA adjusts for multiple comparisons and provides a single indication of which group is statistically significantly different. Caution must be taken in the interpretation of results as the presence of a relationship does not automatically prove causation (Polit & Beck, 2006).

A one-way ANOVA was computed comparing the ARS scores and the CRS scores of the female and male participants. The group size difference is significant (female, $n = 168$; male, $n = 32$). A statistically significant difference between groups was found for the ARS scores only ($F(1,198) = 5.226$, $p = 0.001$).

TABLE A-12 Means and Standard Deviations for LSRQ for Entire Sample

Question	M	SD
Question 1	6.22	1.06
Question 2	2.09	1.51
Question 3	6.58	0.82
Question 4	4.76	1.92
Question 5	5.32	1.65
Question 6	6.06	1.16
Question 7	4.54	2.02
Question 8	2.71	1.86
Question 9	6.70	0.78
Question 10	4.06	1.87
Question 11	6.22	0.99
Question 12	6.44	1.02
Question 13	5.96	1.27
Question 14	6.06	1.14

N = 200

TABLE A-13 Autonomous Regulation Subscale and Controlled Regulation Subscale Means and Standard Deviations by Sample and by Group

	Sample $n = 200$		TBNS $n = 149$		NTBNS $n = 51$	
Score	M	SD	M	SD	M	SD
ARS score	6.26	0.68	6.19	0.68	6.45	0.63
CRS score	4.28	1.05	4.29	1.03	4.22	1.16

This analysis revealed that female participants had higher ARS scores ($m = 6.37$, $sd = 0.60$) than male participants ($m = 5.88$, $sd = 0.92$). No statistically significant difference was determined for the CRS score ($F(1,198) = 2.711$, $p = 0.120$).

A one-way ANOVA of ARS scores, CRS scores, and participant age revealed a statistically significant difference between groups related to ARS scores only ($F(31,168) = 1.595$, $p = 0.033$). Table A-14 presents the means and standard

TABLE A-14 Autonomous Regulation Subscale and Controlled Regulation Subscale Means and Standard Deviations by Age

Variable		Autonomous		Controlled	
		M	SD	M	SD
Age					
19	(n = 3)	6.95	.08	4.38	.68
20	(n = 24)	6.33	.46	4.43	.93
21	(n = 31)	6.14	.60	4.50	.93
22	(n = 25)	6.15	.61	4.27	1.08
23	(n = 14)	6.27	.57	4.37	1.08
24	(n = 9)	5.75	1.24	3.89	.74
25	(n = 10)	5.90	.87	3.66	1.39
26	(n = 4)	6.36	.75	4.96	1.11
27	(n = 2)	6.36	.10	4.14	1.21
28	(n = 5)	6.74	.38	4.00	1.06
29	(n = 3)	6.67	.33	4.29	1.24
30	(n = 8)	6.45	.93	4.30	1.01
31	(n = 6)	5.90	.81	3.95	.96
32	(n = 5)	6.40	.74	4.00	.93
33	(n = 8)	6.54	.49	4.23	1.36
34	(n = 2)	7.00	.00	5.29	.00
35	(n = 3)	6.62	.36	4.57	.80
36	(n = 6)	6.05	.30	3.83	1.10
37	(n = 4)	6.61	.48	5.18	.77
38	(n = 3)	6.76	.41	5.00	.25
40	(n = 3)	6.33	.59	4.48	1.86
42	(n = 2)	6.29	1.01	4.71	2.02
43	(n = 1)	6.86	—	3.14	—
44	(n = 5)	6.34	.60	4.09	1.12
45	(n = 2)	6.29	.61	5.29	.81
46	(n = 3)	6.00	.94	3.76	1.84
47	(n = 2)	5.71	.20	4.07	.10
48	(n = 1)	3.86	—	2.00	—
49	(n = 2)	6.86	.20	5.21	.51
51	(n = 1)	7.00	—	2.71	—
52	(n = 2)	6.21	.30	2.93	.30
55	(n = 1)	6.57	—	3.43	—

N = 200

deviations by age for the ARS score and the CRS score. Further post-hoc analysis with Tukey's Honestly Significant Difference (HSD) was not possible because of the presence of groups with fewer than 2 cases. Post-hoc was conducted with a simple linear regression. The regression equation was not significant for either the ARS score or the CRS score for age (F (1, 198) + 3.62, $p = 0.057$), with an R2 of 0.13.

An additional one-way ANOVA of ARS scores, CRS scores, and number of dependent children was conducted, which revealed a statistically significant difference between groups related to ARS scores only (F (5,194) = 2.830, $p = 0.017$). Further post-hoc analysis with Tukey's HSD was not possible because one group was limited to fewer than 2 cases. Post-hoc was again conducted with a simple linear regression. The regression yielded a statistically significant result for the number of dependent children. A statistically significant regression equation was found for ARS based on the number of dependent children: (F (1,198) = 5.815, $p = 0.017$), with an R2 of .029. Participants' predicted ARS scores were 6.179 + 116 for each dependent child.

Section II

Further data analysis of ARS scores, CRS scores, and family structure revealed a statistically significant difference between groups related to ARS scores only (F (2,197) = 4.421, $p = 0.01$). Post-hoc analysis with the Tukey's Honestly Significant Difference (HSD) was conducted to determine where the difference existed. This analysis revealed that participants in a family without children had statistically significantly lower ARS scores ($m = 6.15$, $sd = 0.73$) than participants in a one-parent family structure ($m = 6.45$, $sd = 0.073$) and participants in a two-parent family structure ($m = 6.43$, $sd = 0.55$). No statistically significant difference was determined for the CRS score (F (1,198) = 2.711, $p = 0.120$).

Additional data analysis was limited to the review of the means and standard deviations of the independent variables of interest collected via the DDCT. These variables included sex, ethnicity, marital status, family structure, previous healthcare experience, current GPA, number of hours spent independently on school work per week, number of hours spent in collaboration on school work per week, the number of hours employed per week, years since previous degree, and previous degree GPA. Tables A-15 to A-18 report these findings.

Summary

This chapter presented the research findings of this cross-sectional study and explained the findings in relation to the posed research questions. The researcher used Microsoft Excel, SPSS Version 15, and R-Project software to

TABLE A-15 Autonomous Regulation Subscale and Controlled Regulation Subscale Means and Standard Deviations by Demographic Variable Including Sex, Ethnicity, Marital Status, and Family Structure

Variable	Autonomous		Controlled	
	M	SD	M	SD
Sex				
Female (n = 168)	6.37	0.60	4.33	1.02
Male (n = 32)	5.88	0.92	4.01	1.21
Ethnicity				
Caucasian (n = 154)	6.23	0.69	4.32	1.01
African-American (n = 37)	6.38	0.66	4.03	1.18
Hispanic (n = 3)	5.71	0.14	4.57	1.87
Asian (n = 2)	6.36	0.71	4.71	1.21
Other (n = 4)	6.29	0.58	4.79	1.01
Marital Status				
Single	6.21	0.67	4.39	1.09
Married	6.38	0.68	4.13	0.99
Divorced	6.14	0.72	4.07	1.03
Widowed	—	—	—	—
Family Structure				
No children	6.15	0.73	4.34	1.05
Two-parent family	6.43	0.55	4.17	1.07
One-parent family	6.45	0.73	4.19	1.10

N = 200

complete the data analysis required for this study. The descriptive statistics were provided and interpreted. A one-way ANOVA was conducted to determine the existence of differences in academic self-regulation in two distinct groups of nursing students. The initial results lead to follow-up analysis, which included further descriptive statistics and the performance of simple linear regression to determine the prediction of subscale scores based on the additional independent variables of age and the number of dependent children. Statistically significant findings will be further discussed in Chapter V.

TABLE A-16 Autonomous Regulation Subscale and Controlled Regulation Subscale Means and Standard Deviations by Demographic Variable Including Previous Healthcare Experience, Current GPA, and Number of Independent Study Hours per Week

Variable	Autonomous		Controlled	
	M	*SD*	*M*	*SD*
Previous Healthcare Experience				
Yes (*n* = 107)	6.30	0.71	4.18	1.09
No (*n* = 93)	6.21	0.64	4.39	1.02
Current GPA				
2.0 – 2.49 (*n* = 1)	5.85	—	4.14	—
2.5 – 2.99 (*n* = 39)	6.26	0.57	4.51	1.04
3.0 – 3.49 (*n* = 93)	6.26	0.64	4.27	1.11
3.5 – 4.0 (*n* = 67)	6.26	0.79	4.14	0.99
# of Hours Spent in Collaboration on School Work per Week				
< 5 (*n* = 4)	5.82	1.00	3.68	0.92
6 to 10 (*n* = 21)	6.12	0.6	3.83	1.13
11 to 15 (*n* = 38)	6.24	0.81	4.5	1.14
16 to 20 (*n* = 59)	6.28	0.61	4.42	0.89
21 to 25 (*n* = 29)	6.31	0.62	4.48	1.12
26 to 30 (*n* = 30)	6.22	0.72	4.15	1.27
> 30 (*n* = 26)	6.34	0.69	3.93	0.82

N = 200

CHAPTER V: SUMMARY OF RESULTS, DISCUSSION OF FINDINGS, IMPLICATIONS AND RECOMMENDATIONS

The purpose of this study was to determine if there was a difference in self-regulation behaviors (autonomous vs. controlled) in two distinct groups of nursing students: (a) traditional baccalaureate nursing students, and (b) non-traditional baccalaureate nursing students (licensed nurses who have previously completed a diploma or associate degree nursing program and are returning to nursing school to obtain a baccalaureate degree). Research participants were nursing students in a baccalaureate nursing program at one southeastern public Alabama university.

TABLE A-17 Autonomous Regulation Subscale and Controlled Regulation Subscale Means and Standard Deviations by Demographic Variable Including Number of Collaborative Study Hours per Week and Number of Hours Employed per Week

Variable	Autonomous		Controlled	
	M	*SD*	*M*	*SD*
# of Hours Spent in Collaboration on School Work per Week				
< 5 (*n* = 61)	6.19	0.73	4.16	1.11
6 to 10 (*n* = 43)	6.27	0.53	4.44	0.93
11 to 15 (*n* = 28)	6.37	0.45	4.45	0.95
16 to 20 (*n* = 19)	6.38	0.64	4.41	1.20
21 to 25 (*n* = 15)	6.23	1.01	4.6	1.09
26 to 30 (*n* = 14)	6.36	0.72	4.13	1.09
> 30 (*n* = 20)	6.11	0.8	3.76	1.02
# of Hours Employed per Week				
0 (*n* = 83)	6.26	0.6	4.38	0.96
1 to 10 (*n* = 16)	5.91	1.03	3.94	1.00
11 to 20 (*n* = 42)	6.16	0.7	4.36	1.07
21 to 30 (*n* = 13)	6.35	0.55	4.04	1.26
31 to 40 (*n* = 44)	6.41	0.65	4.22	1.19
> 40 (*n* = 2)	6.79	0.3	3.79	0.51

N = 200

TABLE A-18 Autonomous Regulation Subscale and Controlled Regulation Subscale Means and Standard Deviations by Demographic Variable: Years Since Previous Degree

Variable	Autonomous		Controlled	
	M	*SD*	*M*	*SD*
Years Since Previous Degree				
No previous degree	6.15	0.62	4.3	0.96
1 to 3 years	6.24	0.87	4.22	1.17
4 to 5 years	6.54	0.64	4.32	1.21
6 to 10 years	6.33	0.52	4.02	1.04
11 to 15 years	7	0	5.27	0.86
> 15 years	6.17	0.57	3.88	1.14

N = 200

The following research questions were explored in this study:

1. Is there a statistically significant difference in academic self-regulation behaviors (autonomous versus controlled) in the following two distinct groups of nursing students: Traditional baccalaureate nursing students and non-traditional baccalaureate nursing students (licensed nurses who have previously completed a diploma or associate degree nursing program and are returning to nursing school to obtain a baccalaureate degree)?
2. Are there significant differences in the following demographic characteristics between the same two groups of baccalaureate nursing students: Age, sex, ethnicity, marital status, family structure, number of dependent children, previous healthcare experience, current GPA, number of hours in independent study per week, number of hours studying collaboratively per week, number of work hours per week, and number of years since previous degree?

This chapter serves as a summation of this research project. The conclusions reached from the analysis of the data will be presented and discussed as they relate to the posed research questions. The implications for nursing education and higher education will be discussed and recommendations for further research will be offered.

Summary of Results

Nurse educators must understand the uniqueness of nursing student subgroups in order to better serve these student groups and support the academic development of critical thinking and self-directed learning strategies (Billings & Halstead, 2005; Cowman, 1998; Magena & Chabeli, 2005; Välimäki et al., 1999). This study explored the existence of possible differences in academic motivation between the following two distinct student subgroups: Traditional baccalaureate nursing students and non-traditional baccalaureate nursing students.

The research questions posed in this study were answered. Question 1 of the research study is as follows: Is there a statistically significant difference in academic self-regulation behaviors (autonomous versus controlled) in the following two distinct groups of nursing students: Traditional baccalaureate nursing students and non-traditional baccalaureate nursing students (licensed nurses who have previously completed a diploma or associate degree nursing program and are returning to nursing school to obtain a baccalaureate degree)? Yes, there was a statistically significant difference in scores on the LSRQ completed by this sample. Analysis of the data through the computation of a one-way Analysis of Variance (ANOVA) revealed that the participants in the NTBNS group had higher autonomous regulation subscale (ARS) scores than participants in the TBNS group. No statistically significant difference was determined for the controlled regulation subscale (CRS) scores.

Question 2 posed the following question: Are there significant differences in the following demographic characteristics between the same two groups of baccalaureate nursing students: Age, sex, ethnicity, marital status, family structure, number of dependent children, previous healthcare experience, current GPA, number of hours in independent study per week, number of hours studying collaboratively per week, number of work hours per week, and number of years since previous degree? These demographic variables data collected with the Demographic Data Collection Tool (DDCT) were further analyzed by the use of a one-way ANOVA to determine if a statistically significant difference existed and follow-up post-hoc analysis was performed as warranted by the initial results. This analysis revealed that female participants had higher ARS scores than male participants. Age was statistically significant in relation to ARS scores; however, post-hoc analysis did not reveal where the difference existed. Participants' scores on the ARS increased for each dependent child in the household. Family structure impacted ARS scores; specifically, participants in family without children had lower ARS scores than participants in a one-parent family structure and participants in a two-parent family structure.

Further review of the means and standard deviations on the ARS scores in relation to the demographic variables revealed the following revelations: a) African-American and Asian students reported a higher ARS score than other minorities; b) married students had higher ARS scores than single students or divorced students; c) students heading up single-parent family households and two-parent households reported higher ARS scores than students without children; d) students with previous healthcare experience reported a higher ARS score than those students with no prior healthcare experiences; e) students who spent more than 30 hours a week in independent study of nursing content reported higher ARS subscores than whose studied less; f) the highest mean scores on the ARS were reported for students who were employed more than 40 hours per week; and g) students with a previous degree showed increased mean ARS scores in comparison with students who were pursuing their first degree.

There was no significant variance in ARS scores for collaboration with nursing studies or years since previous degree. Of interest were the identical mean scores for ARS scores for participants in following three GPA ranges: 2.5 to 2.99, 3.0 to 3.49, and 3.5 to 4.0. One participant with a self-reported GPA between 2.0 and 2.49 had a significantly lower mean ARS score of 5.85; however, no conclusions can be drawn from this difference as the sample was limited to one participant.

Discussion of Findings

There were several limitations of this study. These limitations will be presented prior to exploring the implications of this study's findings. This study was limited to the use of one student body population from one southeastern public Alabama university, which resulted in a limited convenience sampling of 215 voluntary participants. Fifteen participants did not fully complete the DDCT and the data from these participants was removed from the sample resulting in a sample size of 200. This sample size exceeded the desired minimum of 30 participants per group (Polit & Hungler, 1999); however, an increased sample size would strengthen the power of this study. The inequality of student classification groups (TBNS: $n = 149$, NTBNS: $n = 51$) is inherent in convenience sampling as there is no assurance of equality when using a convenience sampling.

The timing of the completion of the LSRQ and the DDCT varied tremendously throughout the sample. Five student groups were surveyed, two groups of NTBNSs and three groups of TBNSs. Data collection time frames for TBNS students were as follows: (a) Group 1 collected at the end of five semesters immediately prior to graduation; (b) Group 2 collected at the end of the second semester; and (c) Group 3 collected within the first two weeks of the first semester in upper graduate study. Data collection time frames for NTBNS students were as follows: (a) Group 1 collected at the end of three semesters of curriculum and immediately prior to graduation and (b) Group 2 collected at the beginning of the first of three semesters of curriculum. In summary two groups were surveyed within the first semester, one group was surveyed mid-semester, and two groups were surveyed just prior to graduation. This factor is a major limitation and may have negatively contributed to the reported variances. Bruner (1964) purported that most learners are initially dependent on extrinsic motivation at the beginning of a learning activity. As the learner develops an understanding of the value of the knowledge or content and interest increases, there may be a shift toward intrinsic motivation. Students just entering the nursing curriculum may not have internalized the value of the content in relation to future endeavors. It is prudent to recognize that the internalization of the value of the content would be much different at the end of the curriculum than at the beginning or shortly thereafter. In addition, returning previous degree students, NTBNSs, may have higher scores because they have a starting point on which to anchor the acquisition of new knowledge and recognize the value of the content presented in the curriculum.

The validity of self-reporting may be impacted by student concern with faculty evaluation of the LSRQ survey results. Students may have been compelled to answer the survey tool in the manner that they thought was desirable as opposed to strictly and honestly answering the survey questions. In addition to the concern about sample size, non-traditional baccalaureate nursing students (NTBNS) (n = 51) comprised only one-fourth of the sample, while traditional baccalaureate nursing students (TBNS) comprised three-fourths of the sample (n = 149). This may also impact the generalizability of the research findings.

The lack of ethnic diversity in this convenience sample may also contribute to the limitation of the research findings. The ethnicity of the sample included 154 Caucasians (77%), 37 African-Americans (18.5%), three Hispanics (1.5%), two Asians (1%), and four participants who indicated "other" (2%). In addition, the gender diversity of the sample consisted of 168 female participants (84%) and 32 male participants (16%). The American Association of Colleges of Nursing Research and Data Center (2007) report the race/ethnicity percentages for the generic baccalaureate nursing programs in the state of Alabama in 2006 to be as follows: Caucasian 79.6%, African-American 16%, Hispanic 1.2%, Asian 2.4%, and other 0.7%. Nationally, males in baccalaureate nursing programs account for 10.0% of nursing school graduates (NLN, 2008). This sample demographic for ethnicity and sex is similar to the enrollment data of the nursing student body population at this southeastern public Alabama university for the past five years and closely parallels the diversity within nursing programs within the state of Alabama; however, a sample with increased diversity would increase the generalizability of the study findings on a national level.

Another significant limitation of the study is directly related to student age. The age range of the participants was from 19 to 55 years with a mean age of 27.79 years, a mode of 21 years, a median of 24 years, and a standard deviation of 8.44. These statistics indicate that the majority of participants were young adults. The LSRQ was developed to assess the learning self-regulation of the adult learner. The NLN (2006) reports that 43% of all pre-licensure nursing graduates in 2006 were over the age of 30 and 16% were over the age of 40. The mean age of this sample, 27.79 years, limits the ability to generalize these findings to the nursing student population at large.

While there is a statistically significant difference between autonomous self-regulation in the student groups, it was not possible to determine which individual factors may have contributed to the group differences. The research results, however, did add to the body of knowledge regarding adult learning self-direction. The LSRQ (Williams & Deci, 1996) was initially designed for use with adult learners to assess learning motivation on two scales: Controlled regulation (external regulation or introjected regulation) and autonomous regulation (identified regulation or intrinsic regulation). These two levels of regulation are both categorized under external motivation; however, the differentiation of academic self-regulation between these two categories serves as the transitional point as the learner moves from extrinsic to intrinsic motivation (Williams & Deci). This tool has been utilized to assess adult learners in various college courses to include organic chemistry (Williams & Deci) and organ systems (Black & Deci, 2000). The successful modification of the LSRQ to reflect nursing school curriculum as a whole, as opposed to merely one course, and the subsequent confirmation of instrument reliability as ensured by the performance of a Cronbach's alpha test of internal consistency on the instrument, further legitimizes this survey tool for use in additional programs of study.

The variable of age as a predictor of self-regulatory behaviors such as cognitive maturity, use of learning strategies, metacognition, and motivation have revealed that older undergraduate students are generally more self-aware, demonstrate greater self-regulation, and report both intrinsic and extrinsic motivation (Alexander, Murphy, Woods, Duhon & Parker, 1997; Gadzella, Stephens, & Baloglu, 2002; Justice & Dornan, 2001; Kasworm, 2003; Smedley, 2007). Academic self-regulation has been reported by previous investigators to be higher in older students (Smedley, 2007); however, Knowles (1980) acknowledged that many mature adults remain extrinsically motivated in the learning environment. The findings of this research study indicated that age was not a significant contributing factor related to autonomous regulation for this sample of nursing students. While this finding cannot be automatically applied to the population, it does add to the discussion.

Gender differences have been found to relate to variances in motivation as a result of variation in enjoyment of the learning task and variations in response to reward contingencies; however, these variations are common across all individuals and have not been directly linked to an individual's sex (Deci, Mims, & Koestner, 1983). This sample consisted of 168 females (84%) and 32 males (16%). While the females reported higher ARS scores, these findings may reflect an inadequate male sample to make a strong analysis. This is a limitation that is directly linked to the use of convenience sampling.

Many researchers have encouraged additional research focusing on individual adult learner variances, the impact of motivational factors on student success in the formal learning environment, and the relationship of age, degree persistence and intrinsic motivation (Alexander & Murphy, 1999; Bye, Pushkar. & Conway, 2007). Tutor (2006) reported that academic self-regulation is a significant predictor of academic success. The investigation of demographic characteristics revealed that there are specific life factors that may positively contribute to higher autonomous regulation. These factors include marital status, parenthood, fulltime employment, previous healthcare experience, and routinely spending more than 30 hours a week in independent study of nursing content. When looking at single factors, the factors may seem coincidental; however, when viewed in relation to the demands of nursing school curriculum, students presenting with these life factors must be highly motivated to successfully complete the nursing curriculum and earn the baccalaureate degree. The results of this study support the inclusion of these students into nursing academia. Often nursing faculty view students with multiple life responsibilities as distracted and may negatively assume that these students are less engaged and less motivated. These research findings argue that additional life roles and responsibilities contribute to increased autonomous regulation.

Within this sample, 39 of 51 (76.5%) NTBNS were parents and 38 of 149 (25.5%) TBNS were parents, a difference of over one-half. It could be argued that employment pursuits and monetary rewards are not solely extrinsic values but contribute to the intrinsic motivation that compels the student who is a spouse or parent to contribute to the needs of the family. Parenthood and the provision of sufficient economic family resources is a major motivator; however, there are many nursing students who are young, single and childless who are just as highly autonomously regulated and highly motivated. While this sample size is limited, educators would be wise to consider that the findings of this research study support the argument that life factors may, in fact, be more contributory to academic self-regulation than student degree choice (associate degree versus baccalaureate degree). It is imperative that nurse educators recognize the unique challenges facing all nursing students and resist discrediting a student's commitment to learning automatically because they are satisfying multiple life roles.

Myers (1999) asserted that associate degree nurses may demonstrate higher intrinsic motivation because the successful attainment of a nursing degree would help to solve acute problems such as the need for economic stability. Myers further argued that baccalaureate students are typically younger and seek degrees in nursing due to the "extrinsic value of employment pursuits and monetary rewards" (1999, p. 92). Delaney and Piscopo (2004) investigated the motivation of NTBNSs to obtain a baccalaureate nursing degree and reported several motivational factors which include the desire to compete in the work environment and experience professional advancement and personal growth. While this research study does demonstrate a difference in academic self-regulation between TBNS and NTBNS, the information gained cannot support or refute the claims of the cited research.

While this study focused on identifying group differences in academic self-regulation, the information provided on contributory factors may further the understanding of the importance of support attainment of increased autonomous regulation for nurse educators as well as nursing students. Multiple research studies have concluded that learners who are autonomously regulated derive psychological benefits such as better learning outcomes, better task performance, better behavioral performance, increased self-efficacy, increased mood, positive coping strategies and increased enjoyment of learning (Black & Deci, 2000; Ryan & Connell, 1989; Grolnick & Ryan, 1987). Burton, Lydon, D'Alessandro, and Koestner (2006) suggested that intrinsic motivation and the accompanying interest and enthusiasm predict academic performance; therefore, nurse educators should strive to progress along the continuum of academic self-regulation in an effort to improve student learning outcomes.

Multiple opportunities exist for educators to support academic motivational progression from controlled to autonomous as proposed in self-determination theory (Svinicki, 2004). Nurse educators can increase self-directed learning for all through the implementation of many different strategies. Learner self-motivation is increased when the learner has academic support from the educator (Dornan, Hadfield, Brown, Boshuizen, & Scherpbier, 2005). This support should include organizational support, the provision of opportunities for student learning in an optimal learning environment. Pedagogic support should include providing learning opportunities to increase self-regulation by allowing students to contribute to the decision-making process concerning learning objectives and learning strategies, collaboration to establish assignment deadlines, promoting individualization of the course learning activities, providing accurate and timely scholastic feedback, and offering instructional guidance and explanation of content (Fink, 2003; Svinicki, 1999). In addition, affective support can assist students as they transition to a more independent and self-directed learning style. This includes nurturing the student through the process, recognizing and encouraging increased learner autonomy, providing appropriate feedback, and modeling the values of self-regulation through all student–faculty interactions (Svinicki, 2004).

Implications

While life factors such as family and work demands and economics concerns may pose barriers for nursing students to continue academic pursuits (Birks, Chapman, & Francis, 2006; Thompson, 1992; Zuzelo, 2001), it is these factors which may increase academic self-regulation. Nurse educators are challenged to view the totality of the individual and recognize their unique life factors and appreciate how these life factors may contribute to the development of a highly motivated, self-regulated learner. While it is not possible to fully extrapolate this study's findings to the entire nursing student population, these findings should cause nurse educators to pause and consider their biases. "Married with children" and/or "fully employed" may predict the student's academic self-regulation in the future. The automatic concern for these students' abilities to succeed may be superseded by the recognition of their ability to self-regulate their learning.

Faculty understanding and recognition of possible differences in academic self-regulation across nursing student groups may assist nursing faculty in supporting student learning endeavors and, as a consequence, increase the number of nursing graduates by limiting the number of students lost to attrition resulting from academic failure. Various methods of supporting student learning self-regulation include formally integrating goal formation, self-monitoring of academic progress, and self-evaluation of learning outcomes into course activities (Schunk & Ertmer, 2000). In addition, modeling self-regulation behaviors in the classroom and during student/faculty interactions can support student development of academic self-regulation.

These research findings add to the body of knowledge documenting variances in nursing student academic self-regulation and provide nurse educators with concrete data on which to base educational decisions regarding content delivery methods, student motivation strategies, and learning activities. Nursing educators must understand and recognize possible differences in academic self-regulation which may exist in relation to individual demographics or student classification. These differences should be further considered when developing curriculum outcomes and course activities. Understanding the impact of life factors on variances in academic motivation can facilitate educators in the development of more effective instructional environments and learning activities.

Educators in higher education, regardless of the discipline, can benefit from these findings by gaining a greater understanding of the complexity of self-regulation and the importance of the role of the educator. The educator must consider the effectiveness of the planned course activities and strive to support academic self-regulation through the proper selection of supportive learning materials, learning activities, and classroom interactions (Azevedo & Cromley, 2004; Barnett, 2000; Porath & Bateman, 2006). In addition, instructional scaffolding through the use of mentoring, journaling, providing timely evaluations and specific feedback, and ensuring a nurturing learning environment that accepts the adult student and values their life experiences and unique characteristics can enhance student self-regulation.

Recommendations

While these research findings have contributed to the body of knowledge regarding academic self-regulation and differences in nursing student groups, replication of this study could confirm these research findings. Changes in the study design to include administering surveys at a specific point of time in the curriculum (beginning, midway point or end) would increase the validity of the findings. An alternative that looks at three groups of students, junior-level traditional nursing students and senior-level traditional nursing students as well as non-traditional baccalaureate nursing students, may reveal additional differences not captured in this study. Additional changes which would strengthen the findings include increasing the sample size, balancing the number of participants in the groups, using more than one student population by sampling other school of nursing, and modifying the DDCT to capture more specific demographic data as opposed to ranges of data.

Further research should be conducted to explore academic self-regulation differences in different learning environments such as hybrid and web-based courses, faculty use of technology to promote increased academic self-regulation, and the effectiveness of faculty introduced self-regulation approaches to enhance student transition to autonomous regulation. In addition, further exploration into the effectiveness of the nurse educator roles in the development and promotion of academic self-regulation strategies is warranted.

Summary

A shift toward intrinsic motivation occurs as learners develop an understanding of the value of knowledge or content (Knowles, Holton, & Swanson, 2005). As undergraduate students progress move into their major field of study and begin to study content they value, intrinsic motivation increases. This holds true for all of higher education, not just in nursing education. External factors in the learning environment, both negative and positive, such as feedback, social support, and the presence of external motivators can contribute to or inhibit academic motivation. Educators must consider the unique needs of the individual student and the theoretical constructs of self-directed learning, self-regulation, and learning motivation and the use of educational strategies and support methods to promote and enhance student integration of content value and progression toward intrinsic motivation. Recognition of differences in student groups' academic self-regulation can assist educators by broadening their understanding of the differences between groups and possible contributing factors. This understanding may enhance educational decisions regarding content delivery methods, student motivation strategies, and learning activities.

Nursing is a demanding scientific educational discipline requiring students to develop academic self-regulation beyond the requirements of many other fields of study. This factor, combined with the recent paradigm shift from teacher-centered teaching to learner-centered learning, requires nurse educators to understand the uniqueness of individual students and the varying needs of different nursing student subgroups. Nurse educators must develop a knowledge base concerning how to best serve nursing students during the academic development of critical thinking and self-directed learning strategies (Billings & Halstead, 2005; Cowman, 1998; Magena & Chabeli, 2005; Välimäki et al., 1999).

This research can by used to better serve both traditional and non-traditional baccalaureate nursing students by helping nurse educators recognize differences in learning motivation resulting from life characteristics. Nursing faculty should strive to provide learning opportunities which promote self-directed learning and offer appropriate supportive feedback in an effort to assist nursing students in the internalization of the value of the content and their individual move toward intrinsic motivation. Through these efforts, nursing educators, indeed, all educators may be more successful in developing supportive student learning environments and thus increase the number of graduates by limiting the number of students lost to attrition resulting from academic failure.

REFERENCES

Alexander, P. A. (1995). Superimposing a situation-specific and domain-specific perspective on account of self-regulated learning. *Educational Psychologist, 30*(4), 189–193.

Alexander, P. A., & Murphy, P. K. (1999). Learner profiles: Valuing individual differences within classroom communities. In P. L. Ackerman, P. C. Kyllonen, & R. D. Roberts (Eds.), *Learning and individual differences: Process, trait, and content determinant* (pp. 413–430). Washington, DC: American Psychology Association.

Alexander, P. A., Murphy, P. K., Woods, B. S., Duhon, K. E., & Parker, D. (1997). College instruction and concomitant changes in students' knowledge, interest, and strategy use: A study of domain learning. *Contemporary Educational Psychology, 22*, 125–146.

Alkhasawneh, I. M., Mrayyan, M. T., Docherty, C., Alashram, S., & Yousef, H. Y. (2008). Problem-based learning (PBL): Assessing students' learning preferences using VARK. *Nurse Education Today, 28*(5), 572–579.

American Association of Colleges of Nursing. (2001). The baccalaureate degree in nursing as minimal preparation for professional practice. *Journal of Professional Nursing, 17*(5), 267–269.

American Association of Colleges of Nursing. (2006). *Student enrollment rises in U.S. nursing colleges and universities for 6th consecutive year.* Retrieved November 29, 2008, from http://www.aacn.nche.edu/Media/NewsReleases/06Survey.htm

American Association of Colleges of Nursing Research and Data Center. (2007). *Enrollments in generic (entry-level) baccalaureate programs by state and race/ethnicity, Fall 2006.* Retrieved November 28, 2008, from http://www.aacne.nche.edu/IDS/pdf/GENBACENROLL06.pdf

Anderson, L. W., & Krathwohl, D. R. (Eds.). (2001). *A taxonomy for learning, teaching, and assessing: A revision of Bloom's Taxonomy of Educational Objectives.* New York: Addison Wesley Longman, Inc.

Artino, A. R. (2007). Self-regulated learning in online education: A review of empirical literature. *International Journal of Instructional Technology and Distance Learning.* Retrieved November 29, 2008, from http://itdl.org/Journal/Jun_07/article01.htm

Auburn University Montgomery. *About AUM.* Retrieved November 2, 2008, from http://www.aum.edu/Administration/University_Relations/About_AUM/index .aspx?id=2796

August-Brady, M. M. (2005). The effect of metacognitive intervention on approach to and self-regulation of learning in baccalaureate nursing students. *Journal of Nursing Education, 44*(7), 297–304.

Azevedo, R., & Cromley, J. G. (2004). Does training on self-regulation learning facilitate students' learning with hypermedia? *Journal of Educational Psychology, 96*(3), 523–535.

Bahn, D. (2007). Orientation of nurses towards formal and informal learning: Motives and perceptions. *Nurse Education Today, 27,* 723–730.

Bandura, A. (1971). *Social learning theory.* New York: General Learning Press.

Bandura, A. (1976). Modeling theory. In W. S. Sahakian (Ed.), *Learning: Systems, models and theories* (2nd ed.) (pp 391–409). Chicago: Rand McNally.

Bandura, A. (1986). *Social foundations of thought and action: A social cognitive theory.* Englewood Cliffs, NJ: Prentice Hall.

Bandura, A. (1997). *Self-efficacy: The exercise of control.* New York: W. H. Freeman.

Bandura, A. (2000). Health promotion from the perspective of social cognitive theory. In P. Norman, C. Abraham, & M. Connor (Eds.), *Understanding and changing health behavior: From health beliefs to self-regulation* (pp. 299–339). Amsterdam: Hardwood Academic Publishers.

Barnett, J. E. (2000). Self-regulated reading and test preparation among college students. *Journal of College Reading and Learning, 31*(1), 42–53.

Barr, R. B., & Tagg, J. (1995). From teaching to learning: A new paradigm for undergraduate education. *Change, 27*(6), 13–25.

Billings, D. M. & Halstead, J. A. (2005). *Teaching in nursing: A guide for faculty* (2nd ed.). St. Louis, MO: Elsevier Inc.

Birks, M., Chapman, Y., & Francis, K. F. (2006). Baccalaureate nursing studies: Voyaging towards discovery. *International Journal of Nursing Practice, 12,* 267–272.

Black, A. E., & Deci, E. L. (2000). The effects of instructors' autonomy support and students' autonomous motivation on learning organic chemistry: A self-determination theory perspective. *Science Education, 84,* 740–756.

Bloom, B. (Ed.) (1971). *Taxonomy of educational objectives: The classification of educational goals.* New York: D. McKay.

Boekaerts, M. (1995). Self-regulated learning: Bridging the gap between metacognitive and motivation theories. *Educational Psychologist, 30*(4), 195–200.

Boshier, R. (1971). Motivational orientations of adult education participants: A factor analytic exploration of Houle's typology. *Adult Education, 21*(2), 3–26.

Boshier, R., & Collins, J. B. (1985). The Houle topology after twenty-two years. A large-scale empirical test. *Adult Education Quarterly, 35*(3), 113–130.

Brockett, R. G. (1985). The relationship between self-directed learning readiness and life satisfaction among older adults. *Adult Education Quarterly, 35*(4), 210–219.

Brockett, R. G. & Hiemstra, R. (1991). *Self-direction in adult learning: Perspectives on theory, research, and practice.* New York: Routledge.

Brookfield, S. D. (1990). *The skillful teacher: On technique, trust and responsiveness in the classroom.* San Francisco: Jossey-Bass.

Brookfield, S. D. (1994). Adult learning: An overview. In T. Husén, & T. N. Postlethwaite (Eds.), *International encyclopedia of education* (2nd ed.) (pp. 163–168). New York: Pergamon Press.

Brookfield, S. D. (2006). *The skillful teacher: On technique, trust, and responsiveness in the classroom* (2nd ed.). San Francisco: Jossey-Bass Publishers.

Bruner, J. S. (1964). Some theorems on instruction illustrated with reference to mathematics. In E. R. Hilgard & H. R. Richey (Eds.), *Theories of learning and instruction: The 63rd yearbook of the National Society for the Study of Education* (pp. 306–335). Chicago: University of Chicago Press.

Buerhaus, P. I., Staiger, D. O., & Auerbach, D. I. (2008). Implications of an aging registered nurse workforce. *Journal of the American Medical Association, 283*(22), 2948–2954.

Burton, K. D., Lydon, J. E., D'Alessandro, D. U., & Koestner, R. (2006). The differential effects of intrinsic and identified motivation on well-being and performance: Prospective, experimental, and implicit approaches to self-determination theory. *Journal of Personality and Social Psychology, 91*(4), 750–762.

Bye, D., Pushkar, D., & Conway, M. (2007). Motivation, interest, and positive affect in traditional and nontraditional undergraduate students. *Adult Education Quarterly, 57*(2), 141–158.

Caffarella, R. S. (1983). Fostering self-directed learning in post-secondary education. The use of learning contracts. *Lifelong Learning, 1*(2), 7–10.

Caffarella, R. S. (1993). Self-directed learning. *New directions for adult and continuing education, 57,* 25–35.

Campbell, W. E., & Smith, K. A. (Eds.) (1997). *New paradigms for college teaching.* Edina, MN: Interaction Book Company.

Campaniello, J. A. (1988). When professional nurses return to school: A study of role conflict and well-being in multiple-role women. *Journal of Professional Nursing, 4,* 136–140.

Cameron, J. (2001). Negative effects of reward on intrinsic motivation—limited phenomenon: Comment on Deci, Koestner, and Ryan (2001). *Review of Educational Research, 71*(1), 29–42.

Cameron, J., & Pierce, W. D. (1994). Reinforcement, reward, and intrinsic motivation: A meta-analysis. *Review of Educational Research, 64*(3), 363–423.

Candy, P. (1991). *Self-direction for lifelong learning.* San Francisco: Jossey-Bass Publishers.

Cassazza, M. (2006). Self-regulation. In P. Sutherland & J. Crowther (Eds.), *Lifelong Learning: Concepts and Contexts* (pp. 146–157). New York: Routledge.

Cervone, D. (1993). The role of self-referent cognitions in goal setting, motivation, and performance. In M. Rabinowitz (Ed.), *Cognitive science foundations of instruction* (pp. 57–95). Hillsdale, NJ: Lawrence Erlbaum Associates.

Chou, P., & Chen, W. (2008). Exploratory study of the relationship between self-directed learning and academic performance in a web-based learning environment. *Online Journal of Distance Learning Administration, 9*(1). Retrieved November 29, 2008, from http://www.westga.edu/~distance/ojdla/spring111/chou111.html

Cooley, M. C. (2008). Nurses' motivations for studying third level post-registration nursing programmes and the effects of studying on their personal and work lives. *Nurse Education Today, 28,* 588–594.

Cowman, S. (1998). The approaches to learning of student nurses in the Republic of Ireland and Northern Ireland. *Journal of Advanced Nursing, 28*(4), 899–910.

Crain, W. (2004). *Theories of development: Concepts and applications* (5th ed.). Upper Saddle River, NJ: Prentice Hall.

Cronk, B. C. (2008). *How to use SPSS: A step-by-step guide to analysis and interpretation* (5th ed.). Glendale, CA: Pyrczak Publishing.

Cross, K. P. (1981). *Adults as learners: Increasing participation and facilitating learning.* San Francisco: Jossey-Bass Publishers.

Cross, K. P. (1991). The renaissance in adult learning. *The Community Services Catalyst, 21*(4). Retrieved November 24, 2008, from http://scholar.lib.vt.edu/ejournals/CATALYST/V21N4/cross.html

Delaney, C., & Piscopo, B. (2004). RN-BSN programs: Associate degree and diploma nurses' perceptions of the benefits and barriers to returning to school. *Journal for Nurses in Staff Development, 20*(4), 157–161.

Deci, E. L. (1971). Effects of externally mediated rewards on intrinsic motivation. *Journal of Personality and Social Psychology, 18,* 105–115.

Deci, E. L., Koestner, R., & Ryan, R. M. (2001). Extrinsic reward and intrinsic motivation in education: Reconsidered once again. *Review of Educational Research, 71*(1), 1–27.

Deci, E. L., Mims, V., & Koestner, R. (1983). Relation of reward contingency and interpersonal context of intrinsic motivation: A review and test using cognitive evaluation theory. *Journal of Personality and Social Psychology, 45*(4), 736–750.

Deci, E. L., & Ryan, R. M. (1985). The General Casuality Orientations Scale: Self-determination in personality. *Journal of Research in Personality, 19,* 109–134.

Deci, E. L., & Ryan, R. M. (2000a). *Intrinsic motivation and self-determination in human behavior.* New York: Plenum.

Deci, E. L., & Ryan, R. M. (2000b). The "what" and "why" of goal pursuits: Human needs and the self-determination of behavior. *Psychological Inquiry, 11*(4), 227–268.

Deci, E. L., Schwartz, A. J., Sheinman, L, & Ryan, R. M. (1981). An instrument to assess adults' orientations toward control versus autonomy with children: Reflections on intrinsic motivation and perceived competence. *Journal of Educational Psychology, 73,* 642–650.

Delaney, C., & Piscopo, B. (2004). RN-BSN programs: Associate degree and diploma nurses' perceptions of the benefits and barriers to returning to school. *Journal for Nurses in Staff Development, 20,* 157–163.

Dohm, A., & Shniper, L. (2007, November). Employment outlook: 2006–16. Occupational employment projections to 2016. *Monthly Labor Review,* 86–125.

Dornan, T., Hadfield, J., Brown, M., Boshuizen, H., & Scherpbier, A. (2005). How can medical students learn in a self-directed way in the clinical environment? Design based research. *Medical Education, 39*(5), 356–364.

Ertmer, P. A., Newby, T. J., & MacDougall, M. (1996). Students' responses and approaches to case-based instruction: The role of reflective self-regulation. *American Educational Research Journal, 33*(3), 719–752.

Evensen, D. H., Salisbury-Glennon, J. D., & Glenn, J. (2001). A qualitative study of six medical students in a problem-based curriculum: Toward a situational model of self-regulation. *Journal of Educational Psychology, 93*(4), 659–676.

Fleming, N. D. (2006). *Teaching and learning styles: VARK strategies* (2nd ed.). Christchurch, New Zealand: The Digital Print and Copy Center.

Fink, L. D. (2003). *Creating significant learning experiences: An integrated approach to designing college courses.* San Francisco: Jossey-Bass, Inc.

Fisher, M., King, J., & Tague, G. (2001). Development of a self-directed learning readiness scale for nursing education. *Nurse Education Today, 21,* 516–525.

Gadzella, B. M., Stephens, R., & Baloglu, M. (2002). Prediction of educational psychology course grades by age and learning style scores. *College Student Journal, 36*, 62–69.

Gall, J. P., Gall, M. D., & Borg, W. R. (2005). *Applying educational research: A practical guide* (5th ed.). New York: Pearson.

Garrison, D. R. (1997). Self-directed learning: Toward a comprehensive model. *Adult Education Quarterly, 48*(1), 18–33.

Goleman, D. (1995). *Emotional intelligence.* New York: Bantam Books.

Goleman, D. (1998). *Working with emotional intelligence.* New York: Bantam Books.

Green, C. (1987). Multiple role women: The real world of the mature RN learner. *Journal of Nursing Education, 26*, 266–271.

Greveson, G. C., & Spencer, J. A. (2005). Self-directed learning: The importance of concepts and contexts. *Medical Education, 39*(5), 348–349.

Grolnick, W. S., & Ryan, R. M. (1987). Autonomy in children's learning: An experimental and individual difference investigation. *Journal of Personality and Social Psychology, 52*, 890–898.

Guglielmino, L. M. (1977). *Development of an instrument to assess readiness for self-directed learning.* (Doctoral dissertation, University of Georgia), *Dissertation Abstracts International, 38*, 11A.

Hammann, L. (2005). Self-regulation in academic writing tasks. *International Journal of Teaching and Learning in Higher Education, 17*(1), 15–26.

Harder, M. (2008). How do rewards and management styles influence the motivation to share knowledge? (SMG Working Paper #6). *Center for Strategic Management and Globalization, Copenhagen Business School*, Fredericksberg, Denmark.

Harvey, B. J., Rothman, A. I., & Frecker, R. C. (2006). A confirmatory factor analysis of the ODDI Continuing Learning Inventory (OCLI). *Adult Educational Quarterly, 56*(3), 188–200.

Hiemstra, R. (Ed.) (1985). Self-directed adult learning: Some implications for facilitators (Occasional Paper #3). Syracuse, NY: Syracuse University, Adult Education Program.

Hiemstra, R., & Judd, R. (1978). *Identifying "success" characteristics in self-directed adult learners.* Ames, IA: Iowa State University, Adult and Extension Education.

Hoban, J. D., Lawson, S. R., Mazmanian, P. E., Best, A. M., & Seibel, H. R. (2005). The Self-Directed Learning Readiness Scale: A factor analysis study. *Medical Education, 39*(5), 370–379.

Hornick, K. (2008). The R Project for statistical computing. Retrieved September 15, 2008, from http://www.r-project.org/

Hockenberry, M., & Wilson, D. (Eds.) (2007). *Wong's nursing care of infants and children* (8th ed.). St Louis: Mosby.

Houle, C. O. (1988). *Patterns of learning: New perspectives of life-span education.* San Francisco: Jossey-Bass Publishers.

Houser, J. (2008). *Nursing research: Reading, using, and creating evidence.* Sudbury, MA: Jones and Bartlett Publishers.

Hudson, L. K. (1992). *Exploration of the relationship between incentive and selected variables associated with graduate students in nursing.* Unpublished doctoral dissertation, University of Missouri, Columbia.

James, W. B., & Maher, P. A. (2004). Understanding and using learning styles. In M. W. Galbraith (Ed.), *Adult learning methods: A guide for effective instruction* (3rd ed.) (pp. 23–37). Malabar, FL: Kreiger Publishing Company.

Justice, E. M., & Dornan, T. M. (2001). Metacognitive differences between traditional-age and non-traditional-age college students. *Adult Education Quarterly, 51,* 236–249.

Kanfer, R., & Heggestad, E. D. (1999). Individual differences in motivation: Traits and self-regulatory skills. In P. L. Ackerman, P. C. Kyllonen, & R. D. Roberts (Eds.), *Learning and individual differences: Process, trait, and content determinants* (pp. 293–309). Washington, DC: American Psychological Association.

Kasworm, C. (2003). Adult meaning making in the undergraduate classroom. *Adult Education Quarterly, 53*(2), 81–98.

Keating, S. B. (2005). *Curriculum development and evaluation in nursing.* Philadelphia: Lippincott Williams & Wilkins.

Keirns, J. L. (1999). *Designs for self-instruction: Principles, processes and issues in developing self-directed learning.* Needham Heights, MA: Allyn and Bacon.

Knowles, M. S. (1980). *The modern practice of adult education: From pedagogy to andragogy.* Chicago: Follett Publishing Company.

Knowles, M. S. (1984). *The adult learner: A neglected species* (3rd ed.). Houston, TX: Gulf Publishing Company.

Knowles, M. S. (1989). *The making of an adult educator: An autobiographical journey.* San Francisco: Jossey-Bass.

Knowles, M. S., Holton III, E. F, & Swanson, R. A. (2005). *The adult learner: The definitive classic in adult education and human resource development* (6th ed.). Burlington, MA: Elsevier.

Kumrow, D. E. (2005). *A pilot study to investigate the relationship between student self-regulatory resource management strategies and academic achievement in a web-based hybrid graduate nursing course.* Unpublished doctoral dissertation, University of Southern California, Los Angeles.

Kuiper, R. (2005). Self-regulated learning during clinical preceptorship: The reflections of senior baccalaureate nursing students. *Nursing Education Perspectives, 26*(6), 351–356.

Lapeyre, E. (1991). Nursing students' learning styles: A comparison of degree and non-degree student approaches to studying. *Nurse Education Today, 12,* 192–199.

Lee, C. J. (2007). Academic help seeking: Theory and strategies for nursing faculty. *Journal of Nursing Education, 46*(10), 468–475.

Lemcool, K. E. G. (2007). *Effects of coaching on self-regulated learning strategy use and achievement in an entry-level nursing class.* Unpublished doctoral dissertation, University of South Alabama, Mobile.

Lengacher, C. A. (1993). Development of predictive model for role strain in registered nurses returning to school. *Journal of Nursing Education, 32,* 301–308.

Levesque, C., & Pelletier, L. G. (2003). On the investigation of primed and chronic autonomous and heteronomous motivational orientations. *Personality and Social Psychology Bulletin, 29*(12), 1570–1584.

Levesque, C., Zuehlke, A. N., Stanek, L. R., & Ryan, R. M. (2004). Autonomy and competence in German and American university students: A comparative study based on self-determination theory. *Journal of Educational Psychology, 96*(1), 68–84.

Lindeman, E. (1926). *The meaning of adult education.* New York: New Republic.

LoBiondo-Wood, G., & Haber, J. (2006). *Nursing research: Methods and critical appraisal for evidence-based practice* (6th ed). St. Louis, MO: Mosby, Inc.

Locke, E. A., & Latham, G. P. (1990). *A theory of goal setting and task performance.* Englewood Cliffs, NJ: Prentice Hall

Long, H. B. (2004). Understanding adult learners. In M. W. Galbraith (Ed.), *Adult learning methods: A guide for effective instruction* (3rd ed.) (pp. 23–37). Malabar, FL: Kreiger Publishing Company.

Lopez, R. P. (1992). A comparison of generic graduates, dropouts, and current students in a nursing-education program: The influence of selected demographic, academic, and personal characteristics and accessibility variables. (Doctoral dissertation, University of San Francisco), *Dissertation Abstracts International, 54,* 02B.

Magena, A., & Chabeli, M. M. (2005). Strategies to overcome obstacles in the facilitation of critical thinking in nursing education. *Nurse Education Today, 25,* 291–298.

Mansouri, P., Soltani, F., Rahemi, S., Nasab, M. M., Ayatollahi, A. R., & Nekooeian, A. A. (2006). Nursing and midwifery students' approaches to study and learning. *Journal of Advanced Nursing, 54*(3), 351–358.

McEwan, L., & Goldenberg, D. (1999). Achievement motivation, anxiety, and academic success in first year Master of Nursing students. *Nurse Education Today, 19,* 419–430.

Merriam, S. B., & Brockett, R. G. (1997). *The profession and practice of adult education: An introduction.* San Francisco: Jossey-Bass Publishers.

Merriam, S. B., & Simpson, E. L. (1995). *A guide to research for educators and trainers of adults* (2nd ed.). Malabar, FL: Kreiger Publishing Company.

Merriam, S. B. & Caffarella, R. S. (1999). *Learning in adulthood: A comprehensive guide* (2nd ed.). San Francisco: Jossey-Bass, Inc.

Mezirow, J. (1981). A critical theory of adult learning and education. *Adult Education Quarterly, 32*(1), 3–24.

Morstain, B. R., & Smart, J. C. (1974). Reasons for participation in adult education courses: A multivariate analysis of group differences. *Adult Education, 24*(2), 83–98.

Mullen, P. A. (2007). Use of self-regulating learning strategies by students in the second and third trimesters of an accelerated second-degree baccalaureate nursing program. *Journal of Nursing Education, 46*(9), 406–412.

Myers, N. A. (1999). *A study of the learning strategies of metacognition, metamotivation, metamemory, critical thinking, and resource management of nursing students on a regional campus of a large Midwestern university.* (Doctoral dissertation, Ball State University), *Dissertation Abstracts International, 60,* 03B.

National League for Nurses. (2005). *Transforming nursing education.* Retrieved July 8, 2008, from http://www.nln.org/aboutnln/PositionStatements/transforming052005.pdf

National League for Nurses. (2006). *Nursing data review, Academic year 2005–2006: Executive Summary.* Retrieved November 29, 2008, from http://www.nln.org/research/datareview/executive_summary.pdf

National League for Nurses. (2008). *Number of nursing school graudates – including ethnic and racial minorities – on the rise but applications to RN programs dip, reflecting impact of tight admissions.* Retrieved November 29, 2008, from http://www.nln.org/newsreleases/data_release_03032008.htm

Niemiec, C. P., Lynch, M. F., Vansteenkiste, M., Bernstein, J., Deci, E. L., & Ryan, R. M. (2006). The antecedents and consequences of autonomous self-regulation for college: A self-determination theory perspective on socialization. *Journal of Adolescence, 29,* 761–775.

Nilsson, K. E., & Stomberg, M. I. W. (2008). Nursing students motivation toward their studies – a survey study. *BioMed Central Nursing, 7*(6), 1–7.

Ofori, R., & Charlton, J. P. (2002). A path model of factors influencing the academic performance of nursing students. *Journal of Advanced Nursing, 38*(5), 507–515.

Pekrun, R., Frenzel, A. C., Goetz, T., & Perry, R. P. (2007). In R. Pekrun, & P. A. Schutz, *Emotion in education: An integrative approach to emotions in education* (pp. 13–36). New York: Academic Press.

Pintrich, P. R. (2000). The role of goal orientation in self-regulated learning. In M. Boekaerts, P. R. Pintrich, & M. Zeidner (Eds.), *Handbook of self-regulation* (pp. 631–649). San Diego, CA: Academic.

Pintrich, P. R., & Schunk, D. H. (1996). *Motivation in education: Theory, research, and applications.* Columbus, OH: Prentice-Hall, Inc.

Pintrich, P. R., Smith, D. A., Garcia, T., & McKeachie, W. J. (1991). *A manual for the use of the Motivated Strategies for Learning Questionnaire (MSLQ).* Ann Arbor: University of Michigan, National Center for Research to Improve Post-secondary Teaching and Learning.

Pintrich, P., Smith, D., Garcia, T., & McKeachie, W. (1993). Reliability and predictive validity of the Motivated Strategies for Learning Questionnaire (MSLQ). *Educational and Psychological Measurement, 53,* 801–813.

Polit, D. F., & Beck, C. T. (2006). *Essentials of nursing research: Methods, appraisal, and utilization* (6th ed.). Philadelphia, PA: Lippincott Williams & Wilkins.

Polit, D. F., & Hungler, B. P. (1999). *Nursing research: Principles and methods* (6th ed.). Philadelphia: Lippincott Williams & Wilkins.

Porath, C. L., & Bateman, T. S. (2006). Self-regulation: From goal orientation to job performance. *Journal of Applied Psychology, 91*(1), 185–192.

Pringle, D., & Green, L. (2005). Examining the causes of attrition from schools of nursing in Canada. *Canadian Journal of Nursing Leadership.* Retrieved February 1st, 2009, from http://www.longwoods.com/search_results.php?cx =009350451624671198534%3Ahjsn4vtdwj4&cof=FORID%3A11&ie=UTF-8 &domains=www.longwoods.com&q=Examining+the+causes+of+attrition +form+schools+of+nursing+in+Canada&x=0&y=0#718.

Rubin, L. M., McCoach, D. B., McGuire, J. M., & Reis, S. M. (2003). The differential impact of academic self-regulatory methods on academic achievement among university student with and without learning disabilities. *Journal of Learning Disabilities, 36*(3), 270–286.

Ryan, R. M., & Connell, J. P. (1989). Perceived locus of causality and internationalization: Examining reasons for acting in two domains. *Journal of Personality and Social Psychology, 57,* pp. 749–761.

Ryan, R. M. & Deci, E. L. (2000a). Intrinsic and extrinsic motivation: Classic definitions and new directions. *Contemporary Educational Psychology, 25,* 54–67.

Ryan, R. M., & Deci, E. L. (2000b). Self-determination theory and the facilitation of intrinsic motivation, social development, and well being. *American Psychologist, 55*(1), 68–78.

Ryan, R. M., & Deci, E. L. (2006). Self-regulation and the problem of human autonomy: Does psychology need choice, self-determination, and will? *Journal of Personality, 74*(6), 1557–1586.

Ryan, R. M., Koestner, R., & Deci, E. L. (1991). Ego-involved persistence: When free-choice behavior is not intrinsically motivated. *Motivation and Emotion, 15*(3), 185–205.

Ryan, R. M., Mims, V., & Koestner, R. (1983). Relation of reward contingency and interpersonal context to intrinsic motivation: A review and test using cognitive evaluation theory. *Journal of Personality and Social Psychology, 45,* 736–750.

Schmidt, J. T., & Werner, C. H. (2007). Designing online instruction for success: Future oriented motivation and self-regulation. *The Electronic Journal of e-Learning, 5*(1), 69–78.

Schunk, D. H. (1993). *Enhancing strategy use: Influence of strategy value and goal orientation.* Paper presented at the Annual Meeting of the American Educational Research Association. Atlanta, GA: April 12–16. ERIC Document Number 359217.

Schunk, D. H. (2001a). Social cognitive theory and self-regulated learning. In B. J. Zimmerman, & D. H. Schunk (Eds.), *Self-regulated learning and academic achievement: Theoretical perspectives* (2nd ed.) (pp. 125–151). Mahwah, NJ: Lawrence Erlbaum Associates, Inc.

Schunk, D. H. (2001b). *Self-regulation through goal setting.* (ERIC ED462671). Retrieved November 28, 2008, from http://www.eric.ed.gov/ERICDocs/data/ericdocs2sql/content_storage_01/0000019b/80/19/e0/d0.pdf

Schunk, D. H., & Ertmer, P. A. (1999). Self-regulatory processes during computer skill acquisition: Goal and self-evaluative influences. *Journal of Educational Psychology, 91*(2), 251–260.

Schunk, D. H., & Ertmer, P. A. (2000). Self-regulation and academic learning: Self-efficacy enhancing interventions. In M. Boekaerts, P. R. Pintrich, & M. Seidner (Eds.), *Self-regulation: Theory, research, and applications* (pp. 631–649). Orlando, FL: Academic Press.

Schunk, D. H., & Zimmerman, B. J. (1994). *Self-regulation of learning and performance: Issues and educational applications.* Mahwah, NJ: Lawrence Erlbaum Associates.

The Self-Regulation Questionnaire. *Self-determination theory: An approach to human motivation & personality.* (n.d.) Retrieved November 28, 2008, from http://www.psych.rochester.edu/SDT/measures/selfreg.html

Slotnick, H. B., Pelton, M. H., Fuller, M. L., & Tabor, L. (1993). *Adult learner on campus.* Washington, DC: Falmer.

Smedley, A. (2007). The self-directed learning readiness of first year bachelor of nursing students. *Journal of Research in Nursing, 12*(4), 373–385.

Smith, R. M. (1982). *Learning how to learn: Applied theory for adults.* New York: Cambridge University Press.

Straka, G. A., & Hinz, I. M. (1996). *The original Self-Directed Readiness Scale reconsidered.* Paper presented at the 10th International Self-Directed Learning Symposium, West Palm Beach, Florida, March 6–10.

Svinicki, M. D. (Ed.) (1999). Teaching and learning on the edge of the millennium: Building on what we have learned. *New Directions for Teaching and Learning, 80*, 1–111. San Francisco: Jossey-Bass.

Svinicki, M. D. (2004). *Learning and motivation in the post-secondary classroom.* Bolton, MA: Anker Publishing Company, Inc.

Thomas, J. W., & Rohwer, W. D., Jr. (1986). Academic studying: The role of learning strategies. *Educational Psychologist, 21*, 19–41.

Thomas, J. W., & Rohwer, W. D., Jr. (1993). Proficient autonomous learning: Problems and prospects. In M. Rabinowitz (Ed.), *Cognitive science foundations of instruction*, pp. 1–32. Hillsdale, N.J.: Lawrence Erlbaum Associates.

Thompson, D. (1992). Beyond motivation: A model of registered nurses' participation and persistence in baccalaureate nursing programs. *Adult Education Quarterly, 42*(2), 94–105.

Tough, A. (1979). *The adult's learning projects: A fresh approach to theory and practice in adult learning* (2nd ed.). Austin, TX: Learning Concepts.

Tough, A., Abbey, D., & Orton, L. (1982). Anticipated benefits from learning. *Adult Education Quarterly, 32*(3). (Sage Journals Online DOI: 10.1177/074171368203200307). Retrieved from http://aeq.sagepub.com/cgi/reprint/32/3/170-d

Tseng, W., Dornyei, Z., Schmitt, N. (2006). A new approach to assessing strategic learning: The case of self-regulation in vocabulary acquisition. *Applied Linguistics, 27*(1), 78–102.

Tutor, P. T. (2006). *Factors influencing nursing students' motivation to succeed.* Unpublished doctoral dissertation, University of Southern California, Los Angeles, California.

United States Department of Health & Human Services Health Resources and Services Administration. (2004). *What is behind HRSA's projected supply, demand, and shortage of registered nurses?* Retrieved November 28, 2008, from ftp://ftp.hrsa.gov/bhpr/workforce/behindshortage.pdf

Välimäki, M., Itkonen, J., Joutsela, J., Koistinen, T., Laine, S., Paimensalo, M. S., et al. (1999). Self-determination in nursing students: An empirical investigation. *Nurse Education Today, 19*(8), 617–627.

Vallerand, R. J., Pelletier, L. G., Blais, M. R., Brière, N. M., Senécal, C. , & Vallières, E. F. (1992). The Academic Motivation Scale: A measure of intrinsic, extrinsic, and amotivation in education. *Educational and Psychological Measurement, 52*, 1003–1017.

Vallerand, R. J., Pelletier, L. G., Blais, M. R., Brière, N. M., Senécal, C., & Vallières, E. F. (1993). On the assessment of instrinsic, extrinsic, and amotivation in education: Evidence on the concurrent and construct validity of the Academic Motivation Scale. *Educational and Psychological Measurement, 53*, 159–172.

Vansteenkiste, M., Lens, W., & Deci, E. L. (2006). Intrinsic versus extrinsic goal contents in self-determination theory: Another look at the quality of academic motivation. *Educational Psychologist, 41*(1), 19–31.

Vansteenkiste, M., Simons, J., Lens, W., Sheldon, K. M., & Deci, E. L. (2004). Motivating learning, performance, and persistence: The synergistic effects of intrinsic goal contents and autonomy-supportive contexts. *Journal of Personality and Social Pathology, 87*(2), 246–260.

Vincent, J. E. (1992). Exploration of selected academic and demographic factors influencing attrition and retention of baccalaureate nursing students. (Doctoral dissertation, Ball State University), *Dissertation Abstracts International,* 60, 03B.

Walker, C. O., Greene, B. A., & Mansell, R. A. (2005). Identification with academics, intrinsic/extrinsic motivation, and self-efficacy as predictors of cognitive engagement. *Learning and Individual Differences,* 16, 1–12.

Walker, J. T., Martin, T. M., Haynie, L., Norwood, A., White, J., & Grant, L. (2007). Preferences for teaching methods in a baccalaureate nursing program: How second-degree and traditional students differ. *Nursing Education Perspectives, 28*(5), 246–250.

Warkentin, R. W., & Bol, L. (1997). Assessing college students' self-directed studying using self-reports of test preparation. Annual meeting of The American Educational Research Association, Chicago.

Wild, T. C., Enzle, M. E., Nix, G., & Deci, E. L. (1997). Perceiving others as intrinsically or extrinsically motivated: Effects on expectancy formation and task engagement. *Personality and Social Psychology Bulletin, 23,* 837–848.

Williams, G. C., & Deci, E. L. (1996). Internalization of biopsychosocial values by medical students: A test of self-determination theory. *Journal of Personality and Social Psychology, 70,* 767–779.

Williams, G. C., & Deci, E. L. (1998). The importance of supporting autonomy in medical education. *Annals of Internal Medicine, 129*(4), 303–308.

Williams, P. E., & Hellman, C. M. (2004). Differences in self-regulation for online learning between first- and second-generation college students. *Research in Higher Education, 45*(1), 71–82.

Winne, P. H. (1995). Inherent details in self-regulated learning. *Educational Psychologist, 30*(4), 173–187.

Wissmann, J. L. (2002). Metacognition in BSN education contexts: A descriptive collective case study (Doctoral dissertation, University of Kansas, 2002), *Dissertation Abstracts International, 63,* 10A.

Wlodkowski, R. J. (1985). *Enhancing adult motivation to learn: A guide to improving instruction and increasing learner achievement.* San Francisco: Jossey-Bass Publishers.

Young, D. B., & Ley, K. (2000). Developmental students don't know that they don't know—Part I: Self-regulation. *Journal of College Reading and Learning, 31*(1), 54–59.

Zimmerman, B. J. (1989). A social cognitive view of self-regulated academic learning. *Journal of Educational Psychology, 81*(3), 329–339.

Zimmerman, B. J. (1990). Self-regulated learning and academic achievement: An overview. *Educational Psychologist, 25*(1), 3–17.

Zimmerman, B. J. (1995). Self-regulation involves more than metacognition: A social cognitive perspective. *Educational Psychologist, 30*(4), 217–221.

Zimmerman, B. J. (1998). Developing self-fulfilling cycles of academic regulation: An analysis of exemplary instructional models. In D. H. Schunk & B. J. Zimmerman, *Self-regulated learning: From teaching to self-reflective practice* (pp 1–20). New York: Guilford Press.

Zimmerman, B. J. (2001). Theories of self-regulated learning and academic achievement: An overview and analysis. In B. J. Zimmerman and D. H. Schunk (Eds.), *Self-regulated learning and academic achievement: Theoretical perspectives* (2nd ed.) (pp. 1–37). Mahwah, NJ: Lawrence Erlbaum Associates.

Zimmerman, B. J., Bandura, A, & Martinez-Pons, M. (1992). Self-motivation for academic attainment: The role of self-efficacy belief and personal goal setting. *American Educational Research Journal, 29*(3), 663–676.

Zimmerman, B. J., Bonner, S., & Kovach, R. (1996). *Developing self-regulated learners: Beyond achievement to self-efficacy.* Washington, DC: American Psychological Association.

Zimmerman, B. J., & Schunk, D. H. (Eds.) (2001). *Self-regulated learning and academic achievement: Theoretical perspectives* (2nd ed.). Mahwah, NJ: Lawrence Erlbaum Associates.

Zuzelo, P. R. (2001). Describing the RN-BSN learner perspective: Concerns, priorities, and practice influences. *Journal of Professional Nursing, 17*(1), 55–65.

Appendix A-1
Learning Self-Regulation Questionnaire

The following questions relate to your reasons for participating in nursing classes. Different people have different reasons for participating in such a class, and we want to know how true each of these reasons is for you. There are three groups of items, and those in each group pertain to the sentence that begins that group. Please indicate how true each reason is for you using the following scale:

1	2	3	4	5	6	7
not at all true			somewhat true			very true

A. I participate actively in my nursing classes:

_____   1. Because I feel like it's a good way to improve my skills and my understanding of patients.

_____   2. Because others would think badly of me if I didn't.

_____   3. Because learning the content well is an important part of becoming a nurse.

_____   4. Because I would feel bad about myself if I didn't study these concepts.

B. I follow my instructor's suggestions:

_____   5. Because I will get a good grade if I do what he/she suggests.

_____   6. Because I believe my instructor's suggestions will help me nurse effectively.

_____   7. Because I want others to think that I am a good nurse.

_____   8. Because it's easier to do what I'm told than to think about it.

_____   9. Because it's important to me to do well at this.

_____   10. Because I would probably feel guilty if I didn't comply with my instructor's suggestions.

C. The reason that I will continue to broaden my nursing knowledge is:

_____   11. Because it's exciting to try new ways to work interpersonally with my patients.

_____   12. Because I would feel proud if I did continue to improve at nursing.

_____   13. Because it's a challenge to really understand what the patient is experiencing.

_____   14. Because it's interesting to use the nursing process try to identify what needs the patient has.

Appendix A-2
Demographic Data Collection Tool

Student Classification
☐ Junior   ☐ Senior   ☐ EARN

Sex: _____   **Age:** _____

Ethnicity
☐ Caucasian   ☐ Hispanic   ☐ African-American   ☐ Asian   ☐ Other

Marital Status	**Dependent Children**	**# of Dependent**
☐ Single	☐ 2-parent family	**Children** _____
☐ Married	☐ 1-parent family	
☐ Divorced	☐ no children	
☐ Widowed		

Previous Healthcare Experience   **Current GPA**
☐ Yes   _____ 4.00 to 3.5   _____ 2.99 to 2.50
☐ No   _____ 3.49 to 3.0   _____ 2.49 to 2.00

Number of Hours Spent Independently on School Work per Week:

_____ < 5   _____ 16 to 20   _____ > 30
_____ 6 to 10   _____ 21 to 25
_____ 11 to 15   _____ 26 to 30

Number of Hours Spent in Collaboration on School Work per Week:

_____ < 5   _____ 16 to 20   _____ > 30
_____ 6 to 10   _____ 21 to 25
_____ 11 to 15   _____ 26 to 30

Hours Employed per Week:

_____ 0   _____ 11 to 20   _____ 31 to 40
_____ 1 to 10   _____ 21 to 30

Years Since Previous Degree:

_____ 1 to 3 years   _____ 11 to 15 years
_____ 4 to 5 years   _____ > 15 years
_____ 6 to 10 years _____ No previous degree

Previous Degree GPA:

_____ 4.00 to 3.50   _____ 2.99 to 2.50
_____ 3.49 to 3.00   _____ 2.49 to 2.00

Appendix A-3
Recruiting Script

Introduction: Hi, my name is Michelle Schutt. I am a doctoral student at Auburn University and I am conducting a study for my dissertation in partial fulfillment for the education doctorate from Auburn University.

Invitation to Participate: You were selected as a potential participant for a research study entitled "Examination of Learning Self-Regulation Variances in Nursing Students" because you are presently enrolled at the Auburn Montgomery School of Nursing. All of you are invited to participate in this study that will evaluate learning self-regulation. I will study the differences in learning self-regulation across different groups of nursing students.

Agreement to Participate: If you agree to participate, I will need you to read the information letter. Your completion of the survey conveys consent to participate in this research. The information letter states that participants will anonymously complete a two-sided document with one side being a short demographic tool and the opposite side being a short survey and return the survey in a sealed envelope. There will be no future requirements of the participants.

Anticipated Risks: The risks associated with this study are minimal but could include a breach in confidentiality, social discomforts, or feelings of coercion to participate. Should you need to discuss your feelings about participating in this research, you can speak with me, your advisor or someone at the Auburn Montgomery Counseling Center. Contact information for the Auburn Montgomery Counseling Center is attached to the informed consent form.

Confidentiality of Data: All information obtained about you will remain confidential in a locked filing cabinet in Room 315 Moore Hall. The only other individuals who will review the data will be professors in the Auburn University educational doctoral program assisting with data analysis. No identification will be provided on the forms to link the response to an individual student.

How the Study Will Help: Your participation will greatly benefit future nursing students and will support efforts to improve teaching effectiveness in the Auburn Montgomery School of Nursing, other schools of nursing, and education as a whole.

Decision to Participate or Not and Withdrawal of Consent: Your decision whether or not to participate will not prejudice your future relations with Auburn University, Auburn Montgomery, or the Auburn Montgomery School of Nursing.

If you decide to participate, you are free to withdraw your consent and to discontinue participation at any time without penalty. If you decide to withdraw from the study prior to completing the requested demographic tool and survey, please simply do not return these collection tools. Once these tools are collected, your specific response tool will not be retrievable as it will not have your name or an identifying code on it.

If you have questions concerning the study, presently or in the future, I will be happy to answer/address those concerns. You can contact me by email at mschutt1@aum.edu or by phone at (334) 328-4293.

Appendix A-4
IRB Required Alternative
Recruiting Script

NOTE: This script will be used for obtaining informed consent and data collection for two groups of participants: 1) Junior participants during April 2008 and 2) EARN participants during May 2008.

Introduction: Hi, my name is Dr. Debbie Faulk. I am here on behalf of Michelle Schutt, a doctoral student at Auburn University, and I am conducting a study for my dissertation in partial fulfillment for the education doctorate from Auburn University.

Invitation to Participate: You were selected as a potential participant for a research study entitled "Examination of Learning Self-Regulation Variances in Nursing Students" because you are presently enrolled at the Auburn Montgomery School of Nursing. All of you are invited to participate in this study that will evaluate learning self-regulation. I will study the differences in learning self-regulation across different groups of nursing students.

Agreement to Participate: If you agree to participate, I will need you to sign an informed consent form. The form states that you agree to the following:
    Participants will anonymously complete a two-sided document with one side being a short demographic tool and the opposite side being a short survey. There will be no future requirements of the participants.

Anticipated Risks: The risks associated with this study are minimal but could include a breach in confidentiality, social discomforts, or feelings of coercion to participate. Should you need to discuss your feelings about participating in this research, you can speak with me, your advisor or someone at the Auburn Montgomery Counseling Center. Contact information for the Auburn Montgomery Counseling Center is attached to the informed consent form.

Confidentiality of Data: All information obtained about you will remain confidential in a locked filing cabinet in my office in Room 318 Moore Hall until course grades have been entered in Webster in May (August) at which time I will surrender the data collection tools to Mrs. Schutt. The only other individuals who will review the data will be professors in the Auburn University educational doctoral program assisting with data analysis. No identification will be provided on the forms to link the response to an individual student.

How the Study Will Help: Your participation will greatly benefit future nursing students and will support efforts to improve teaching effectiveness in the Auburn Montgomery School of Nursing, other schools of nursing, and education as a whole.

Decision to Participate or Not and Withdrawal of Consent: Your decision whether or not to participate will not prejudice your future relations with Auburn University, Auburn Montgomery, or the Auburn Montgomery School of Nursing.

If you decide to participate, you are free to withdraw your consent and to discontinue participation at any time without penalty. If you decide to withdraw from the study prior to completing the requested demographic tool and survey, please simply do not return these collection tools. Once these tools are collected, your specific response tool will not be retrievable as it will not have your name or an identifying code on it.

If you have questions concerning the study, presently or in the future, I will be happy to answer/address those concerns. You can contact me by email at mschutt1@aum.edu or by phone at (334) 328-4293.

Appendix B

Understanding the Impact of the AACN Endorsement of the DNP: A Systems Analysis Using Effects-Based Reasoning

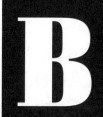

Review the following research project in its entirety. Analyze it to find implementation of each of the steps of the research process.

QUESTIONS TO GUIDE YOUR ANALYSIS

1 What is the research problem? What is the population being studied?

2 Was a hypothesis used or a research question? Was the author's choice appropriate for the type of study implemented? Give your rationale for your answer. Write additional hypotheses or research questions that could have been utilized.

3 Can a theoretical or conceptual framework be identified? If it is not clearly stated, is it implied at some point in the document? Was it an appropriate choice for this project?

4 Was the literature review thorough enough for the topic? Give your rationale for your answer.

5 Was informed consent or an institutional review board utilized in this research project? Was the author's choice to utilize an IRB or not appropriate? Give your rationale for your answer.

6 What type of research design was utilized for this project? How could this project have been implemented differently with a different type of research design?

7 What type of sampling was used in this research project? How could this project have been implemented with a different type of sampling utilized?

8 What type of data collection method was used? Was it the most appropriate one for this study? Give your rationale for your answer.

9 What type of statistical analysis was used with this study? Are there other statistics that could have been utilized but were not selected? Does this study have implications for the population being studied?

10 If you were to replicate this research project, what would you decide to do differently?

Understanding the Impact of the AACN Endorsement of the DNP: A Systems Analysis using Effects-Based Reasoning[1]

Marilyn K. Rhodes, EdD, MSN, RN, CNM
Assistant Professor
Auburn University at Montgomery
Montgomery, Alabama

CHAPTER I: INTRODUCTION

The study of leadership and transformational change balances on an ever changing, complex society. In pursuit of effective leadership, organizations and leaders employ a myriad of leadership methods and styles. To determine method of leadership, an organization must consider the leaders, followers, and the system in which the transformation is to occur. Hughes, Ginnett, and Curphy (1993) define leadership as a "process in which leaders and followers interact dynamically in a particular situation or environment" (p. 107) and state that in the analysis of leadership and leadership effectiveness, one must consider the domains of leader, follower and situation.

When introducing change, variables and outcomes may be uncontrollable. Pullan (2001) states that although change can rarely be controlled, it can be led, requiring leadership to combine elements that do not "easily and comfortably go together" (p. 42). Further, he establishes a new perspective on leading in a culture of change, explaining that change is not linear, but occurs as leaders create coherence through a dynamic event. Pascale, Millemann, and Gioja (2000) describe change within a system as progressing toward chaos. They emphasize that systems cannot be directed along a linear path and unforeseen outcomes are inevitable. "The challenge is to disturb them in a manner that approximates the desired outcome" (p. 6).

O'Toole (1995) describes leadership as the ability to pilot an organization through the "rolling seas in a purposeful and successful manner" (p. xii) for creating or maintaining order amid the turbulence of change. He further states that change alone is inadequate and that entities must be transformed effectively. O'Toole identifies trust as the singular element strong enough to ensure success. He adds that trust must be borne of shared purpose, vision and values with those who are led.

---

[1] Courtesy of Marilyn K. Rhodes, EdD, MSN, RN, CNM.

Roach and Behling (1984) define leadership as "the process of influencing the activities of an organized group toward goal achievement" (p. 46). Some authors describe characteristics of successful leadership while others provide guidance for leading change, prescribing action plans, including specifying phases for implementing change (Bennis, 1994; Kotter, 1996). Pullan (2001) emphasizes that change, ever increasing in complexity, provokes emotions, and that leadership is key in managing the outcomes that change begets.

The current healthcare environment presents many challenges for health-care professionals, as advances in the diagnosis and treatment of illness have introduced change at every level of care. The nursing profession faces challenges including an increasingly elderly population in need of nursing care, an explosion of technology in the work place, and additional roles to fill in the healthcare system. Nursing education adjusts to incorporate these changes, to prepare nurses to care for future generations (Burke, 2004).

In October 2004, amid a severe and growing national nurse and nursing faculty shortage, the American Association of Colleges of Nursing (AACN) set into action a change process by endorsing its position paper to establish the Doctor of Nursing Practice (DNP) as entry-level education for advanced practice nurses (APNs), effective 2015 (AACN, 2004a). The AACN, a nursing organization comprised of 612 deans of nursing schools (AACN, 2007a) states as their mission:

> The American Association of Colleges of Nursing is the national voice for baccalaureate and graduate-degree nursing education. A unique asset for the nation, AACN serves the public interest by providing standards and resources, and by fostering innovation to advance professional nursing education, research, and practice. (AACN, 2004b, n.p.)

This endorsement and subsequent publication of the AACN *DNP Roadmap Report* (AACN, 2006a) and launched a plan for transformational change in nursing education, within a system of systems. This action will affect schools of nursing, university and state educational systems, credentialing systems and health care delivery systems (Fulton & Lyon, 2005). The AACN stated its purpose for introducing this transformational change was to provide a more comprehensive educational preparation for APNs, and the benefits of the DNP are identified by the AACN:

- development of needed advanced competencies for increasingly complex clinical, faculty and leadership roles;
- enhanced knowledge to improve nursing practice and patient outcomes;

- enhanced leadership skills to strengthen practice and healthcare delivery;
- better match of program requirements and credits and time with the credential earned;
- provision of an advanced educational credential for those who require advanced practice knowledge but do not need or want a strong research focus (e.g., clinical faculty);
- parity with other health professions, most of which have a doctorate as the credential required for practice;
- enhanced ability to attract individuals to nursing from non-nursing backgrounds;
- increased supply of faculty for clinical instruction; and
- improved image of nursing. (AACN, 2004a, p. 7)

Although relatively small in number, advanced practice nurses (APN) make significant contributions to the health care of our nation, in the specialties of certified nurse midwives (CNMs), certified registered nurse anesthetists (CRNAs), advanced registered nurse practitioners (ARNPs), and clinical nurse specialists (CNSs) (Phillips, 2006). According to the U.S. Department of Health and Human Services, Health Resources and Services Administration (HRSA), APNs comprise 8.3% of the nursing population (HRSA, 2004). Advanced practice nurses complete educational programs which are accredited by the professional association of that practice specialty (e.g., American College of Nurse-Midwives [ACNM] and American Association of Nurse Anesthetists [AANA]) or by agencies that accredit all nursing programs (National League for Nursing Accrediting Commission [NLNAC] or the Commission on Collegiate Nursing Education [CCNE]). Nationally, approximately 75% of APNs enter advanced practice with a master's degree or post-master's certificate (HRSA, 2004).

Statement of the Research Problem

The AACN endorsement of the Doctor of Nursing Practice initiated a transformational change in the education of advanced practice nurses, for which the AACN cannot influence directly or guarantee the outcomes. For example, the AACN possesses influence over schools of nursing to transform a current master's program into a DNP curriculum, but it does not carry the authority to direct universities to add or remove degree programs (Cartwright & Reed, 2005). As an organization, the AACN may lobby for change in laws to transform state nurse practice acts, but the authority to license advanced practice nurses belongs to state agencies. Likewise, the AACN states that the DNP will command a greater salary, but can guarantee neither job opportunity nor salary range for DNP-prepared practitioners (Fulton & Lyon, 2005).

Since October 2004, the proliferation of literature in nursing journals surrounding the AACN White Paper endorsement illustrates the controversy within the nursing profession (Eisenhauer & Bleich, 2006). The American Nurses Association (ANA) and the National League for Nursing (NLN) questioned the introduction of the degree and its timing, during the nursing and nursing faculty shortage (ANA, 2005; NLN, 2007). The American College of Nurse-Midwives and the American Association of Nurse Anesthetists published position statements that counter this educational mandate. The ACNM revised its position statement on mandatory degree requirements, reiterating that a graduate degree would be required for entry into midwifery practice by 2010 (ACNM, 2006). In 2007, the ACNM published a position statement stating that midwives may enter practice through a "variety of educational programs" (ACNM, 2007, p.1) and the DNP may be one of them, but will not be a requirement. In this statement, the ACNM also states that it has set the standard for midwifery since 1962, that evidence is lacking to support the DNP as a requirement for entry into practice, and there is inadequate data on the cost of the DNP for students and the healthcare system. The ACNM adds:

> Because the educational standards for midwifery education, accreditation and certification have been and continue to be carefully updated, monitored and maintained, the practice of nurse-midwives has well-documented evidence regarding its safety and positive outcomes for women and newborns. ACNM does not support the requirement of the DNP for entry into clinical midwifery practice. (ACNM, 2007, p. 2).

The AANA Interim Position Paper states,

> The AANA cannot, at this time, support AACN's position on the clinical doctorate as entry into advanced practice since our initial review of the proposal raises a number of serious concerns. The AANA encourages professional development for nurse anesthetists up to the doctoral level. However, evidence currently does not support mandatory clinical doctoral degrees for entry into nurse anesthesia practice. (AANA, 2006b, n. p.)

In July 2007, the AANA announced its new position, supporting doctoral education in preparation for nurse anesthetists by 2025 (AANA, 2007).

The debate within the nursing profession over the DNP strikes many chords in the world of education. Fulton and Lyons (2005) raise concerns about whether the DNP will be recognized as a degree worthy of tenure, especially in a research university, should the APN join a university faculty. They also question whether the title will be recognized and achieve parity with other disciplines using similar titles, e.g. MD, JD. Further, they discuss the possibility that those who may have sought a PhD in nursing will instead chose the DNP, diminishing the number of potential PhD students. The discipline of Pharmacy experienced such a trend after the practice doctorate, the PharmD, was required for entry into practice. The cost of establishing the DNP as a degree program with regard to student and faculty time and monetary considerations is largely unknown. Should funding be diverted from prelicensure or graduate programs in place to ease the nursing and nursing faculty shortage, the price of establishing the DNP degree would be unacceptable (Fulton & Lyons, 2005).

Nursing literature regarding the DNP fails to present evidence that master's-prepared APNs are currently performing inadequately in the health care system (Avery & Howe, 2007). In fact, the American Academy of Nurse Practitioners (AANP) published a summary of research reports supporting the quality of nurse practitioner practice (AANP, 2006a). The president of the ACNM stated that based on "decades of evidence" (Carr, 2005, p. 3) graduates of ACNM-accredited programs demonstrated safe and effective care, regardless of their academic degrees. Additionally, there is no evidence that DNP-prepared APNs will be employed or reimbursed to utilize the proposed additional requirements or that health care leaders support the DNP as the sole educational track for entry-level APNs (Fulton & Lyon, 2005). Further, deficiencies in the literature include addressing regulatory issues of nurse providers, the potential for changing APN scope of practice in nursing practice acts (Fulton & Lyon, 2005), and APN programs housed in schools of medicine or allied health (Avery & Howe, 2007).

The length of time from a Bachelor of Science in Nursing (BSN) degree to completing a DNP is estimated at three years of continuous course work or four academic years (AACN, 2006a), which approximately doubles that of a Master of Science in Nursing (MSN) degree. The associated costs of graduate education create additional barriers to education (DeValero, 2001), possibly reducing the number of primary care providers, resulting in reduced access to health care. A survey of midwifery students yielded responses including "might as well go to medical school" (Avery & Howe, 2007, p. 17) if the length and cost of education increased significantly with the DNP requirement. This suggests the possibility exists for a decrease in the midwife model of care, should the DNP preclude some from entering the midwifery profession.

The publication of the AACN White Paper prompted the American Medical Association (AMA) to generate Resolution 211, opposing nurse practitioners using the title doctor. This resolution states that nurses will misrepresent themselves to patients (AMA, 2006a). Creating adversarial relationships between physicians and advanced practice nurses increases the potential for legislative changes restricting not only the use of the term *doctor*, but also restricting the practice of advanced practice nurses (Phillips, 2007). Currently, seven states prohibit the use of the title *doctor* by non-physician providers: Georgia, Illinois, Maine, Missouri, Ohio, Oklahoma, and Oregon (Klein, 2007). More restricted APN practice could further diminish access to care to vulnerable populations.

Background

The AACN endorsement of the DNP as the educational preparation for entry to advanced nursing practice parallels actions by the American Nurses Association over 40 years ago to bring the educational level of entry into professional nursing practice as the baccalaureate degree (Nelson, 2002). Registered nurses comprise the largest single professional discipline within the healthcare system (HRSA, 2004). Unlike most professions, nurses may enter practice after achieving one of three different levels of education and successfully completing a common national licensing examination.

In 1965, the American Nurses Association (ANA) published a position paper in an effort to establish the baccalaureate degree as the sole prelicensure educational track for registered nurses, "Education for those who work in nursing should take place in institutions of learning within the general system of education" (ANA, 1965, p. 107). Their purpose for replacing the prevalent hospital diploma nursing schools was to promote mastery of "a complex, growing body of knowledge and to make critical, independent judgments about patients and their care" (ANA, 1965, p. 107).

The ANA position on nursing education echoed recommendations of the Goldmark Report of 1923. During the age of Progressivism in the United States, the Rockefeller Foundation's Committee for the Study of Nursing Education studied the conditions of nursing education. This study revealed that didactic instruction was unevenly provided and at times absent from hospital schools (Burke, 2004; Cheal, 1999). The Goldmark Report recommended a separation of nursing education and hospitals to improve the quality of nursing care and to promote a professional level of education. Cheal reports that the primary reasons these recommendations were not universally enacted included the social status of women and the absence of support from "professional organizations, colleges and universities, licensing boards, and philanthropies" (1999, n.p.).

Although the Goldmark Report resulted in the advancement of university nursing education, the ANA's effort to establish the baccalaureate degree as entry level for nursing practice prompted "an impassioned debate which continues to frustrate and divide nursing" (Nelson, 2002, n. p.). Jacobs, DiMattio, Bishop, and Fields (1998) report that nurses, hospitals and physicians opposed the educational transformation from the hospital diploma school of nursing education, because it introduced a new and less socially acceptable image of university educated women. In the 21st century, nurses continue the struggle to provide appropriate education to meet the healthcare needs of our nation, while facing challenges of an increasingly complex world. In 2004, nurses entered the nursing profession with diplomas from hospital diploma schools (25.2%), associate degree programs (42.2%), baccalaureate programs (30.5%), and a small number with master's or doctoral degrees (0.5%) (HRSA, 2004).

The greatest increase in education levels among nurses occurred in the group seeking master's degrees. A primary reason supporting this advancement in education was the increased number of advanced practice nurses (HRSA, 2004). HRSA also recorded the trend that progressively more nurses seek baccalaureate and master's degrees beyond their prelicensure education. According to HRSA, the highest levels of education reached by RNs in 2004 were: diploma from hospital schools (17.5%), associate degree (33.7%), baccalaureate degree (34.2%), and master's or doctoral degree (13.0%).

Even as the AACN focuses on the DNP, the master's degree continues to evolve as the primary educational level for entry into advanced practice. The DNP has not been established by all professional organizations as the only approved educational preparation. The American College of Nurse-Midwives (ACNM) will not require the master's level of education for certification until 2010 (ACNM, 2006) and the American Academy of Nurse Practitioners offers adult and family nurse practitioner certification to master's and post-master's education but will allow other practitioners to petition to take the certifying exam (AAPN, n.d.). In 2004, approximately 62% of CNMs, 37% CRNAs, 76% ARNPs, and 97% CNSs entered practice following a master's or post-master's educational program (HRSA, 2004). Currently, 19 states require a master's degree for APN licensure, 23 states and the District of Columbia require a graduate degree or a minimum of a master's degree for licensure, and eight states' regulatory documents do not address educational preparation for APN practice (AACN, 2006a). Perhaps the greatest impetus for graduate education came in 1998, when the Federal Register required the master's degree for reimbursement by the Centers for Medicare and Medicaid Services (CMS) (Code of Federal Regulations, 1998).

As the catalyst for transformational change in nursing education, the AACN established the DNP Roadmap as their leadership tool. The AACN *DNP Roadmap Task Force Report* (AACN, 2006a) states that Rogers' *Diffusion of Innovations* provided the conceptual framework for initiating their vision. This theory is "essentially a social process in which subjectively perceived information about a new idea is communicated from person to person" (Rogers,

2003, p. xx). The AACN regards the transition to the DNP as entry-level education for advanced practice nurses as the next step in the evolution of nursing education (AACN, 2006a). However, given a published date for compliance, this implies a mandate rather than evolution.

In October 2004, the AACN adopted its vision to establish the DNP as entry-level education for advanced practice nursing, by a vote of 160 in favor of and 106 in opposition. This organization also set the date for fruition of its vision as 2015 (Fulton & Lyon, 2005). At the time of the endorsement, there were few DNP programs matriculating students. Amid the debate over the value of the DNP and its establishment as entry-level education for the APN, 78 programs have been developed and an additional 140 schools of nursing are considering DNP programs (AACN, 2008).

In the AACN *DNP Roadmap Task Force Report,* the AACN states that the Commission on Collegiate Nursing Education (CCNE), "an autonomous arm of the AACN" (AACN, 2006a, p. 12) will initiate accreditation of DNP programs. The Secretary of Education first granted the CCNE recognition as an accrediting agency in 2000 (AACN, 2007); the CCNE currently accredits the majority of schools of nursing that produce advanced practice nurses (Avery & Howe, 2007). This document states "programs will need to make decisions regarding advanced practice offerings at the master's level and their viability and ethical standing when the profession has evolved advanced practice education to the doctoral level" (AACN, 2006a, p. 12).

From the perspective of the organization endorsing the DNP, which is also the parent organization that accredits the majority of APN programs, offering a master's degree for advanced practice nursing after 2015 would not be ethical. However, the assertion of ethical behavior is based on the assumption that the nursing profession supports the vision of the AACN and will see it to fruition. The AANA and the ACNM accredit programs for certified registered nurse anesthetists and certified nurse midwives respectively (AANA, 2006a; Varney, 1997). The actions of the AACN may well result in the closure of MSN programs currently producing health care providers, because not all institutions currently granting master's degrees have the capacity or will to create the DNP degree (Fontaine, Stotts, Saxe, & Scott, 2007).

The AACN initiated a transformational change in nursing education; however, according to leadership and change research, it does not have the ability to control or guarantee the outcomes or effects (Pullan, 2001; Pascale et al., 2000). If the DNP endorsement induces actions similar to those following the 1965 ANA position on education, several possible options for advanced practice nurse education could ensue. Directors of APN programs may comply and create DNP programs, though cost and healthcare implications remain unknown. Program directors may ignore the AACN vision and remain accredited or seek accreditation through the National League for Nursing Accrediting Commission (NLNAC), an organization similar to the CCNE. Directors could continue accreditation through specialty professional organizations. Or, similar to the AACN itself, program directors or deans of nursing schools may create a completely new accrediting agency. During the current nursing shortage and nursing faculty crisis, a divisive result of one organization's educational vision could potentially threaten the entire future of nursing (Chase & Pruitt, 2006).

Increasing the educational level of advanced practice nurses should be viewed in a positive light. However, debates persist with regard to the proposed educational benefits of the DNP degree. Implications of implementing the DNP by 2015 reach far beyond the arena of nursing education and have not been adequately addressed for health care leaders outside academia. Clinical APNs, who provide clinical preceptorship for DNP students should hold a doctorate, as programs require at least the same level of education to prepare students. Currently, there are very few doctorally prepared ANPs in purely clinical practice (Avery & Howe, 2007). The American Organization for Nursing Executives (AONE) expresses concerns that nurses will seek master's degrees in other disciplines to avoid the increased time and cost for a DNP. They add that "issues of accreditation, education, certification and licensure related to the advanced practice nurse" (AONE, 2007, n.p.) have yet to be resolved. Concerns raised by the proposed transformation of advanced practice nursing education require examination within a systems approach to transforming health care, as education of APNs constitutes only one facet of advanced nursing practice. State boards of nursing and some state boards of medicine regulate the practices of APNs (Phillips, 2007).

As Pascale et al. (2000) described change within a living system, the AACN's endorsement and plan to achieve the DNP as entry-level education for advanced practice nurses has set in motion a change process that can be described as progressing toward chaos. The nonlinear effects include potential disenfranchisement of APNs and their leadership organizations, increased cost of APN education, a decreased number of graduating APNs, and changes in state regulation and licensing of APNs. Additionally, should collaborative relationships between APNs and physicians erode, fewer APNs may be allowed to practice, decreasing access to care for vulnerable populations. Further, a strain on the nursing faculty could result in a worsening of the nursing shortage. The AACN is challenged to create coherence among stakeholders, working within the system comprised of the higher education system, the APN credentialing systems, the healthcare regulatory system, and the healthcare delivery system (see Figure B-1).

FIGURE B-1 Illustration of the AACN as a system within a system of systems.

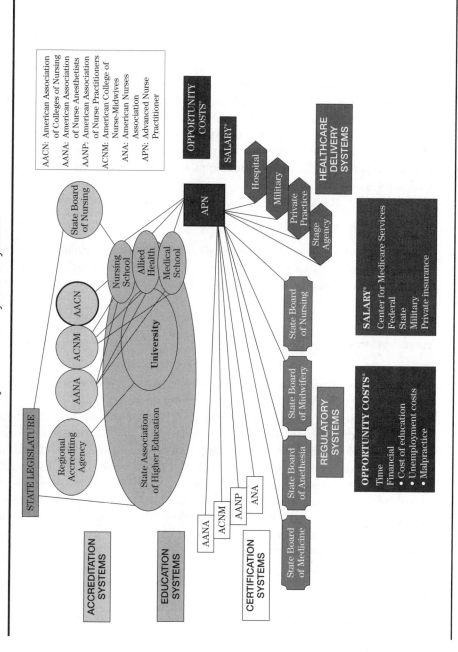

AACN: American Association of Colleges of Nursing
AANA: American Association of Nurse Anesthetists
AANP: American Association of Nurse Practitioners
ACNM: American College of Nurse-Midwives
ANA: American Nurses Association
APN: Advanced Nurse Practitioner

Purpose of the Study

The purpose of this study is to examine the leadership change processes involved in the AACN's effort to transform the entry level of education for advanced practice nurses to the DNP. This researcher believes that transformational leadership best describes AACN's sharing of its vision and empowering members of the AACN to bring that vision to fruition. Illustrating the AACN as a system within a system of systems, the conceptual framework used will examine this process within the domains of leader, followers and situation. Understanding the processes of the leadership of the AACN, comprised of a relatively small number of nurse educators, may allow other professional organizations to examine how this one organization plans to change an educational paradigm that affects many organizational systems and even more individuals within the system of healthcare.

Research Question

What are the effects-based outcomes of introducing transformational change into an open system that will result from the American Association of Colleges of Nursing endorsement of the Doctor of Nursing Practice as sole educational entry to advanced nursing practice?

Assumptions

The AACN's vision of establishing the DNP for entry-level education for advanced nursing practice is based on the intrinsic value of education.

The AACN believes that the DNP will translate into tangible benefits in the practice realm; that extended education, in the form of additional academic degrees, will create a superior health care provider and improve health care.

The intended results of establishing the DNP, according to the Roadmap (AACN, 2006a), depend on first-, second- and third-order effects. First-order effects are the immediate and direct results of AACN actions. Second- and third-order effects include results of intervening variables on the actions of the AACN. For example, establishing a DNP program requires approval of a university board (second-order effect) and sometimes a state higher education organization (third-order effect).

Limitations

The leadership processes were analyzed in only one framework, a systems approach considering the domains of leader, followers and situation. The situation will represent the influence of the AACN as a system, affecting a system of systems.

The leadership analysis examined one primary essential document, the DNP *Roadmap Report.* This report outlines the leadership plan to implement the DNP as the sole educational entry to advanced nursing practice.

The leadership process studied is dynamic; unpublished data may reveal nuances that would influence the analysis.

A limited number of questions were asked of the participants, which cannot address every effects-based outcome initiated by this leadership process.

Merriam (1988) states that in qualitative research, human qualities create limitations, specifically the subjective perceptions of both the interviewees and the researcher.

Definition of Terms

For the purpose of this study the italicized words or phrases are defined:

Leadership: Roach and Behling define leadership as "the process of influencing the activities of an organized group toward goal achievement" (1984, p. 46).

Transformational Leadership: Transformational Leadership is a type of leadership characterized by a leader who explicitly communicates a vision, inspires followers to share and work toward fruition of the vision, and provides resources for developing the personal potential of the follower. Transformational Leadership is most effective in an "empowered dynamic culture" and occurs when a leader "inspires followers to share a vision, empowering them to achieve the vision, and provides the resource necessary for developing their personal potential" (Smith, Montagno & Kuzmenko, 2004, p. 80).

Diffusion of Innovations Theory: The *Diffusion of Innovations* (DOI) is "a social process in which subjectively perceived information about a new idea is communicated from person to person" (Rogers, 2003, p. xv).

Doctoral Degrees recognized by the American Association of Colleges of Nursing:

Doctor of Nursing Practice (DNP): Admits nurses who want to pursue a doctoral degree that focuses on practice rather than research. This practice-focused doctoral program prepares graduates for the highest level of nursing practice beyond the initial preparation in the discipline and is a terminal degree.

Doctor of Nursing (ND) Program: A generic doctoral program with a clinical focus primarily designed for nonnursing baccalaureate-prepared college graduates.

Doctoral (Research-focused) Program: Admits RNs with master's degrees in nursing and awards a doctoral degree. This program prepares students to pursue intellectual inquiry and conduct independent research for the purpose of extending knowledge. In the academic community, the PhD, or Doctor of Philosophy degree is the most commonly offered research-focused doctoral degree. However, some schools for a variety of reasons may award a Doctor of Nursing Science (DNS or DNSc) as the research-focused doctoral degree (Berlin et al., 2005, p. xi).

Advanced Practice Nurse: An Advanced Practice Nurse is:

> a registered nurse (RN) who has met advanced educational and clinical practice requirements beyond the two to four years of basic nursing education required of all RNs. Advanced practice registered nurses include nurse practitioners, clinical nurse specialists, nurse anesthetists, and nurse midwives. (ANA, 2006, n.p.)

Advanced Registered Nurse Practitioner:

> Nurse Practitioners (NPs) include RNs prepared beyond initial nursing education in an NP program of at least 3 months. Approximately 65 percent of NPs have completed a master's degree program and an additional 10 percent have a post-masters certificate as their NP preparation ... Nurse Practitioners may practice independently, or they may work in hospitals, long-term care facilities, and for various health care agencies. Most NPs function primarily as clinicians. NPs may diagnose and treat a wide range of acute and chronic illnesses and injuries, interpret lab results, counsel patients, develop treatment plans, and they may prescribe medication. (ANA, 2006, n.p.)

Certified Nurse Midwife:

> A Certified Nurse midwife (CNM) is an individual educated in the two disciplines of nursing and midwifery, who possesses evidence of certification according to the requirements of the American College of Nurse-Midwives. Midwifery practice as conducted by Certified Nurse-Midwives (CNMs) ... is the independent management of women's health care, focusing particularly on common primary care issues, family planning and gynecologic needs of women, pregnancy, childbirth, the postpartum period and the care of the newborn. The CNM ... practice[s] within a health care system

that provides for consultation, collaborative management or referral as indicated by the health status of the client. CNMs...practice in accord with the Standards for the Practice of Midwifery, as defined by the American College of Nurse-Midwives. (ACNM, 2004, n.p.)

Certified Registered Nurse Anesthetist:

Certified Registered Nurse Anesthetists (CRNAs) provide anesthetics to patients in collaboration with surgeons, anesthesiologists, dentists, podiatrists, and other qualified health care professionals. When anesthesia is administered by a nurse anesthetist, it is recognized as the practice of nursing; when administered by an anesthesiologist, it is recognized as the practice of medicine. CRNAs practice in every setting in which anesthesia is delivered: traditional hospital surgical suites and obstetrical delivery rooms; critical access hospitals; ambulatory surgical centers; the offices of dentists, podiatrists, ophthalmologists, plastic surgeons, and pain management specialists; and U.S. Military, Public Health Services and Department of Veterans Affairs health care facilities. (ANA, 2006, n.p.)

Clinical Nurse Specialist:

Clinical Nurse Specialists (CNS) are licensed registered nurses who have graduate preparation (Master's or Doctorate) in nursing as a Clinical Nurse Specialist. CNSs are expert clinicians in a specialized area of nursing practice. The specialty may be identified in terms of a:

- Population (e.g. pediatrics, geriatrics, women's health)
- Setting (e.g. critical care, emergency room)
- Disease or Medical Subspecialty (e.g. diabetes, oncology)
- Type of Care (e.g. psychiatric, rehabilitation)
- Type of Problem (e.g. pain, wounds, stress)

Clinical Nurse Specialists practice in a wide variety of health care settings. In addition to providing direct patient care, CNSs influence care outcomes by providing expert consultation for nursing staffs and by implementing improvements in health care delivery systems.

Clinical Nurse Specialist practice integrates nursing practice, which focuses on assisting patients in the prevention or resolution of illness, with medical diagnosis and treatment of disease, injury and disability. (National Association of Clinical Nurse Specialists, n.d., pp. 2–3)

Effects-Based Methodology: The basis for defining the term effect is described as "the power to bring about a result" (Mann, Endersby, & Searle, 2002, p. 30). Because one action may bring about a cascade of consequences, Mann et al. define effect as "full range of outcomes, events, or consequences that result from a specific action" (p. 31). A direct or first-order effect is the immediate result of an action, without intervening variables. Additional outcomes, which may be intended or untoward, are indirect or second-, and sometimes third-order effects. The AACN introduced an educational paradigm change into the profession of nursing. Fruition of the AACN vision is based on second and third orders of effects, for which the AACN can neither control nor guarantee the variables or the outcomes.

Social System: Social systems are open systems consisting of "matter, energy and information that are sets of parts with relationships between those parts" (Busch & Busch, 1992, p. 276). A living, negotiated system transacts with the environment, exchanging matter, energy and information (Busch & Busch, 1992). The work of a system allows it to "bring forth" a product of its work (Capra, 1996).

CHAPTER II: REVIEW OF LITERATURE

This review of literature provides the contextual background information required for an analysis of the effects-based outcomes of the AACN's leadership process for transformation. In order to appreciate the many facets involved in an effort to change an educational paradigm, a broad range of subjects is reviewed. In addition, some documents will be examined in the analysis phase of this qualitative research. To provide a basis for analysis, literature on essential concepts will include leadership influencing change, systems, effects-based outcomes, nursing education and regulation, and advanced practice nursing.

Leadership and Change

For the purpose of this study, the researcher defines leadership as "the process of influencing the activities of an organized group toward goal achievement" (Roach & Behling, 1984, p. 46). Most experts on leadership tend to stress the relationship between the leader and followers as the fundamental issue to be understood (Hughes, et al., 1993; O'Toole, 1995; Pullan, 2001). In creating a successful leader–follower relationship, trust is identified as the essential element (Fairholm, 1994; O'Toole, 1995). Meanwhile, Gardner (1993) states that leadership must be based on accepted values shared with followers, which seeks to establish common ground. This author concludes that the essential task of leadership is the establishment, maintenance and renewal of values.

On the topic of change management, Pullan (2001) acknowledges the importance of recognizing emotional reactions of followers, especially when leading change. He states that because change arouses emotions, for good or bad, potential emotional responses must be anticipated in planning change. Pullan describes five components of leading change, describing them as independent and mutually reinforcing. The first component is *moral purpose* or the intention of making a positive difference. A leader must also respect the complexities of the process and demonstrate *understanding change*. In leading change, the leader must purposefully interact and problem solve in *relationship building*. The leader participates in social processes to translate information into knowledge through *knowledge creation and sharing*. Lastly, leaders must tolerate ambiguity and prevent total disequilibrium caused by change in the constant effort of *coherence making*.

Hughes et al. (1993) agree that leaders are most effective when they acknowledge human emotions as well as intellect while seeking to influence followers. They emphasize that leadership and followership are equally important. Hughes et al. define leadership as "a social influence process shared among all members of a group" (p. 8). In this light, the authors express the study of leadership as an "immature science" (p. 64) as they believe researchers have not yet identified the truly important research questions to ask—much less finding any answers to them. This work also considers leadership an art, which encompasses understanding the situation in order to influence others to accomplish common goals.

Regarding the art and science of leadership, Hughes et al. (1993) differentiate between assessing leadership and measuring its effectiveness. In assessing leadership the five most common approaches are "critical incidents technique, interview, observations, paper-and-pencil measures, and assessment centers" (p. 70). The authors recognize that assessment of the leadership process will be more complete when more than one method is employed and the assessment technique should center on the researcher's definition of leadership. In measuring the effects of leadership, Hughes et al. underscore the need to determine if the criteria are affected by actions of the leader or external factors, as well as critically evaluate the criteria for relevance. The authors add that experimental and correlational studies are conducted to test leadership theories, while case studies provide principles for the leadership practitioner.

For the analysis of leadership, Hughes et al. devised a three-factor model as an *interactional framework* for analyzing leadership. The three factors are the leader, the followers and the situation. The leader in the analysis being conducted is the AACN, which is the collective association of its followers represented by individual deans of the member nursing schools. The situation is their endorsement of the DNP as sole education entry level for advanced practice nurses by the year 2015.

FIGURE B-2 Interactional framework for analyzing leadership
(Hughes et al., 1993, p. 92).

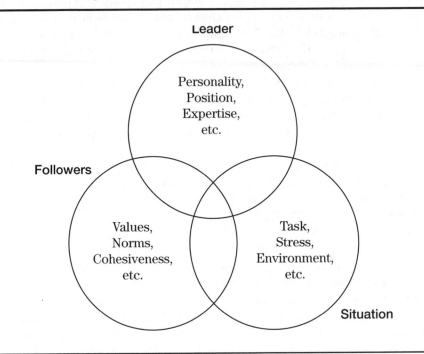

Transformational Leadership

Transformational Leadership is a type of leadership characterized by a leader who explicitly communicates a vision, inspires followers to share and work toward fruition of the vision, and provides resources for developing the personal potential of the follower. Transformational Leadership is most effective in an "empowered dynamic culture" and occurs when a leader "inspires followers to share a vision, empowering them to achieve the vision, and provides the resource necessary for developing their personal potential" (Smith, et al., 2004, p. 80).

The works of Bass and Avolio (as cited in Smith et al., 2004) conceptualize the four behaviors of transformational leadership as idealized influence, inspirational motivation, intellectual stimulation and individualized consideration. In contrast to servant leadership, which is most effective in a static environment, transformational leadership empowers the dynamic culture of the AACN in their process of establishing the DNP as entry-level education for APNs.

FIGURE B-3 AACN interactional framework for analyzing leadership
(Adapted from Hughes et al., 1993).

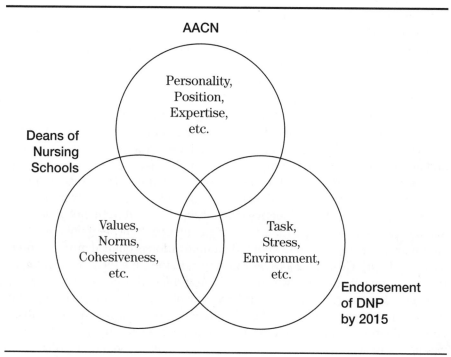

Diffusion of Innovations Theory

The AACN *DNP Roadmap Task Force Report* (2006a) states that Rogers'
Diffusion of Innovations Theory was employed as a framework for informing
and promoting adoption among stakeholders for the AACN's vision of the DNP.
Rogers adds that within the social system where the innovation is introduced,
important factors in its adoption include its compatibility with values, beliefs,
and past experiences. Within the AACN, a system comprised of deans of nursing schools who chose to become members, it is reasonable to infer, for the
most part, that the values and beliefs concerning graduate education are compatible. However, in this case, diffusion is the crux of the matter.

Diffusion is a process by which "(1) an innovation (2) is communicated
through certain channels (3) over time (4) among the members of a social
system" (Rogers, 2003, p. 11). Types of innovations include ideas, practices or
objects. Rogers adds that most innovations have been technological and that
only some have been comprised of information only. In diffusion research,

perceived attributes of innovations, affecting the rate of adoption, include relative advantages—better than previous idea; compatibility—consistency with values, needs, and past experiences; complexity—degree of difficulty to understand or use; "trialability" (p. 16)—ability for experimental research to reduce uncertainty; and observability—results of innovation are visible to others. Moreover, Rogers reminds readers that diffusion and adoption of all innovations are not desirable (e.g. introduction of automated tomato pickers resulted in the loss of business for small farmers).

The communication aspect of innovation is a process whereby the provider of information and the recipient reach a mutual understanding regarding the innovation. Methods of communication include mass media, interpersonal, and more recently, use of the Internet. Although objective research regarding innovation is not immaterial, Diffusion of Innovations (DOI) research indicates that those individuals who are the early adopters of innovations base their acceptance on the subjective evaluation conveyed to them by individuals like themselves, rather than scientific evidence. Interpersonal communication among peers who had adopted an innovation produced more adopters in that network (Rogers, 2003). For example, at the time the AACN endorsed their position papers, there was one DNP program in the nation (AACN, 2004). Although this program did not have APN students matriculating in the specialties of nurse practitioners, anesthetists, midwives or clinical nurse specialists, communication within the AACN membership achieved support for this innovation. There was no evidence, therefore, of the actual benefit of the DNP at the time of endorsement. Nonetheless, and as expected, communication and adoption of an innovation occurs more rapidly when persons involved share attributes (*homophily*) and less when persons do not (*heterophily*) (Rogers, 2003).

The third and fourth elements of the diffusion process involve a time period and targeted members of a social system. For the DNP innovation, the time period began at the AACN's endorsement of its vision in October, 2004. Those immediately targeted included all members of the AACN system. Soon afterward, the DNP taskforce held a series of conferences, meetings, and conference calls outside its system, to gain consensus on the plan to establish the DNP as entry-level education for the advanced practice nurse (AACN, 2006).

Systems Model

Social systems are open systems consisting of "matter, energy and information that are sets of parts with relationships between those parts" (Busch & Busch, 1992, p. 276). The AACN represents an open, social system comprised of deans of schools of nursing (matter). It is also constituted of individual systems, which also comprise the matter of other systems, such as university deans, members of other professional organizations, and representatives to boards of nursing. Within the system, energy facilitates relationships, in the form of research, discussions, and presentations, allowing members of the AACN to understand concepts of the DNP and plan for its implementation by relaying this information to individuals and groups outside the system represented by the AACN. Key expressions of the system in terms of the DNP include the AACN Position Statement, the Essentials document and the DNP Roadmap document. These provide sources of understanding the work (information) of the system, from which the AACN will attempt to produce its product. The energy produced will assist in the implementation of DNP programs and will continue the work of the AACN to promote the DNP as the sole educational entry level for the APN. This represents a significant change in the structure and the life processes of the system.

Capra (1996) describes key criteria of a living system as the pattern of organization, the structure and life process. The membership of the AACN fulfills the criteria of a living system. First, the pattern of organization is a collection of human systems. The human systems build relationships within the AACN, creating the structure of the organization—these human systems are deans of schools and colleges of nursing and therefore also create structures of other organizational systems. The life process of this system incorporates the activity of injecting energy and information into the system, processing it, and producing guidelines for the education of nurses. According to Capra, the AACN will "bring forth" as a result of a properly functioning system the universally accepted policy of the DNP as educational preparation for APNs.

As a living system, the AACN also meets requirements for a negotiated system, as illustrated by Busch and Busch in *Sociocybernetics* (1992). This type of system transacts with the environment, exchanging matter, energy and information. These transactions act as catalysts, which allow external influences to enter into the system, becoming a part of the work of the AACN. For example, a catalyst would be the attendance of any one dean, who may also be a member of a university committee that approves new programs. Physically, as that dean enters the system, she brings with her the matter that is her person as well as perspectives from her environment outside the AACN. The information she brings includes her knowledge of educational administration and research, as well as information from all life experiences. As a result, the dean will infuse energy as she communicates with others and participates in the discussions of the AACN, as well as transacts with the university new program committee by communicating the perspective of the committee.

In the manner of negotiated systems as expressed by Busch and Busch (1992), the AACN will transact with other systems in the realms of health care, education, and regulation. While fulfilling the primary function of the

AACN, producing guidelines for baccalaureate and graduate nursing education, it exerts authority over schools of nursing, producing a direct effect on types of programs offered. As systems, schools of nursing produce nurses, including advanced practice nurses. Because the accrediting body of the AACN, the Commission on Collegiate Nursing Education (CCNE), accredits 566 member schools (AACN, 2007), the result of its vision for advanced practice nursing brings with it potential consequences of loss of accreditation, should the school continue to offer master's degrees instead of replacing an established program with the DNP program.

Colleges or schools of nursing are also systems, comprised of teachers, students, curriculum, and administrators (matter). These processes of relationships among the elements express energy in the form of curriculum delivery, teaching and learning, and exchanging information with the university, a system subsuming the nursing school system. Schools of nursing also interface with other systems, such as specialty APN accrediting bodies, university accrediting organizations, and the state boards of nursing. As a result of the energy, or work, of the system, the schools of nursing will bring forth graduates who will successfully complete the licensure process and become members of the health care delivery system (see Figure B-1).

Effects-Based Outcomes

After the Cold War, the United States military adopted the concept of Effects-Based Operations (EBO), a framework for achieving the desired outcome of a specific action. Smith defines an effect as "a result of impact created by the application of military or other power" (Smith, 2002, p. 111). He emphasizes that the application of power could be political, especially because military power is used as a component of our nation's power. Smith further describes effects-based operations as "series of stimulus and response interactions" (p. 113). He adds that the challenge in planning an effects-based operation is to determine the stimulus which will yield the desired response, or effect.

The twenty-first century required military thinking to adapt to a broad spectrum of operations. In essence, EBO represents actions "designed to achieve specific effects that contribute directly to desired military and political outcomes" (Mann et al., 2002, p. 1). Historically, the military pursued objectives with one primary result measured, the target. Objectives were selected with less emphasis on creating the conditions for achievement and perhaps inadequate attention was paid to collateral effects. Mann et al. describe EBO methodology to address effects in the achievement of military objectives as well as the evaluation of the results of actions.

Mann et al. (2002) proposed Effects-Based Operations Theory to be incorporated into planning, executing and assessing military operations. This process includes both political and military agencies. The collapse of the Soviet Union and the end of the Cold War required modification in the defense of the United States because threat to national security changed radically. During the Cold War, the major threat was nuclear annihilation, so stated by the leaders of the Soviet Union. Today, instead of one major, organized threat, Mann et al. state the politicians and military services must be prepared to counter different ideologies. Many threats are not directly sponsored by legitimate nations and are not guided by the Just War Tradition, a concept established on moral imperatives, which provides international guidance for declaring and conducting war (Christopher, 2004).

Newly identified military responsibilities include protection from international terrorist groups, criminal organizations, and drug cartels. Current military operations illustrate the need for "interservice, interagency, and international coordination, as well as highly sophisticated understanding of the direct, indirect , intended, and unintended consequences of all actions taken" (Mann et al., 2002, p. 9). As an example, the authors describe how actions taken to stop the drug production or money laundering in one country led these activities to move to another country.

Other activities involving military resources include responding to humanitarian crises, specifically human suffering due to national instability or natural disasters. At times, humanitarian operations have included combat. Success in these situations requires the collective effort of joint military, interagency, and international organizations to answer immediate humanitarian needs, and create the foundation for sustained improvement and improved humanitarian conditions. EBO establishes a framework for addressing the planning, execution, and assessment of such operations (Mann et al., 2002).

In addition to military operations, Mann et al., (2002) address the application of EBO in the business world. Paralleling geopolitical changes, economic globalization and technological advances have changed international commerce, decreasing some barriers to international economics and presenting challenges and vulnerabilities unknown until now. The Internet offers real-time exchange of information but brings the vulnerability of cyber attack from hackers. Agencies with long term economic relationships with the United States may find themselves suddenly in a political setting no longer friendly to our nation. One example of an unintended consequence is an embargo against one nation that causes a negative impact upon other nations, who are also partners in international trade. EBO offers a construct to address such issues in the planning phase of either establishing business ties or creating a political policy for trade restriction.

Smith extends the discussion of effects-based operations by examining the nature of first-order effects in terms of "what is done...[and] how it is done" (2002, p. 236). The examination of what an initial action represents and how it has been executed become the basis for the extended analysis. In this regard, the "nature of the power used to undertake the action" (p.238) is most revealing. Smith posits that the power chosen "will tell observers a great deal about the action itself and the direction of any continuing chain of interactions" (p. 238) into a larger system of systems.

For the purpose of achieving success across the entire spectrum of engagement, whether political, military, or humanitarian actions, the Air Force and the Department of Defense established effects-based methodology to plan, execute, and assess operations (Mann, et al., 2002). The purpose of this work is to apply this framework to the leadership process of the AACN in its endorsement of the DNP. Evidence-based methodology will illustrate the planning, execution, and assessment of the outcomes of this leadership process.

Nursing Education

Throughout history, nurses have cared for the sick and dying from many different levels of educational preparation and social status (Burke, 2004). Military action, specifically the Crimean War in 1854–1855 and the Civil War in 1861–1865, necessitated improvement in medical and nursing care. In 1860, Florence Nightingale established the Nightingale Training School for Nurses at St. Thomas's Hospital in England, creating the modern model for nursing education where formal didactic instruction was added to an apprenticeship to prepare nurses (Berman, Snyder, Kozier, & Erb, 2008; Burke, 2004). The Belleview Training School for Nurses, Connecticut Training School for Nurses, and the Boston Training School for Nurses introduced the Nightingale model of nursing education to the United States. This provided the dominant method for educating nurses for nearly a hundred years (Burke, 2004). These schools were operated independently from hospitals, but were affiliated for clinical practice.

Unlike medical schools, the early nursing schools lacked the financial backing and endowments offered to sustain them (Gardenier, 1991). Before the turn of the century, they were forced by economic need to become dependent upon their affiliated hospitals. Gardenier states that schools of nursing became "captive of the medical community, fully controlled by the hospital" (p. 20). As economically profitable subordinates of hospitals, the number of nursing training programs increased rapidly, reaching 432 schools in 1900 and 1129 in 1910 (Burke, 2004). During the proliferation of nurse training, the early diploma programs focused more on providing service to the hospital, with less attention given to the formal education of nurses (Berman et al., 2008). Early nursing education lacked the formality of standardized curriculum and the quality of education varied widely throughout the country. The American Society of Superintendents of Training Schools for Nursing, formed in 1893, worked to improve and standardize the quality of instruction for nurses and initiated the first university affiliation with Teachers College, Columbia University (Gardenier, 1991). Gardenier states that although nursing was acceptable for proper women, it was viewed by society as a vocation and not a career. Women who wished to receive a university education in classical studies did so for the sake of becoming more educated wives and mothers, not in preparation for a career. The American Society of Superintendents of Training Schools for Nursing published *A Curriculum for Schools of Nursing* in 1917 and *A Curriculum Guide for Schools of Nursing* in 1937 (Burke, 2004). The standardization of curriculum was a first step in the professionalization of nursing.

In 1923, the Rockefeller Foundation's Committee for the Study of Nursing Education, called the "Goldmark Study," studied the conditions of nursing education. This committee identified the conflict of interest within the hospital administrations' control of nursing education and the hospital service of nursing students (Burke, 2004). Burke reports the recommendations of this landmark study included university affiliations for nursing education, specific training for nursing educators, licensing of nurses to ensure quality and safety, and financial support for nursing education to promote autonomous governance. The Goldmark Study is credited with the national movement to move nursing education to universities and the development of nursing as a profession. At the time of the report, there was one baccalaureate nursing program at the University of Minnesota (Berlin et al., 2008). Immediately following the release of the Goldmark Report, baccalaureate programs began accepting nursing students at Yale School of Nursing and the Frances Payne Bolton School of Nursing at Case Western Reserve University (Maraldo, Fagin, & Keenan, 1988).

However, the Goldmark Report failed to produce an upsurge of baccalaureate program development. In the mid-1920s there were only 25 university programs with a combined enrollment of 368 students, compared to hospital diploma programs with enrollments of more than 75,000 students (Maraldo et al., 1988). Soon the Great Depression created a surplus of nurses, and the motivation to move nursing education to the university was lost.

The surplus of nurses became a nursing shortage at the end of World War II. Interest in nursing education grew with the immediate need for nurses to resume work in low-paying hospitals (Maraldo et al., 1988). With funding from the Russell Sage Foundation, Lucille Brown studied the conditions and education of nurses. The resulting Brown Report recommended nursing education take place in universities and that a national accreditation system be developed to oversee nursing education. After this research, private foundations began to support nursing education, as well as promote the transition of the American Society of Superintendents of Training Schools for Nursing into the National League for Nursing, in order to accredit nursing education. Additionally, the Nurse Practice Act, passed in 1943, provided public funding for nursing education (Burke, 2004).

During the next three decades, many university nursing programs began to educate nurses, as did programs in junior colleges. Graduates of the junior, or community, colleges were awarded associate degrees in nursing. This concept in nursing education allowed students degrees in only two years and became immediately, immensely popular. "By 1981, half of the new nurses were being graduated from associate degree programs, a third from baccalaureate programs, and less than a fifth from diploma (hospital) programs" (Maraldo et al., 1988, p. 133). In addition to accrediting programs, the NLN encouraged the development of the master's degree in nursing. These programs allowed development in nursing research and specialization for educators and research. The first master's degree was conferred in psychiatric nursing at Rutgers University in 1954 (Berman et al., 2008).

The first doctoral degree conferred to nurses was the Doctorate of Education, established at Columbia University in 1924 (Courtney, Galvin, Patterson, & Shortridge-Baggett, 2005). In 1934, New York University offered a Doctor of Philosophy (PhD) in nursing (Waldsperger-Robb, 2005). By the 1960s, several nursing doctorates were recognized. The first clinical doctorate established was the Doctor of Nursing Science (DNS or DNSc) (Berman et al, 2008). Since then several types of nursing doctoral programs have developed, including the Nursing Doctorate (ND) and the newest, the Doctor of Nursing Practice, the DNP (Berman et al., 2008).

Regulation of Nurses

At its inception in the United States, nursing was marked by the struggle of nurse leaders to bring quality and standardized education to the profession of nursing (Burke, 2004). Members of the American Society of Superintendents of Training Schools for Nurses collaborated to improve and standardize the quality of nursing education. Their mission included improving the quality of life for nursing students, in the hospital setting as well as their basic living conditions. In 1896, a group of nursing leaders founded the Nurses Associated Alumnae of the United States and Canada. Their goal was to "strengthen the union of existing nursing organizations, to elevate nursing education, and to promote ethical standards" (Gardenier, 1991, p. 10).

The Nurses Associated Alumnae of the United States and Canada held their first convention in 1898. In step with the organizational progressive thrust of the time, they identified the need for regulation to combat the labeling of graduates from questionable nursing programs as *trained nurses* (Gardenier, 1991). At the end of the 19th century, nursing programs varied widely both in quality of instruction and time to completion, which ranged from six months to two years. The Nurses Associated Alumnae recommended licensure for all trained nurses to protect the public from untrained and poorly trained individuals. Gardenier reports that in 1903, nursing leaders in New York advocated, and were the first to gain, state legislation to regulate the profession.

Legislation for nursing was modeled after extant laws regulating physicians. New York's law specified requirements for a Board of Nurse Examiners, comprised of five nurses selected by the Board of Regents, along with testing of nurse candidates for licensure. "The strength of the bill was in the Board of Regents' power to determine the proper standards of training schools for nurses. Its weakness, however, unlike medicine, lay in its permissive compliance" (Gardenier, 1991, p. 11). Later corrected, this early New York law allowed programs to ignore its provisions. Following New York, all states enacted nurse practice acts by 1923, establishing legal status for the nursing profession in the United States.

The Advanced Practice Nurse

Advanced nursing practice began in the late 19th century when nurses answered the call from surgeons to provide their "undivided attention" to anesthetized patients, as the morbidity and mortality associated with anesthesia was unacceptably high (AANA, 2006, n.p.). Formal nurse anesthesia education was established in the United States in 1909 (AANA, 2005) and was introduced internationally in 1914 in preparation for casualty care in World War I. After the war, the demand for nurse anesthesia programs grew exponentially.

Established in 1931, the American Association of Nurse Anesthetists has been responsible for education, standards of practice, and certification of nurse anesthetists, currently representing 28,000 CRNAs. The AANA initiated certification in 1945 and recertification in 1978. The American Association of Nurse Anesthetists began accrediting nurse anesthetist programs in 1952 and became recognized by the U.S. Department of Education as the accrediting authority for nurse anesthetists in 1955 (AANA, 2006).

The first nurse midwifery practice in the United States was established in 1925 to improve the health of mothers and babies in the mountains of Kentucky. Brought from the United Kingdom, nurse midwives worked first in rural areas, then in medically underserved areas in New York City. Although efforts were made to educate nurses in the discipline of midwifery in the early 1920s, American nurse midwifery education officially began in 1931 at the Lobenstine Midwifery Clinic, Inc., in New York City, formerly named the "School of the Association for the Promotion and Standardization of Midwifery" (Varney, 1997, p. 9). Throughout their history, nurse midwives recorded their contributions toward improvement of maternal and infant health (Carr, 2005).

The American Association of Nurse-Midwives was established in 1929 and evolved into the American College of Nurse-Midwives (ACNM). Incorporated in 1955, it now represents nearly 13,000 CNMs, with over 7,000 active members. This professional organization defined nurse midwifery and set goals for the organization. These goals included the development and evaluation of standards of care for women and infants and the education of midwives, as well as the accreditation of educational programs and the promotion of research. The additional goal was to establish the "college as a leader and major resource in the development and promotion of high quality care for women and infants, nationally and internationally" (Varney, 1997, p. 19; HRSA, 2004). The ACNM Division of Accreditation is recognized by the U.S. Department of Education as the accrediting authority for certified nurse midwives (ACNM, 2005).

In 1965, the University of Colorado Health Sciences Center (UCHSC) launched the nurse practitioner career field when it initiated a pediatric nurse practitioner course of study utilizing an interdisciplinary faculty that included nursing, medicine and related health fields. Sixty pediatric nurse practitioners graduated from the four-year funded project, leading the way for the school of nursing to expand the nurse practitioner program into other specialties. Additionally, the founders became consultants for other universities in the establishment of additional programs (Tropello, 2000). advanced registered nurse practitioners numbered 116,447 in 2005 (Phillips, 2006), representing twelve specialties (AANP, 2004).

The primary accrediting authority for ARNP programs is the Commission on Collegiate Nursing Education, the autonomous agency of the AACN. Some programs are accredited by NANLAC, affiliated with the National League for Nursing. Unlike midwifery and nurse anesthetist programs, nurse practitioner and clinical nurse specialist programs are not accredited by specialty agencies beyond the schools of nursing.

Because there are twelve subspecialties within the ARNP title, there are many professional organizations which represent this advanced practice nurse category. The American Academy of Nurse Practitioners, established in 1985, represents 90,000 ARNPs and offers certification for adult nurse practitioners and family nurse practitioners (AANP, 2005). The Nurse Practitioner Healthcare Foundation (NPHF) has as its mission "to improve the health status and quality of care through nurse practitioner (NP) innovations in education, research, health policy, service and philanthropy" (NPHF, 2006). In addition, the American Nurse Credentialing Center (ANCC), the credentialing body of the American Nurses Association, offers certification for nurse practitioners as well as clinical nurse specialists (ANCC, 2006).

The clinical nurse specialist is an advanced practice nurse who, having earned a graduate degree in nursing, is described as an expert clinician. The CNS may work in the role of educator, or provide direct clinical practice, research, consultation or administration (Henderson, 2004). According to the National Association of Clinical Nurse Specialists (NACNS), there are approximately 69,000 CNSs of which approximately 14,500 are also educated and employed as nurse practitioners. Clinical nurse specialists may seek certification through the ANCC or through specialty organizations, specifically, the American Association of Critical Care Nurses, the Rehabilitation Nursing Certification Board, and the Oncology Nursing Certification Corporation. The National Association of Clinical Nurse Specialists came into existence in 1995 for the purpose of unifying CNSs and promoting the contributions of CNSs and advanced practice nursing (NACNS, n.d.a).

By definition, all clinical nurse specialists enter practice with at least a master's degree. However, other advanced practice nurses may enter the APN role having graduated from programs awarding a post-baccalaureate certificate. According to the Health Resources and Services Administration (2004), 76% of nurse practitioners completed a master's degree, 62 % of CNMs were prepared at that level of education, and only 37% of CRNAs entered practice with a master's or post-master's degree with 58% of CRNAs entering practice with a post-RN certificate.

Endorsement of the Doctor of Nursing Practice Degree

AACN's endorsement of its vision of establishing the DNP as entry-level education for advanced practice nurses is reminiscent of the American Nurses Association (ANA) resolution of 1965, declaring the minimum educational level for professional nurses as the baccalaureate in nursing degree. Similar to the AACN decision, the ANA published this resolution to increase the entry-level education, stating that the delivery of health care and the provision of nursing care had evolved into an increasingly complex endeavor. In 1965, the percentage of nurses nationally with baccalaureate degrees as the highest level of education attained was 29.6 % (Nelson, 2002, n.p.); that percentage has grown to 34.2% (HRSA, 2004). The 1965 ANA resolution resulted in drastically reduced numbers of diploma nursing schools and an increase in baccalaureate programs. It did not, however, prevent the proliferation of associate degree nursing programs or the philosophical chasm between baccalaureate nurses and nurses with nursing diplomas or associate degrees (Nelson, 2002).

Although health care has become increasingly complex and nurses continue to adapt to new challenges, the education required for entry into practice remains hospital diploma programs, the Associate Degree in Nursing (ADN) in community colleges, and the Bachelor of Science Degree in universities. The American Nurses Association refers to nurses with the Baccalaureate degree as professional nurses whereas those with ADNs or Diplomas are referred to as technical nurses. When the ANA published their position statement in 1965, it was their intention that nurses with ADN and Diploma degrees would continue education to complete the BSN degree (Nelson, 2002). Although the number of nurses with diplomas decreased and those with baccalaureate degrees as entry-level education continued to increase, in 2004 only 30.5% of entry-level nurses earned baccalaureate degrees, 25.2% diploma nurses, 42.2% associate degrees, and 0.5% entered nursing with master's or doctoral degrees (HRSA, 2004).

Soon after the publication of the American Nurses' Association position statement on entry-level education for nurses, the American Association of Colleges of Nursing was established in 1969:

> to answer the need for a national organization dedicated exclusively to furthering nursing education in America's universities and colleges. Representing nursing education programs at 592 public and private universities and colleges, AACN serves the public interest by assisting deans and directors to improve and advance nursing education, research, and practice. (Fang et al., 2006, p. ix)

The accrediting division of the AACN, the CCNE is one of two accrediting agencies for colleges or schools of nursing, although the ACNM and the AANA accredit programs for CNMs and CRNAs.

The AACN *Essentials of Doctoral Education for Advanced Nursing Practice* (AACN, 2006b) states the AACN Task Force on the Practice Doctorate in Nursing created the policy statement over the period of two years. Members of this task force included representatives from universities considering the DNP, those who currently offered the DNP, "a specialty professional organization" (p. 4), and nursing administrators. The AACN membership, comprised of deans of baccalaureate and higher degree nursing programs, adopted the final position statement in October 2004 (AACN, 2004a). Of the nearly 600 schools of nursing which comprised the membership of the AACN at that time, only 266 deans were present and authorized to vote on this issue. Assistant deans were not allowed to vote, nor was proxy or absentee voting permitted. The vote was recorded as 160 in favor of and 106 opposed to the DNP (Fulton & Lyon, 2005). Additionally, the AACN division of accreditation, the Commission on Collegiate Nursing Education (CCNE), declared that, "only practice doctoral degrees with the Doctor of Nursing Practice (DNP) title will be eligible for CCNE accreditation (AACN, 2005).

In establishing the DNP as the entry-level degree for nurse practitioners, the AACN vision statement carries implications for every university offering a degree for advanced practice nursing, numerous nursing and health care organizations, and innumerable individuals providing and receiving health care. Having published their position statement, the AACN conducted hearings from September 2005 to January 2006, as well as a conference, to "provide opportunities for feedback from a diverse group of stakeholders" (2006a, p. 5). Stakeholders include health care organizations, professional organizations representing APN specialties, interdisciplinary health care providers, schools of nursing not accredited by the AACN, federal and state legislators, and more than 168,000 APNs (Philips, 2006). The AACN mandate to establish the DNP as the entry level of advanced practice nurses by 2015 may not have the support needed to reach fruition. This places the nursing profession, once again, at odds over nursing education. In order to examine the potential for success in implementing the DNP by 2015, one must examine the leadership process of the AACN as a system, within a system of systems.

Conclusion

The American Association of Colleges of Nursing introduced a transformational change into a system of systems. The outcomes of this action remain largely unknown and may have many effects on the larger health care system. This analysis of the AACN leadership process will examine leadership, change, systems, use of the diffusion of innovations approach, and issues within nursing, and will be framed within effects-based methodology.

CHAPTER III: METHODOLOGY

Research provides a structure for purposeful inquiry and the development of new knowledge. To this end, qualitative research explores phenomena that describe, explain or create understanding (Freebody, 2003). Merriam describes a qualitative case study as "an intensive, holistic description and analysis of a bounded phenomenon such as a program, an institution, a person, a process, or a social unit" (1988, p. xiv). According to Stake, a qualitative case study should develop a "greater understanding of a case" (1995, p. 16), while an instrumental case study provides a qualitative illustration of a specific issue (Creswell, 2005).

Merriam (1988) explains that a case study design does not follow one specific course of action, since the exploration and analysis can develop and change as the study progresses. The primary methods of data collection for case studies commonly involve interviews and questionnaires, observation, mining data from documents, and audiovisual materials (Creswell, 2005). Freebody adds that the "case study methodology uses multiple data collection and analytic procedures" (2003, p. 63). In case study research, methodological triangulation refers to combining multiple methods of data collection such as interviews, questionnaires, and documents, which provides internal validity (Merriam, 1988).

Research Design

This instrumental case study illustrated a leadership process by examining the introduction of a transformational change into a system of systems. Specifically, the researcher employed a qualitative case study of the leadership process demonstrated by the American Association of Colleges of Nursing regarding their endorsement of the Doctor of Nursing Practice degree. This organization introduced a transformational change of the entry-level educational degree for advanced practice nursing into one system within a much larger multiple system construct. The study of this leadership process took place within the context of a system of systems (Figure B-1). Hughes et al. (1993) describe three components of leadership, the leader, followers and situation. In this case study, the leader and followers consisted of AACN, as a unified body and its membership, deans of schools of nursing, respectively. The situation encompasses the introduction of this change into the education systems, accreditation systems, certifying systems, regulatory systems, and healthcare delivery systems. The complexity of the situation lends itself appropriately to a qualitative inquiry of the leadership process.

As documents were examined and interviews were conducted, the leadership process of the AACN (situation) was analyzed as an interconnected system, within a system of systems, illustrating the potential effects of its endorsement of the Doctorate of Nursing Practice for all advanced practice nurses by 2015. The system of systems into which the vision had been introduced is comprised of five major categories of systems: accrediting, education, certifying, regulatory, and health care delivery.

Within the set of accrediting systems, the Commission on Collegiate Nursing Education, which is the accrediting division of the AACN, is one of several organizations that accredit nursing programs (AACN, 2006a). The AANA and ACNM establish standards and accredit programs to educate nurse anesthetists and nurse midwives (AANA, 2006a; ACNM 2004). In addition to the accreditation of nursing schools, regional organizations customarily accredit universities to which the schools of nursing belong. The education system may be comprised of one private institution with a single nursing school—or may be as complex as a state university system with many member schools.

Certifying systems include organizations that recognize that the graduate education offered is appropriate for APNs, and provide certification to individual APNs having demonstrated competence on a standardized examination (AANA, 2006a; AANP, n.d.; ACNM 2004). Two of the certifying bodies also encompass accrediting authority for APN specialties, the AANA and the ACNM. Each state possesses at least one agency responsible for the safe practice of APNs; usually this is the state's board of nursing. In five states, boards of medicine in conjunction with boards of nursing authorize the professional practice of APNs (Phillips, 2007), and in some states, boards of anesthesia or boards of midwifery regulate APNs (Avery, 2007). In addition to systems influencing the effects of the DNP policy, other factors which become the *environment* of the situation include time, financial and malpractice considerations.

Data Collection

Data collection for this study was derived from organizational documents, pertinent literature reviews, and interviews. Documents examined included those published by the AACN, (state) Nurse Practice Acts, position statements by advanced practice nursing organizations, regulatory documents, and public health care policies. Journal articles responding to the proposed transformational change by the AACN provided perspectives of nursing professionals, independent of a particular organization. Documents selected were either public domain and accessed via the Internet on non-secured websites, or published in professional journals.

After approval from the Spalding University Ethics Committee, interviews were requested from a purposeful sample of nursing and health care professionals. A maximal variation sampling included representatives of systems affected by the actions of the AACN. Specifically, those interviewed included a dean of a nursing school, one director of nursing, executive members of national nursing organizations, and advanced practice nurses, representing CRNAs, CNMs, ARNPs and CNSs, one of whom who had recently earned a DNP degree. The diversity of the sample interviewed reflected the diversity within the nursing profession and provided multiple perspectives of the effects of the introduction of the transformational change by the AACN within the system of systems.

Confidentiality Human Rights Protection

Individuals meeting criteria were invited to participate and provided the researcher with a signed Informed Consent Agreement. Risks to the individual were considered minimal, not exceeding those encountered in one's daily life. Although no direct benefits to participants were identified, benefits to the profession of nursing and leadership may result from their contributions. To ensure anonymity, data were presented in group form to ensure identifying information could not be linked to a participant's data. Three of the eight interviews were conducted in person and the remainder by telephone. The length of the interviews averaged one hour and were recorded then transcribed by the researcher. All materials will remain in a locked area in the home office of the researcher for a period of five years. The Ethics Committee request and approval are found in Appendix D.

Effects-Based Methodology for Analysis

This researcher applied the use of a specific method of analysis in the education of advanced practice nurses in an effort to illuminate the complexities of educational leadership within interconnected systems. Effects-based outcomes refer to results of one action; first order of effects indicate the result is a direct consequence to the action taken. Second-order effects require the intervention of one variable and third-order effects result from more than one intervening variable. Although defined as systems in terms of organizational dynamics, this study considered professional organizations such as the AANA as singular entities, as unitary actors within one of the five major systems described. As such, the unitary response of organizations were examined in an effects-based methodology.

Mann et al. define *effect* as the "full range of outcomes, events, or consequences that result from a specific action" (Mann, et al., 2002, p. 31). A direct or first-order effect is the immediate result of a single action, without intervening variables. The immediate result may then generate additional consequences which may be intended or unintended, and described as second- or even third-order effects.

As an organization that creates standards for nursing education, the AACN can direct change in nursing programs because this organization is the same agency that accredits nursing programs. The AACN does not possess the authority to create doctoral programs, as this is the purview of universities and sometimes state higher education agencies. Neither does the AACN regulate the profession of nursing, as that is the responsibility of state boards of professional practice. However, its scope of influence may well shape the future for advanced practice nursing.

Hughes et al. (1993) define leadership as a process where "leaders and followers interact dynamically in a particular situation or environment" (1993, p. 107). This researcher identifies the AACN as the leader, and the deans of nursing schools as followers. The endorsement of the DNP constitutes the situation, and the environment is the system of systems as depicted in Figure B-1. According to Pullan (2001), having introduced the proposed transformational change, the leader cannot control the variables or the outcomes resulting from this action. He adds that change is not linear, but rather a dynamic event, requiring the leader to associate unlikely elements. At best, the leader can pilot an organization through the "rolling seas in a purposeful and successful manner" (O'Toole, 1995, p. xii) toward its goal of the stated change.

In this case study, the *trigger* action is the AACN's endorsement of the DNP as entry-level education for advanced practice nurses. The first-order variable is not amenable to control by the AACN. This variable encompassed the initial reactions to this event leading to a discourse among professionals most directly affected by this proposed change, as evidenced in the discussions in nursing literature. The first-order effect includes organizational responses (actions) that reflect the dynamics of its members. Within this first order of effects, deans of nursing schools agreed or declined to develop a DNP program or deferred the decision until a future time. Professional organizations supported or challenged this proposed change by publishing position statements or organizations chose to defer making a decision to support or challenge.

The second order of effects depends on variables encountered after nursing schools decided whether or not to develop DNP programs, and after professional organizations published position statements on the DNP. Such variables included the classification of a university, university success with other practice doctorates, and nursing schools' available funding for designing DNP proposals for presentation to university administrations. Another example of a variable following a second-order effect was the interaction among member APNs within specific professional organizations resulting from position statements of support or challenge to the proposed DNP.

Third-order effects are identified as the consequences of variables following second-order effects. For example, a university administration must choose to accept or refuse a proposal for a DNP program within its nursing school. Likewise, professional organizations may petition regulatory agencies to support the current level of education for licensure for APN practice or add the DNP as an additional academic degree for entry to practice. If a professional organization provides certification for practice, it must create policy that allows DNP graduates to apply for certification, create policy to allow only DNP graduates to apply, or modify current policy to allow graduates of different levels of education to apply for certification. The following illustration depicts one sequence of effects from the AACN introduction of this transformational change. This simple algorithm addresses only three potential effects. The only effect developed in this figure was that which leads to the fruition of the AACN vision.

Interview Questions

The interview questions were based on those presented by the American Nursing Association in September 2005 while discussing concerns about the AACN's introduction of the DNP. Permission was granted to adopt these questions and alter them as needed for this study. They are divided into categories to reflect first, second and third orders of effects or outcomes. Answers to the questions were sought through document review, interviews, and review of pertinent literature.

First Order:
1. Are educators deciding that there is a gap in clinical practice: that they feel there needs to be a practice doctorate, rather than responding to a study that demonstrates the need?
2. What empirical evidence exists to support the development of the DNP?
3. Will those with a DNP be tenured/equitable within the university setting or become second class citizens in the academic environment?

Second Order:
4. Who is going to teach DNP students since the role is considered advanced practice?
5. Will there be confusion if master's degree programs still exist? Should those programs be phased out now?

Third Order:
6. What is the cost of the DNP in regard to the economics of the profession?
7. Has there been a financial analysis performed of the impact on universities by eliminating the master's program?
8. What research demonstrates that nursing service can bear the additional cost associated with hiring someone with a DNP? If such evidence is missing, will AACN or another organization conduct such an analysis? Why or why not?

FIGURE B-4 Effects-based outcomes with adjacent potential outcomes.

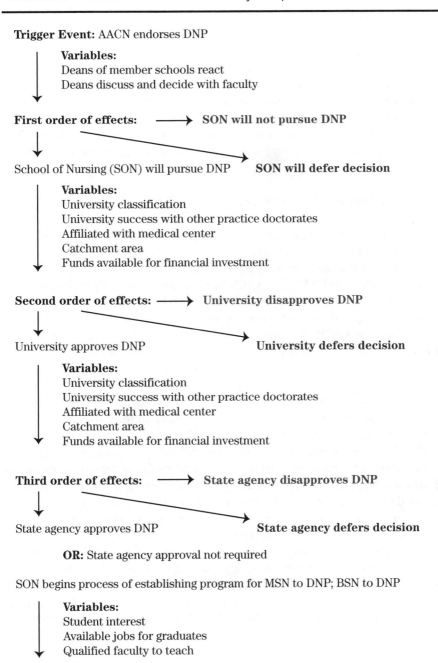

Trigger Event: AACN endorses DNP

    Variables:
    Deans of member schools react
    Deans discuss and decide with faculty

First order of effects: ⟶ **SON will not pursue DNP**

School of Nursing (SON) will pursue DNP   **SON will defer decision**

    Variables:
    University classification
    University success with other practice doctorates
    Affiliated with medical center
    Catchment area
    Funds available for financial investment

Second order of effects: ⟶ **University disapproves DNP**

University approves DNP   **University defers decision**

    Variables:
    University classification
    University success with other practice doctorates
    Affiliated with medical center
    Catchment area
    Funds available for financial investment

Third order of effects: ⟶ **State agency disapproves DNP**

State agency approves DNP   **State agency defers decision**

    OR: State agency approval not required

SON begins process of establishing program for MSN to DNP; BSN to DNP

    Variables:
    Student interest
    Available jobs for graduates
    Qualified faculty to teach

9. Has there been a cost benefit analysis of how the DNP will affect cost of nursing faculty?

… *how the DNP will affect cost of educating DNP-prepared advanced practice nurses?*

… *how the DNP will affect cost of care provided by DNP-prepared advanced practice nurses?*

10. How would state nurse practice acts and regulatory language need to change upon implementation of the DNP?

11. What will be the role of credentialing bodies? Will those entities need to create certification mechanisms and new specialty exams for DNPs?

CHAPTER IV: PRESENTATION AND ANALYSIS OF THE DATA

This research examined the leadership change processes involved in the initiative by the American Association of Colleges of Nursing (AACN) to transform the entry-level educational requirement for advanced practice nurses to the Doctor of Nursing Practice (DNP). The AACN introduced this paradigm change into a system of systems. This change has and will continue to produce effects that can neither be controlled nor guaranteed by the AACN. By examining the leadership processes of the AACN, an organization comprised of a relatively small number of nurse educators, the researcher sought a greater understanding of how this one organization could effect a change of an educational paradigm involving many systems and even more individuals within the health care system.

Primary sources of data included published documents of nursing organizations, specifically the *AACN Position Statement on the Practice Doctorate in Nursing* (2004a), the *DNP Roadmap Task Force Report: October 20, 2006* (AACN, 2006a), and position statements from national nursing organizations. Eight individuals were interviewed, selected from executive members of national organizations representing the profession of nursing, one nursing school dean, one nurse administrator, one individual from each of the four APN specialties (clinical nurse specialist, nurse anesthetist, nurse midwife, and nurse practitioner) and one APN who had earned the DNP degree. Data were collected from pertinent literature, representing secondary data sources.

The researcher identified national nursing and advanced practice nursing organizations that had published position statements on the DNP (Table B-1), included available professional literature and limited the number of interviewees to the description given here. Participants were selected to include a maximum variation sample of categories of individuals most directly affected by the action of the AACN. Literature was selected to present the most varied perspectives on the DNP initiative as well as sentinel documents, which were cited in subsequent publications. The data collected demonstrate integration of similar data or the *emergence of regularities* representing a theoretical guideline for ending this phase of the research (Merriam, 1988).

Findings

Interview questions for this research were analyzed within the framework of Effects-Based Outcomes, to illustrate first, second, and third orders of effects derived from the introduction of the proposed paradigm change. First-order effects are those which result directly from the introduction of the paradigm change by the AACN. The system into which the change was introduced generated variables and produced planned and unplanned outcomes, which created subsequent variables and outcomes, described as second- and third-order effects. Findings are presented and discussed within the context of effects-based outcomes.

Eleven questions selected from those posed by the American Nurses Association on the DNP organized and explored the data from organizational documents, participant interviews, and pertinent literature. Questions were grouped to demonstrate orders of effects within the data from each of the research areas. The researcher acknowledges that each question may not be addressed by every organization, participant or author(s) of pertinent literature. Triangulating data for this case study provided internal validity (Merriam, 1988).

First-Order Effects

The introduction of the Doctor of Nursing Practice as the sole entry educational preparation for advanced practice nurses by the American Association of Colleges of Nursing represents the trigger action for effects-based outcomes and the basis for this case study. First-order effects include outcomes resulting directly from this action, specifically, the acceptance, rejection, or deferral of the DNP initiative. In order for a school of nursing or organization to accept, reject or defer decision on the concept of the DNP, factors for consideration and reasoning are included in the following questions:

> Are educators deciding that there is a gap in clinical practice: that they feel there needs to be a practice doctorate, rather than responding to a study that demonstrates the need?

> What empirical evidence exists to support the development of the DNP? (ANA, 2005, n.p.)

TABLE B-1 Professional Nursing Organization Documents Included in Case Study

Organization	Membership
American Association of Colleges of Nursing (AACN)	Deans of colleges of nursing offering baccalaureate and graduate nursing degrees
American Nurses Association (ANA)	All nurses
American Organization of Nurse Executives (AONE)	Nurse administrators
Association of Faculties of Pediatric Nurse Practitioners (AFPNP)	Pediatric family and school, nurse practitioner nursing educators
National League for Nurses (NLN)	Deans of colleges of nursing offering all nursing degrees and all nurse educators
National Organization of Nurse Practitioner Faculties (NONPF)	Nurse practitioner nursing educators
American Academy of Nurse Practitioners (AANP)	All nurse practitioners Certified registered nurse practitioners (CRNPs)
American Association of Nurse Anesthetists (AANA)	Certified registered nurse anesthetists (CRNAs)
American College of Nurse–Midwives (ACNM)	Certified nurse–midwives (CNMs)
American College of Nurse Practitioners (ACNP)	All nurse practitioners Certified registered nurse practitioners (CRNPs)
National Association of Clinical Nurse Specialists (NACNS)	Clinical nurse specialists (CNSs)
National Association of Nurse Practitioners in Women's Health (NPWH)	Nurse practitioners providing primary care to women
National Association of Pediatric Nurse Practitioners (NAPNAP)	Pediatric nurse practitioners (PNPs) Certified pediatric nurse practitioners (CPNPs)
National Conference of Gerontological Nurse Practitioners (NCGNP)	Nurse practitioners providing primary care to older adults

Organizational Documents: Developing the DNP

American Association of Colleges of Nursing

The DNP Roadmap document (AACN, 2006a) discusses the utilization of Rogers' Diffusion of Innovations Theory to introduce the DNP initiative into the health care system. Rogers (2003) states that this process involves the communication of an innovation through social channels over a period of time. According to the AACN white paper, clinical practice doctoral nursing programs have been a focus of discussion in educational circles, beginning with the introduction of the Nursing Doctorate (ND) in 1979. At the time of the DNP initiative endorsement in October 2004, there were four ND programs, two of which offered entry into practice tracks to both pre-licensure nursing and advanced practice nursing (AACN, 2004a). Additionally, other practice-focused doctorates established in 1999 admitted post-master's students with expertise in areas of advanced practice nursing in programs granting the Doctor of Nursing Science (DNSc) and the DNP. These programs offered specialization in executive management and population-based clinical practice. Following Rogers' Diffusion of Innovations Theory, the practice doctorate initiative was first communicated, or initially triggered, among members of the AACN, sharing information on the perceived benefits of the DNP.

In its position statement on the DNP, the AACN (2004a) references several reports published by the Institute of Medicine (IOM) regarding the quality of health care in the United States, including *To Err is Human: Building a Safer Health System* (IOM, 1999), *Crossing the Quality Chasm* (IOM, 2001), and *Health Professions Education: A Bridge to Quality* (IOM 2003). These reports analyzed preventable deaths and morbidity caused by health care providers and institutions as well as made recommendations for improving quality and safety of health care in the United States. The most specific recommendation regarding education is found in *Health Professions Education: A Bridge to Quality,* "All health professionals should be educated to deliver patient-centered care as members of an interdisciplinary team, emphasizing evidence-based practice, quality improvement approaches, and informatics" (IOM, 2003, p. 3). Although the IOM discusses problems within the health care system and provides recommendations to improve quality in health care, the reports do not directly address advanced practice nurses, nor do they indicate a pressing need to transform the current master's degree preparation to the doctorate level. Many of the recommendations by the IOM are appropriate for nurse response, but do not specifically provide empirical evidence to support the DNP.

The Roadmap document also cites work by the National Research Council (NRC), "The need for doctorally prepared practitioners and clinical faculty would be met if nursing could develop a new nonresearch clinical doctorate, similar to the MD and PharmD in medicine and pharmacy, respectively" (NRC, 2005, p. 74). The statement is made within a context to allow nurses with research doctorates to focus on research, not practice or teaching. The NRC goes on to suggest strategies to produce nurse scientists at a younger age, who would have longer careers in research. Suggested changes include incorporating the master's degree curriculum into a PhD program for the purpose of creating the most expeditious route to creating nurse scientists and to encourage potential nurse scientists to seek a PhD with or without clinical experience in order to extend the tenure of their career in research.

The AACN and the National Organization of Nurse Practitioner Faculties (NONPF) conducted a collaborative study revealing an increase in the amount of time devoted to didactic and clinical education in APN educational programs. From 1995 to 2000 the average number of contact hours in theory courses increased by 72 hours and time in the clinical areas increased by 36 hours, without an increase in academic credit hours. This requirement was based on "the growing complexity of health care, burgeoning growth in scientific knowledge, and increasing sophistication of technology" (AACN, 2004a, p. 7). This document also states that the amount of time APN students matriculate in programs far exceeds that of other disciplines. However, this study did not address a gap in clinical practice or observe that advanced practice nurses had practiced below expected standards.

The AACN position paper refers to one survey conducted by the University of Kentucky to test the marketability of the DNP. In 1999, prior to launching the DNP program, the university mailed questionnaires to 385 executives in health care settings, including acute, long-term care and public health agencies. The response rate of 29% yielded 68 respondents indicating they would be interested in hiring nurses with the DNP degree. Stated differently, 17.8% of those surveyed responded favorably regarding the employment of DNP-prepared professionals. Respondents provided examples of work titles for DNP nurses as "Vice President for Clinical Services, Program Director, Vice President for Patient Care, Chief Executive Officer, Health Officer or Commissioner, Quality Improvement Director, Director of Clinical Services, Clinical Information Technology Specialist, Direct Care Clinician, and Faculty Member" (AACN, 2004, p. 8). In fact, only one of the ten potential positions included direct patient care, which is the primary role of advanced practice nurses.

National Organization of Nurse Practitioner Faculties

In its *Statement on the Practice Doctorate in Nursing*, the NONPF (2006) states that the DNP is anticipated to become the standard for nurse practitioner education and supports the development of the DNP, as evolutionary progress in the education of nurse practitioners. However, this organization recommends gradually advancing toward the DNP as the sole educational level, rather than meeting a deadline for transition from master's to doctoral educational preparation for nurse practitioners. Finally, this organization accepted the DNP to become the level of preparation for nurse practitioners, a clear first-order effect.

National League for Nursing

In a position paper on the transformation of nursing education, the National League for Nursing (NLN) acknowledged the absence of evidence for establishing the DNP as the sole entry-level educational requirement for advanced practice nurses. This organization also requested that creating new practice roles for nurses, changing curriculum and adding content to current programs be evidence-based (NLN, 2005). Responding to the actions of the AACN, the NLN made comments on the education of nurses but neither accepted nor rejected the DNP as the sole entry point into APN practice and encouraged further research to support the advancement of nursing education.

American Nurses Association

Another flagship nursing organization, the American Nurses Association (ANA), published a list of questions delineating concerns about creating the DNP as the sole entry point into practice for APNs. These questions addressed concerns in the areas of education, practice, economics, regulation, and credentialing. In the organization's first position statement in 1965, it proposed the baccalaureate degree as the sole educational preparation for nurses, which was discussed earlier in this document. In the forty-plus years since this position, only 30.5% of nurses enter the profession with baccalaureate degrees (HRSA, 2004). As the organization representing all nurses in the United States, it has chosen to remain neutral, neither acceping nor rejecting the DNP as the only entry-level education for advanced practice nursing (ANA 2005).

American Association of Nurse Anesthetists

Although the two longest established organizations representing both nurses and nursing education have chosen to remain neutral at this point, most national organizations representing advanced practice nursing have published positions declaring support or non-support of the DNP as the sole entry-level education for APNs. One of the oldest APN organizations is the American Association of Nurse Anesthetists, established in 1931. Representing CRNAs, the AANA has provided certification since 1945 (AANA, 2008) and accreditation of educational programs since 1952 (AANA, 2006a). In February 2006, the AANA published an interim position in opposition to the DNP as entry-level preparation for CRNAs, stating:

> evidence currently does not support mandatory clinical doctorate degrees for entry into nurse anesthesia practice. The AANA will make a decision on this matter following stakeholder input, data collection and analysis, and a thorough assessment of the potential impact of requiring clinical doctoral education the profession and the public we serve. (2006b, n.p.)

Later in 2006, the AANA posted a background statement on its website citing a lack of opportunity to be involved with the preparatory work for the AACN white paper on the DNP. It also noted a similar problem with planning activities to explore the proposed mandate of the DNP (AANA, 2006c). In its definitive position statement, adopted July 2, 2007, the "AANA supports doctoral education for entry into nurse anesthesia practice by 2025" (AANA, 2007, p. 1). This position extends the first-order effect, sought by the AACN, by a decade. In its rationale for this position, the AANA describes advancing the educational level of CRNAs throughout its history and proposes the DNP to ensure that CRNAs remain the "best-prepared, safest anesthesia providers possible" (p. 1). However, the statement does not offer empirical evidence in support of the DNP.

American College of Nurse-Midwives

Inadequate evidence to support the DNP is the primary rationale stated in the American College of Nurse-Midwives (ACNM) Division of Accreditation Statement on Midwifery Education (ACNM, 2005). Established in 1929, this professional organization of nurse midwives establishes and maintains standards for education and practice. The ACNM defines a nurse midwife as "a person educated in the two disciplines of nursing and midwifery" (ACNM, 2005, p. 1). The ACNM also supports and accredits educational programs, and certifies direct entry midwives designated as certified midwives (CMs). Educated in the discipline of midwifery, CMs are educated and held to the same standards of practice as CNMs. The U.S. Department of Education recognized the ACNM as an accrediting body in 1982, even though it began accrediting nurse midwifery education in 1962. To this end, the Division of Accreditation states:

> ■ Whereas the ACNM Division of Accreditation has over 40 years of expertise in setting standards of accreditation for midwifery education programs and has been recognized by the U.S. Department of Education since the early 1980s;

- Whereas the ACNM DOA bases its evaluation of midwifery education programs on ACNM Core Competencies, Standards of Practice, and the regularly conducted ACC/AMCB task analysis of midwifery practice;
- Whereas all ACNM DOA accredited programs based on the above documents have decades of evidence of preparation of successful graduates in all aspects of midwifery, including leadership, political action and service to women and childbearing families regardless of terminal degree; and
- Whereas the ACNM DOA and its members recognize the increasing public need for midwifery care and the national and global shortage of midwives,
- Whereas there is inadequate evidence to document the advantages of a practice doctorate in the provision of care to women and childbearing families, especially in an era of rising health care and educational costs, therefore:

The ACNM Division of Accreditation:

1. Continues to support a **variety of educational pathways** leading to professional midwifery education, including direct entry, prior nursing preparation, and accelerated/combined nursing and midwifery education;
2. Supports and promotes the **development of independent schools of midwifery,** in affiliation with institutions of higher learning, where the determination of content and terminal outcomes is based on competencies needed for full-scope midwifery practice including leadership, business, and teaching; and
3. Recognizes that among the variety of educational pathways, the Doctor of Nursing Practice may be one option for some nurse-midwifery programs, but **does not 'support the DNP as a <u>requirement</u>** for midwifery education. (ACNM, 2005)

The ACNM position statement on the DNP acknowledges potential educational benefits of the DNP, however,

> no data are available addressing the need for additional education to practice safely as a midwife. Indeed there are decades of evidence that graduates from ACNM Division of Accreditation (DOA) accredited midwifery education programs, regardless of terminal degree, are safe, cost-effective care providers of maternity and women's health care.

> ... ACNM does **not** support the requirement of the DNP for entry into clinical midwifery practice. (ACNM, 2007, n.p.)

National Association of Clinical Nurse Specialists

The National Association of Clinical Nurse Specialists (NACNS) "founded in 1995, exists to enhance and promote the unique, high value contribution of the clinical nurse specialist to the health and well-being of individuals, families, groups, and communities, and to promote and advance the practice of nursing" (NACNS, n.d.b). The NACNS published a white paper on the DNP in April 2005. This document is a result of an analysis conducted by the NACNS and expresses areas of concern from an organizational perspective. The following comments address the interview questions on a perceived gap in clinical practice, a need for the DNP, and empirical evidence for the development of the DNP:

- The AACN Proposal represents a major professional paradigm shift in nursing practice and education that warrants extensive dialogue from stakeholders. Opportunities for collegial dialogue in regional and national meetings should precede a change of this magnitude.
- There is a lack of consensus from specialty and other professional organizations about how the DNP proposal will complement the nursing profession.
- There are no studies showing that doctorally-prepared advanced practice nurses have better outcomes than master's-prepared advanced practice nurses.
- The nature of additional knowledge infused into the DNP curricula versus the knowledge in the present MSN curricula is not known.
- Current evidence supports the safety of CNSs and other advanced practice nurses in providing high quality and cost effective advanced practice nursing.
- Harm data about care provided by CNSs and other advanced practice nurses prepared at the master's level does not exist according to the American Nurses Association Malpractice Data Bank.
- It is unclear how the proposed DNP will contribute to increased patient safety as there have been no studies done to support this premise.
- Decisions to initiate this major paradigm shift were not derived from an extensive nursing practice analysis, but from one group of advanced practice professionals.
- The proposed DNP was developed with limited input from a full range of higher education organizations such as private universities or smaller universities that cannot offer doctoral degrees. (NACNS, 2005)

As a result of this analysis, the NACNS responded to the AACN's leadership proposed first-order effect for the DNP, stating "NACNS remains neutral about the proposed DNP until our concerns can be resolved and our questions answered" (NACNS, 2005, p. 5). Further work by the NACNS is published in a 2007 document entitled *A Vision of the Future for Clinical Nurse Specialists*, which states

NACNS believes that the master's degree is an appropriate level of education for entry into practice as a CNS. Although the knowledge and competencies needed for beginning CNS practice can be developed within the number of credit hours in a typical master's program, it does not preclude an entry into CNS practice at the doctoral level. (NACNS, 2007)

Nurse Practitioner Roundtable

The advanced practice group categorized as nurse practitioners is subdivided into nurse practitioner specialties. Seven nurse practitioner organizations comprise the Nurse Practitioner Roundtable (NPR) for the purpose of addressing nurse practitioner issues, collaborating efforts and presenting a unified position (NPR, 2008). Several of these groups have published individual position statements. The NONPF position statement has already been discussed and the remaining groups will be discussed in turn. They include: the American Academy of Nurse Practitioners, the American College of Nurse Practitioners, the Association of Faculties of Pediatric Nurse Practitioners, the National Association of Nurse Practitioners in Women's Health, the National Association of Pediatric Nurse Practitioners, the National Conference of Gerontological Nurse Practitioners, and the previously mentioned National Organization of Nurse Practitioner Faculties.

The Nurse Practitioner Roundtable statement entitled *Nurse Practitioner DNP Education, Certification and Titling: A Unified Statement* dated June 2008 was posted on June 16, 2008. In this document the coalition addressed the role of the nurse practitioner in the treatment of patients and described strategies of patient-centered care, including advocacy, coordination of care, therapeutics and evaluation. This document describes NP education as building on a foundation of sciences across multiple disciplines as well as the art and science of nursing. Although the document does not provide empiric evidence for the DNP as sole entry-level educational requirement for nurse practitioners, it does state:

> Current master's and higher degree nurse practitioner programs prepare fully accountable clinicians to provide care to well individuals, patients with undifferentiated symptoms, and those with acute, complex chronic and/or critical illnesses. The DNP degree more accurately reflects current clinical competencies and includes preparation for the changing health care system. It is congruent with the intense rigorous education for nurse practitioners. This evolution is comparable to the clinical doctoral preparation for other health care professionals. (2008)

The American Academy of Nurse Practitioners (AANP), incorporated in 1985, is the "largest and only full-service professional membership organization in the Unites States for NPs of all specialties" (AANP, 2006b, n.p.). Its mission includes promoting nurse practitioner practice, education and research and advancing health care by informing health care policy, both nationally and internationally. This organization does not accredit programs but provides certification for nurse practitioners (AANP, 2007a). The AANP posted a discussion paper on the development of the DNP. This document described the primary objectives for the development of the DNP to create parity with other health care disciplines and to provide a degree commensurate with the number of required academic credit hours. This discussion paper, revised in 2007, stresses the importance of avoiding disenfranchisement or denigration of master's-prepared nurse practitioners (AANP, 2005; AANP 2007b). Although supportive of the DNP, the AANP document does not offer empirical evidence for developing the DNP. However, this organization published two documents providing empirical evidence on the safety and quality of nurse practitioner health care provided primarily by master's prepared nurse practitioners (AANP, 2006a; AANP, 2007c).

The American College of Nurse Practitioners (ACNP), established in 1993, is an "advocacy organization dedicated to ensuring a solid policy and regulatory foundation that enables Nurse Practitioners to continue providing accessible, high quality healthcare to the nation" (AANP, n.d.b). Its members include individual student and practicing nurse practitioners as well as national and state NP organizations. The ACNP position on NP education states that standards of education and practice must be based on "accountability and outcome based research" (ACNP, n.d.a). This position statement does not address the DNP nor any other academic credential.

The Association of Faculties of Pediatric Nurse Practitioners (AFPNP) is "a national organization of nursing educators who teach in pediatric, family and school nurse practitioner programs, and who work together on relevant practice and educational issues" (AFPNP, 2005).

Although there is no position statement on the DNP, a copy of *Philosophy, Conceptual Model and Terminal Competencies for the Education of Pediatric Nurse Practitioners* has been requested via email. However, at this writing, the researcher has not received a response.

An organization comprised of nurse practitioners with different NP specialties, the National Association of Nurse Practitioners in Women's Health (NPWH) represents NPs who provide care to women in both primary care and women's health specialty practices. The mission of the NPWH is to "assure the provision of quality health care to women of all ages by nurse practitioners" (NPWH, 2007, n.p.). The NPWH acknowledges the value of increased knowledge and recognizes the DNP as an option for nurse practitioners. The position statement addresses first-, second- and third-order effects. Information applicable to determining first-order effects notes the following:

- The mechanism for educating NPs in specialty areas is unclear. Recommendations regarding increasing clinical practicum hours in NP preparation are not supported by existing evidence.
- In the absence of evidence of superior patient outcomes, we cannot support the DNP as the entry to practice requirement for NP practice. Rather we continue to encourage and support existing NP programs to meet existing national requirements and sustain sound and rigorous programs in providing NP education. (NPWH, 2007, n.p.)

The National Association of Pediatric Nurse Practitioners (NAPNAP) has as its mission to promote "optimal health for children through leadership, practice, advocacy, education and research" (NAPNAP, 2004). The NAPNAP position statement on the DNP, adopted April 13, 2008 supports the DNP as entry-level education for advanced practice nurses. However, NAPNAP (2008) acknowledges that challenges for implementing this initiative include time to actualize the DNP, potential for additional costs, no guarantee for increase in salary, and variability in the transition from master's to DNP. Although this document cites the Institute of Medicine and Pew commission, it does not offer empirical evidence that there is a gap between education and clinical practice. NAPNAP believes that:

- The changing demands of the nation's complex health care environment require that PNPs [pediatric nurse practitioners] have the highest level of scientific knowledge and practice expertise possible.
- The DNP is a future oriented goal for PNP practice entry.
- The DNP is the terminal degree for professional practice representing the highest level of clinical competence.
- The DNP graduate is prepared to be an expert clinical practitioner and faculty member.
- The DNP will incorporate the scope of practice as outlined in the *Pediatric Nursing: Scope &Standards of Practice* document (NAPNAP & SPN, in press).
- Master's prepared PNPs will continue to be valued.
- Those who choose to acquire the DNP may do so over time; articulation programs should be provided.
- It is not necessary for all Masters prepared PNPs to acquire a DNP.
- It is important to monitor the practice doctorate and its impact on practice, education, regulation and certification. (NAPNAP, 2008, n.p.)

In concluding, the white paper states that the practice doctorate "prepares PNPs to provide leadership in coordination of care and improvement of methods of health care delivery for children and complements the research focused nursing doctorates" (n.p.).

The Nurse Practitioner Roundtable also includes the National Conference of Gerontological Nurse Practitioners (NCGNP). The NCGNP represents NPs who provide care for older adults. The stated goals of this organization include the promotion of communication and collaboration among health care providers, the support of quality care and research regarding older adults, and the promotion of professional development for APNs. This organization has not published an individual organizational position on the DNP (NCGNP, n.d.)

American Organization of Nurse Executives

Another nursing specialty organization that expressed clear first-order effects is the American Organization of Nurse Executives (AONE). Its position statement on the DNP states that AONE:

> identified the lack of an analysis detailing the need for and the efficacy of a practice doctorate across all aspects of the care continuum ... AONE supports the Doctorate of Nursing Practice (DNP) as a terminal degree option for practice-focused nursing. However, AONE, at this time, believes nursing masters' degree programs in both specialty and generalist courses of study should be retained. (AONE, 2007, p. 2)

Interviews: Developing the DNP

Eight individuals were interviewed for this work and chosen to achieve a maximal variation sample, representing systems affected by the DNP initiative. The interviewees included executives from national nursing organizations, representatives from nurse administration, nurse education administration, each of the four advanced practice nursing specialties and an advanced practice nurse who had earned a DNP. In order to protect the anonymity of the participants, the category of representation will not be identified in the following discussion:

> Are educators deciding that there is a gap in clinical practice: that they feel there needs to be a practice doctorate, rather than responding to a study that demonstrates the need?

> What empirical evidence exists to support the development of the DNP? (ANA, 2005, n.p.)

Participants overwhelmingly agreed that the impetus for the paradigm change was from educators instead of clinical practice. One respondent stated "there is a huge disconnect between academia and the practice arena." None interviewed were aware of any systematic study to support changing the entry-level educational requirement of the APN from a master's degree. One respondent commented "I don't need a DNP to do my job." Three replied that nurse providers are held to the highest standards of practice and that the degree neither defines the role of the APN, nor would change the expected outcomes. Further, they indicated there was no appreciable evidence in the clinical outcomes of nurse providers with master's degrees and post-baccalaureate certificates. One APN stated that published research in at least one specialty supports equal outcomes from care provided by master's degree and baccalaureate-prepared advanced practice nurses.

Two respondents posited the Institute of Medicine (IOM) studies as support for the proposed paradigm change. However, another stated that the AACN's inclusion of the IOM studies was coincidental to the rationale for the DNP, and had been added to the discussion after the AACN proposal for the DNP was drafted. Two participants responded that the DNP-prepared APN may be better skilled to implement evidence-based practice. Three questioned the lack of evidence that specified markers or outcomes data that could be used to measure a higher caliber of performance in the provision of health care.

In the discussion concerning support for the DNP, five respondents discussed the need for parity with other health care professions, with regard to level of educational degrees and in credit hours to earn the master's degree. Two described the proposed DNP as "following other professions" and jumping "on the bandwagon" to create parity in degrees. Four of the respondents indicated that the change in degrees would make a difference in relating to other disciplines; one stated that it would cause confusion and potential conflict with medical doctors; two stated the role of the clinical-focused practitioner would not change, one replied that the DNP would not change the role or the governance of an APN in the health care setting as APNs "practice under medical staff bylaws."

Regarding credit hours, one participant stated that the number of hours to convert one specialty's degree from a master's degree to a practice doctorate would require the addition of only one semester to align with AACN guidance. Another responded that 24 months of study was reasonable to prepare for the role of an APN, but indicated that further study in pharmacology and additional classes with other health care disciplines are needed. One participant emphatically stated that educators proposed the DNP initiative precisely for the purpose of offering academic equity for the amount of class time and clinical hours required of APN students as well as granting faculty and schools of nursing recognition for the amount of effort required to provide APN education. This person added that courses proposed by the AACN are not germane to the APN in clinical practice and that most APNs will remain in clinical settings; that more science-focused courses, such as genetics or advanced microbiology should be added not "administrative stuff."

In responding to the second question, participants unanimously stated that there is no empirical evidence to support the development of the DNP. Comments included, "none," "no evidence of absolute entry to practice," "no compelling evidence," and "there is no indication that the DNP will improve care … not sure who or why the push." Although one responded that it seemed the DNP was "thrust upon us" this respondent also added that although there may be no change in the outcomes of APN care, there might be a role for the DNP-prepared APN in replacing medical doctors who are "unwilling or unable" to address the disparity of health care needs of vulnerable populations.

Professional Literature: Developing the DNP

This portion of the data analysis includes literature in peer-reviewed nursing journals, expressing perspectives from individual authors. Information retrieved from these sources demonstrates the Diffusion of Innovations as the AACN DNP Roadmap document described for dissemination of the DNP initiative. Many of the references reviewed the same articles discussed in this analysis and nearly all cited the organizational documents discussed earlier in this chapter. It is important to note that all articles that provided author information were written by nurse educators, not clinicians. This is not surprising, given that professional literature is dominated by academia. However, this finding provides an answer to the first question that it is indeed nursing educational leaders who proposed the future of advanced nursing practice:

> Are educators deciding that there is a gap in clinical practice: that they feel there needs to be a practice doctorate, rather than responding to a study that demonstrates the need?

> What empirical evidence exists to support the development of the DNP? (ANA, 2005, n.p.)

While authors debated whether evidence exists to support the DNP initiative, only two surveys of clinical APNs were included in the discussion. Lenz, identified as chair of the AACN Task Force on the Practice Doctorate in Nursing (Lenz, 2005), describes a study presented at the State of the Science Conference, Washington, DC in 2002:

In order to ascertain the extent to which actively practicing NPs perceived gaps in their formal education and to identify potential areas for curricular emphasis, Columbia University researchers conducted a national mailed survey. Results from 2303 NPs revealed that although formal education provided the basis for their skills in patient diagnosis and management (in a majority of cases supplemented by subsequent on-the-job training), gaps existed in relation to cross-site practice, credentialing, use of information technology, evidence as a basis for practice, policy, synthesis and application of knowledge at a high level, and multiple aspects of practice management. Although they expressed a desire for more education about these topics, few anticipated obtaining more formal education; because they did not believe existing research-focused doctoral programs to be particularly relevant. (Lenz, Mundinger, Clark, Hopkins, & Lin, 2000, as cited in Lenz, 2005, n.p.)

One other journal article referenced a "telephone FNP graduate survey, [that provided] considerable support" (Brown, et al., 2006) for the development of the DNP program at the University of Washington. However, details of this survey were not discussed in this description of the development of a DNP program.

In searching for evidence to support the DNP, Chase and Pruitt (2006) describe the leadership accomplishments of master's-prepared APNs in influencing legislation resulting in increased autonomy in practice, prescriptive authority and obtaining admitting privileges in hospitals. They state this new degree does not address the profession's most critical need to produce nursing faculty. Also, the authors posit that the AACN's mandate for the practice doctorate is premature as the DNP has not been adequately evaluated in terms of its worth for the profession and the health care system.

The nursing profession has, until fall 2004, accepted that the master's degree in nursing prepares nurses to be competent providers of advanced practice nursing. Certifying bodies have performed extensive job analyses, developed certification examinations, and are credentialing master's-prepared nurses in advanced practice roles. State boards of nursing, albeit with a good bit of variety, credential advanced practice nurses with the master's degree to practice in the expanded role. In the absence of evidence that competence is lacking, a variety of programs should be available to students seeking advanced preparation. (Chase & Pruitt, 2006, p. 157)

Fulton and Lyon (2005) indicate that the primary impetus for this degree generates from the leadership of two educational organizations, the AACN and NONPF and has not received adequate input from other stakeholders, including advanced practice nurses. The authors add that these leaders imply that master's-prepared APNs are not safe, though there is no literature to support this; in fact, current literature supports the safety and effectiveness of master's-prepared APNs. Fulton and Lyon add there is no evidence to support that the DNP-prepared clinician will improve health care outcomes, a third-order effect, and question the issue of academic parity when there is insufficient data to indicate improved health care since the establishment of other practice doctorates. They state, "Nationally, the intellectual capital exists to solve the current and future health care dilemmas. What is lacking is the political will to make needed changes" (Fulton & Lyon, 2005, n.p.). Continuing in this vein, McKenna (2005) states there can be "no rational argument against the education of nurses for a complex and often life-saving undertaking being at an advanced level" (p. 245). However, Apold (2008) continues:

> Although it is intuitively appealing that educational requirements and standards will address the Institute of Medicine's concerns about patient safety and health care quality, there is no evidence that the DNP addresses these issues. Studies relating educational preparation and quality at the entry level do support that more and different education results in higher quality. These data are not generalizable to advanced practice, and the suggestion that better patient care will result from this preparation, although intuitively appealing, has not been made on the basis of evidence. (n.p.)

Upvall and Ptachcinski (2007) discussed one of the justifications for the DNP, parity with other health care professionals, and suggested lessons that nurses can learn from the pharmacists. The authors explored similarities and differences of the DNP for advanced practice nurses and the PharmD for pharmacists. The PharmD requirement resulted from need for educational preparation when "pharmacotherapy became an increasingly important component of health care. The unique body of knowledge in pharmacology, pharmacokinetics, and clinical pharmacotherapy filled a gap that was not being met" (p. 317). Parity with other disciplines and educational advancement were secondary effects of greater involvement in pharmaceutical care.

Second-Order Effects

The first-order effects of the introduction of the DNP included acceptance, rejection or deferral of the DNP; all were the direct results of the *trigger* action of the introduction of the DNP as entry-level education for APNs. Variables introduced beyond nursing schools and organizations determine subsequent outcomes. Second-order effects include consequences outside schools of nursing and professional nursing organizations. For the purpose of this study, questions posed by the American Nurses Association create the framework for determining variables and potential outcomes after a school of nursing has decided to pursue the doctor of nursing practice degree. The following questions are discussed to determine variables introduced by the health care system and potential second-order outcomes resulting from schools of nursing having accepted the DNP initiative and working to bring it to fruition:

> Who is going to teach DNP students since the role is considered advanced practice?
>
> Has there been a cost benefit analysis of how the DNP will affect cost of nursing faculty?
>
> Has there been a cost benefit analysis of how the DNP will affect cost of educating DNP prepared advanced practice nurses?
>
> Will those with a DNP be tenured/equitable within the university setting or become second class citizens in the academic environment? (ANA, 2005, n.p.)

Organizational Documents: Faculty Considerations

Questions identifying second-order of effects are addressed by the American Association of Colleges of Nursing in the position paper and the Roadmap document, stating that DNP students should ideally be taught by doctorally prepared individuals, within the nursing discipline as well as others in health care, informatics and public policy. One suggestion by the AACN was to offer DNP courses to current faculty during the university program approval, so that once the degree had been established, those faculty could become the school's first graduates. The AACN recommends those who wish to teach concentrate education in clinical expertise, but add additional courses in pedagogy during or at the completion of the DNP. Since clinical expertise is stressed, all DNP students will require clinical preceptors; AACN suggestions included utilizing APNs with either a master's or doctoral degree other than the DNP until a critical mass of DNP graduates would be available to act as clinical faculty (AACN, 2006a).

The AACN also addresses costs and benefits to students, educational institutions and to society. Although the leadership of the AACN recognized that costs will increase, it argued that the proposed benefits of the practice doctorate will justify the cost. In addressing the length of study, the AACN Roadmap document recommends that "post-baccalaureate DNP programs be three calendar years, or 36 months of full-time study including summers, or four years on a traditional academic calendar (AACN, 2006a, p. 11). The AACN states that there is no evidence to support suggestions that nurses are unwilling to accept the additional costs, including tuition and deferred income resulting from increased time out of the workforce as a result of a longer educational program.

These leaders also maintained that "the growing presence of a second-degree nursing student population provides evidence that, increasingly, the potential nursing student is willing to incur significant costs provided a clear benefit is visualized in terms of career opportunities and earning potential" (AACN, 2006a, p. 16). The AACN Roadmap document counters the increased cost of the program with the benefits of "a more sophisticated skill set and acquiring specialized expertise, which is highly desirable and presents a larger range of opportunities for employment or enhanced earning potential" (p. 17). Further, this document recommends potential resources to assist students financially, including working to obtain federally funded traineeships, teaching assistantships, scholarships, paid internships, military scholarships and deferments, and working as support staff in nurse-managed clinics.

The AACN acknowledges that the primary cost of graduate programs is the cost of faculty, as ideally all will hold an earned doctoral degree. Suggestions to meet the challenge of increased costs include following the medical education model by establishing strong relationships with community DNPs to act as clinical faculty and mentors. Additionally, developing faculty practices provide clinical opportunities for students and income for faculty support. A source of limited funding, the AACN recommends seeking changes to lift restrictions on doctoral degrees from the Department of Health and Human Services Title VIII program. The AACN recognizes that the increased number of credit hours required in the DNP program will generate income for the university. Lastly, the AACN recommends institutional support and community advocacy for the program as evidenced by employing DNP graduates and providing additional resources for the DNP program (AACN, 2006a).

Regarding societal costs and benefits, the AACN states:

> The growing recognition that nurses prepared with graduate degrees are important resources for health care delivery and access to needed services will require a focused approach to ensure that the number of nurses prepared for this level does not diminish. As academic programs begin transitioning to the DNP, efforts to assist master's degree nurses in acquiring the DNP could delay the production of new advanced nursing clinicians. Schools must focus on ensuring the production of additional nurses prepared at the advanced level and maintaining a robust production capacity that maintains the current graduation level. (AACN, 2006a, p. 18)

In the discussion on the academic standing of the DNP-prepared university faculty member, the AACN describes scholarship for the nursing profession within the Boyer framework, which consists of discovery, teaching, application and integration, which supports the DNP role (AACN, 2006a). The AACN suggests different faculty appointment options to provide flexibility for the DNP faculty member to participate in teaching and practice. The DNP Roadmap document states that the possibility of tenure depends on the mission of the university and the precedence of other practice doctorates and that "Tenure policies should not dictate the educational preparation for advanced nursing practice" (p. 15).

The examination of second-order effects of this initiative by the AACN leadership reveals an uneven response by national nursing organizations. Of the professional organizational position statements studied, only that of the National Association of Clinical Nurse Specialists offer data concerning cost/ benefits of the DNP in terms of faculty or university costs or the status of the DNP in academia. The NACNS states:

> Consistent with nationally approved standards that preceptors must have a degree greater than that of the student, master's prepared CNSs, as well as other advanced practice nurses, will not be considered qualified to precept doctoral students who are obtaining a practice doctorate. (NACNS, 2005, p. 3)

In addition, the NACNS points to a more difficult second-order effect outcome with regard to costs and benefits of the DNP education; this document adds:

> From an academic perspective, the cost and affordability of shifting current master's level curricula to the proposed DNP have not been determined. From a student perspective, costs in relation to increased tuition, time, and reduced income while enrolled in a lengthy program have not been determined. We also do not know if post-graduation salaries for CNSs as well as other advanced practice nurses will offset the increased educational costs. (NACNS, 2005, p. 3)

Moreover, the NACNS expressed concern that DNP-prepared faculty may experience tenure and promotion difficulties, especially in the absence of other professional practice doctorates within the university faculty.

Interviews: Faculty Considerations

Second-order effects were explored with study participants by asking the following questions:

> Who is going to teach DNP students since the role is considered advanced practice?
>
> Has there been a cost benefit analysis of how the DNP will affect cost of nursing faculty?
>
> Has there been a cost benefit analysis of how the DNP will affect cost of educating DNP prepared advanced practice nurses?
>
> Will those with a DNP be tenured/equitable within the university setting or become second class citizens in the academic environment? (ANA, 2005, n.p.)

All eight individuals interviewed responded that doctorally prepared individuals should teach doctoral students, primarily those with PhD and DNS degrees. Five respondents commented that there are a limited number of DNPs graduated who are eligible to teach; one pointed out that DNP graduates will need to seek additional preparation in order to become educators, creating a delay in the teaching availability of the DNP in academia. Four participants stated that master's-prepared APNs will be required to provide adequate numbers of clinical faculty to supervise during the many clinical hours required in APN curricula.

One of the master's-prepared APNs, currently in full-time clinical practice, holds a faculty appointment with a college of medicine. This APN provides didactic and clinical instruction to family practice residents and stated that her experience and master's degree are accepted by the residents. However, the interviewee expressed doubt that nurses seeking a DNP will tolerate learning from a master's-prepared APN, given the respondent's "experience within nursing hierarchy."

The next two questions on the cost benefit analysis regarding how the DNP will affect cost of nursing faculty and educating DNP-prepared APNs are addressed together. As a group, the interviewees were not aware if any such analyses had been performed on these topics. One participant discussed experience in difficulty in recruiting master's-prepared faculty APNs and the expectation that recruiting DNP faculty would be even more difficult and more expensive. Another interviewee stated that the faculty cost would remain the same, arguing that a clinical faculty member would be paid the same regardless if the educational preparation was master's degree or DNP. The DNP-prepared APN stated that DNP faculty would cost more, since upon earning the DNP, a raise in pay was granted in recognition of the degree and in expectation

that responsibilities for this faculty position would increase. This person high- •
lighted the additional cost incurred while faculty members work to develop a
DNP program, adding to the cost of nursing faculty.

On the topic of cost of educating DNP-prepared APNs, all eight participants
remarked that this included an increase in students' time in school, time out
of the workforce and increased tuition, and one person added an increase in
the amount of student loans. Two participants stated this would not be a cost
to the school or program, because there would be no change in credit hours
taught, "one student for four years or two students for two years." This interviewee added, however, if students do not wish to attend a four-year program,
the overall enrollment would drop, creating an unintended second-order effect
for the school. Another stated that, especially in private institutions, the cost
would be passed along to the student in tuition. One individual added that
a master's degree is attainable, but a four-year program would decrease the
number of APNs, because increased time in school, time out of the workforce,
and the increased cost of education would create barriers many potential APNs
could not overcome.

As the discussion turned toward the issue of tenure embodied in the question, will those with a DNP be tenured/equitable within the university setting,
not one of the participants responded affirmatively. Three provided qualifiers:
obtaining tenure and equity will depend on strength of the school of nursing,
culture of the university, and on the university and its mission. Three respondents replied: "absolutely not," "as a DNP, I am not offered a tenure track,"
and "easily a second class citizen" for what is considered a "made-up degree."
The first participant had inquired about the DNP and was told the DNP would
not be considered a terminal degree within the school of nursing nor would
it fill the requirement for tenure. The DNP-prepared participant stated tenure
was not an option and that only a few faculty in that institution were tenured;
most worked on one-year contracts. A recently assessed PhD-prepared APN
was granted a three-year contract. The third respondent expanded by saying
the PhD is the standard for considering academic requirements, adding that
the DNP holds less credibility, which is "not right or wrong—it just happens."

One of the APN participants, who recently earned a master's degree, offered
an interesting observation in this area of second-order effects. The "old school"
professors, the respondent noted, viewed the DNP as "robbing from the PhDs"
by obtaining a doctoral degree that did not require adequate research, yet
would gain doctoral status. The younger, "more modern instructors" thought
the DNP was equitable and should be widely accepted in academia. This
respondent posited a generational difference in valuing academic achievement.

Another participant shared an historical perspective of the nursing profession's journey to attaining equal status in universities and that the idea that

nursing science was worthy of the PhD. This respondent stated that gaining equal standing in academia was a "hard won fight" and may be diminished if more nurses chose the DNP rather than the PhD, resulting in loss of academic status for the profession of nursing. This person also added that if tenure is critical to an individual, the PhD would be the recommended degree. Moreover, the move to the DNP is an effort to keep up with the health care industry tendency to evolve continually, so "ten years from now, who knows?"

The last respondent answered about tenure, "I just don't care, I will have a job." This APN added that tenure is an issue for the AACN leadership to address, but did not believe it would be a problem. Additionally, this person posited that tenure is a concept that would not last in education, and therefore certainly would not be a problem for future DNP-prepared faculty.

In discussing requirements for tenure, two participants commented on the role of research in nursing. They both acknowledged the centrality of publishing in peer-reviewed journals. One who had been a principal investigator as a master's-prepared APN did not experience difficulty in obtaining grants for research. However, this respondent added, "but not from a national source." Moreover, they both recognized the role of the PhD-prepared nurse in publishing research and creating knowledge for the profession of nursing, adding the DNP-prepared nurse would not meet criteria for this essential role.

Professional Literature: Faculty Considerations

In order to collect pertinent data regarding second-order effects, answers to the following questions were sought from nursing literature:

> Who is going to teach DNP students since the role is considered advanced practice?
>
> Has there been a cost benefit analysis of how the DNP will affect cost of nursing faculty?
>
> Has there been a cost benefit analysis of how the DNP will affect cost of educating DNP prepared advanced practice nurses?
>
> Will those with a DNP be tenured/equitable within the university setting or become second class citizens in the academic environment? (ANA, 2005, n.p.)

Professional nursing literature on the DNP offers several answers to the question of who will teach DNP students since the role is considered advanced practice. Lenz (2005) states that nearly all nursing schools planning to offer the DNP will face challenges regarding faculty requirements, acknowledged the current faculty shortage and added that there is a steady graduation of PhD nurses, but there is need for increased production of doctorally prepared nurses. Lenz adds that the DNP provides "ideal preparation for clinical teaching" (n.p.). Early DNP programs were established in universities that offered research doctoral degrees, availing doctorally prepared faculty to teach DNP students.

Clinton and Sperhac (2006) and Draye, Acker, and Zimmer (2006) recommend current master's-prepared APN faculty complete courses toward the DNP degree during the program's development, then teach as DNP-prepared APNs. Several authors offered the creation of partnerships between institutions (Lenz, 2005) offering master's degrees and those that offer the DNP for "more efficient use of limited faculty resources by better leveraging regional faculty talents, rather than competing among schools for limited faculty resources" (Hathaway, Jacob, Stegbauer, Thompson, & Graff, 2006, p. 493).

Dracup, Cronewell, Meleis, and Benner (2005) expressed concern that the "adoption of the DNP will lead to a future where nurses with DNPs teach all the clinical courses in a curriculum and PhD-prepared faculty (with PhDs in disciplines other than nursing) teach doctoral students and research courses" (p. 180). Chase and Pruitt (2006) pointed out that many universities currently employ master's-prepared APNs to teach in master's degree programs. Avery and Howe (2007) cautioned that extending another year to a clinical practice course of study further increases demands on community faculty by adding a third cohort of APN students into a saturated network of clinical faculty. Issues of who will teach and the cost of DNP faculty are addressed by Fulton and Lyon (2005):

> The impact of adding another degree with more credit hours on already scarce faculty resources is not known. Consistent with nationally approved standards that preceptors must have a degree greater than that of the student, master's prepared advanced *practice* nurses may not be considered qualified to precept doctoral students who are obtaining a *practice* doctorate. This need to precept DNP students will pull doctorally prepared nurses in yet another direction. (n.p.)

Fulton and Lyon explain that neither the costs of transforming the master's degree curricula into that for a doctoral program nor the costs to the student have been adequately addressed.

Turning toward programmatic concerns, Cartwright and Reed (2005), in providing policy and planning advice to universities planning to develop a DNP program, state:

The move to the DNP is a resource-intensive decision, which in most cases will require additional resources as well as redeployment of existing ones. This may include realigning faculty roles and reassigning faculty time, reallocating resources within the nursing college and other academic units, and generating increased revenues. (n.p.)

The literature does not address a cost benefit analysis of how the DNP will affect cost of nursing faculty and students per se, but most discuss the anticipated increased cost of doctorally prepared faculty as well as increased cost to students. Because it is projected that the DNP-prepared APN will graduate with a skill set beyond that of one earning a master's degree, some authors agree that a DNP graduate "will have the ability to demonstrate their worth" (Clinton & Sperhac, 2006, p. 13) and expect a higher salary than a master's-prepared APN. However, all agree that a higher salary is not guaranteed, that salary will be market driven. There is no data to suggest the salary will be different from that of a master's-prepared APN (Avery & Howe, 2007; Chase & Pruitt, 2006; Fulton & Lyon, 2005; Sperhac & Clinton, 2004). According to Upvall and Ptachcinski (2007), the difference in salaries in 2004 between baccalaureate-prepared and PharmD pharmacists was 0.7%.

Along this line of investigation, the cost to the student includes increased time in the program, increased tuition and increased loss of income due to deferred earnings (Avery & Howe, 2007; Dracup et al., 2005; Fulton & Lyon, 2005). DNP students will pay up to 100% more financial costs than those seeking master's degrees. Chase and Pruitt (2006) question what type of financial aid will be available to students who may pay as much as $100,000 for tuition in a post-baccalaureate DNP program. Authors Avery, Howe, and Chase and Pruitt suggest that students will chose medical school rather than a four-year practice doctorate in nursing, given the higher salaries of physicians and the income gained in residency programs.

The Directors of Midwifery Education (DOME) of the American College of Nurse-Midwives surveyed nurse midwifery students about their perceptions of the DNP and its effects on midwifery education and practice. Among questions asked was that of opportunity and financial investment. Of the 147 participants, 65 (49%) responded they would not have applied to a midwifery program had a doctorate been required and 67 (51%) would have applied to a practice doctorate program. Reasons provided for negative replies included "30 responses for the option 'could not afford the tuition,' 24 for the option 'unable/unwilling to spend 3–4 years in school,' 38 for 'might as well go to medical school,' and 18 selections for 'other'" (Avery & Howe, 2007, p. 17).

Much of the debate on the DNP addresses the issues of tenure and academic equity for DNP-prepared faculty. Brown (2005) states that an individual with an ND is unlikely to earn tenure and that after six years of practice, this individual was "unable to achieve true parity clinically or academically" (p. 467). Lenz (2005) states that tenure for DNP-prepared faculty depends on "institutional policy and scholarly productivity" (n.p.). Cartwright and Reed (2005) discuss the possibility of DNP-prepared faculty meeting tenure requirements based on more recently developed concepts of scholarly activity. These authors stress that each institution will decide if the degree and the individual meet local standards for tenure and add that "there is a groundswell of support for changing promotion and tenure guidelines to accommodate the broader definition of scholarship" (n.p.).

In a related publication, Meleis and Dracup (2005) discuss the potential problem within a university if the DNP-prepared faculty become the majority of nursing faculty:

> In most U.S. universities, membership in the academic Senate is granted to faculty members who hold tenured professorial ranks with the requirement of a PhD. Many DNP-prepared faculty will be excluded from the "Senate" of universities, and thus will be excluded from having a voice and a vote in decision making pertaining to educational and faculty policies. Faculty members with the DNP, getting neither tenured positions nor Senate membership, will be barred from dialogues and discussions pertaining to their educational role. By developing a professional practice doctorate and a research doctorate, we are creating a second-class citizenship in universities and we are enhancing the potential of marginalization of one group by another group. (n.p.)

While some predict whether DNPs will earn tenure, others question if DNP faculty are prepared to produce scholarly work required to seek tenure. Fulton and Lyon (2005) posit that faculty with practice doctorates may lack the skill set required for teaching and scholarship and "may be set up for failure in a university setting" (n.p.). McKenna (2005) warns "without an adequate background in the knowledge and skills necessary for teaching and scholarship, these people [practice doctorate graduates] may be set up for failure in the University setting" (p. 246).

Dracup et al. (2005) discuss the future of nursing scholarship should the DNP be equated with the PhD and its effects on the nursing profession from both university level and on a national level:

We also worry that the DNP will mean that our university-based faculties will not be vibrant PhD prepared faculties with the research training necessary to lead interdisciplinary research teams and to be Principal
Investigator's (PI's) and co-PI's with faculties of other schools. If a high
percentage of nursing faculties have DNPs rather than PhDs, they will take
secondary roles in the advancement of science in the university community
and the profession will lose the hard-won rights to autonomy and leadership
in academe. This is a particularly important loss as the National Institutes
of Health directs PhD-prepared scientists to optimize opportunities to col-
laborate in scientific discovery in its recent Roadmap Initiative. (p. 179)

Organizational Documents: Closing Master's Degree Programs

Turning to second-order effects within the greater university system, the discussion centers on, "Will there be confusion if master's degree programs still
exist? Should those programs be phased out now? (ANA, 2005, n.p.). In its
position paper on the DNP, the American Association of Colleges of Nursing
discussed the confusion within the nursing profession as well as the public
regarding the Nursing Doctorate (ND), an "entry-level practice doctorate analogous to the MD" (AACN, 2004a, p. 4). The first practice doctorate for nursing
did not provide a nursing specialty nor were the role and competencies of the
ND clearly defined. The issue that caused the most confusion was the lack of
differentiation between entry-level and advanced practice degree.

To prevent confusion with regard to the DNP, the AACN established the
DNP as a post-master's or post-baccalaureate degree and as entry-level education for advanced practice nursing roles. After 2015, the master's degree would
be appropriate only for nurse generalists. The AACN Roadmap document states
"Specialty focus master's level programs will be phased out as transition to
DNP programs occurs" (AACN, 2006a, p. 12). The document continues, stating
that the accrediting arm of the AACN will continue to accredit master's degree
programs for APNs as well as develop accreditation for DNP programs. "In the
future, however, programs will need to make decisions regarding advanced
practice offerings at the master's level and their viability and ethical standing
when the profession has evolved advanced practice education to the doctoral
level" (AACN, 2006a, p. 12). The AACN does not address the financial impact
on universities by eliminating APN master's programs.

The National Organization of Nurse Practitioner Faculties (NONPF) pre-
dicts the DNP will become the standard educational level for entry into practice for nurse practitioners as an evolutionary process. The NONPF does not
recommend closing master's degrees nor does it address economic impact on
universities if such programs are eliminated. "NONPF does not support any

finite deadline by when NP programs should be at doctoral level preparation but instead encourages NP educators to continue to sustain the highest quality programs to prepare NPs for clinical practice" (NONPF, 2006, n.p.)

The American Nurses Association prepared a handout with questions and concerns that formed a guideline for discussion in 2005. From this list, questions were selected to provide the framework for collecting data. (ANA, 2005). The National League for Nursing expresses concern about the DNP-prepared APN as an educator upon graduation but offers no further information for the purpose of this research (NLN, 2005; NLN, 2007). The American Association of Nurse Anesthetists (2007) published a position statement stating "The AANA supports doctoral education for entry into nurse anesthesia practice by 2025" (n.p.). This organization does not further address the remainder of the questions explored for this research.

Representing CNMs, the American College of Nurse-Midwives does not address closing master's degrees and states that it does not support the DNP as the sole entry-level educational requirement into midwifery practice (2007). The National Association of Clinical Nurse Specialists states that in 2005, there were 351 schools of nursing that offered master's degrees and 91 offering PhD programs. The position statement on the DNP states "Some existing CNS programs, as well as other advanced practice nursing programs, may need to close because they are not permitted by state statute to offer doctoral education or may lack the fiscal or faculty resources" (NACNS, 2005, p. 3). This organization acknowledges that the financial impact on universities in the transition from master's to DNP programs is unknown.

The Nurse Practitioner Roundtable addresses the transition from master's degree to DNP as an evolution; this organization does not make a recommendation to close master's programs, nor does it address economic impact on universities (NPR, 2008). Three member organizations of the Roundtable, the American Academy of Nurse Practitioners, the American College of Nurse practitioners, and the National Association of Women's Health address neither confusion potential of continuing of the master's degree nor financial impact on universities. Another member of the NPR, the National Association of Pediatric Nurse Practitioners (NAPNAP) supports the AACN position on the DNP. However it goes on to state that master's-prepared PNPs will continue to be valued and that is not necessary for all master's-prepared PNPs to acquire a DNP. This organization does not address financial impact for universities with regard to a transition from master's to the DNP.

When the American Organization of Nurse Executives (2007) published its position statement on the DNP, it stated, "AONE supports the Doctorate of Nursing Practice (DNP) as a terminal degree option for practice-focused nursing. However, AONE, at this time, believes nursing masters' degree programs in both specialty and generalist courses of study should be retained" (AONE, 2007, n.p.). AONE does not address closing master's degree programs or impact on universities.

Interviews: Closing Master's Degree Programs

One of the most contentious issues surrounding this transformational initiative by the AACN centers on the closing of existing master's degree programs for APNs. Addressing this issue are the questions: "Will there be confusion if master's degree programs still exist? Should those programs be phased out now?" (ANA, 2005, n.p.). Six respondents replied no, one replied yes, that the master's programs should phase out over time, and one had no position on this question. Four participants noted that the number of DNP programs in existence was inadequate and growing too slowly to replace current master's programs preparing APNs. Two respondents expressed doubt that BSN-prepared nurses will be interested in a four-year program to become an APN; both of these individuals would choose medical school over a four-year APN program. One interviewee added the return on the investment of a DNP education for advanced practice nursing is less than that of a master's degree because there is a ceiling on salaries for APNs, stating that potential APN students could go to medical school, make "a lot more money" and have "none of the hassles" that APNs endure for the privilege to care for patients.

An additional insight on second-order effects surrounding the issue of closing master's programs, one respondent stated "that would be jumping the gun" considering nursing did not have a "good history of making the BSN entry level education." This individual went on to note that it would be "very presumptuous" to do away with master's programs because nursing could not meet the need for APN nurses with the DNP programs. Another participant stated that nursing had not learned from its past allowing "so many" levels of education for entry to nursing practice. This person encouraged a transition plan to "avoid disenfranchisement" of currently practicing master's-prepared APNs, and suggested reviewing the New York state model for education for teachers, where teachers must obtain a master's degree within five years to continue teaching. The respondent added that "predicated on a growing body of evidence" baccalaureate-prepared nurses improve patient outcomes and that the BSN is the proper entry degree for nursing.

The reference to the entry-level requirement to join the nursing profession was addressed by another interviewee, stating there is already confusion; since students "still don't understand the program they are learning in will have a different result, school of nursing versus university." The respondent continued,

"I used to think that physicians, had it right, you're a doctor—you're a doctor, then I learned that there were different entry levels for them, some are DOs, [doctors of osteopathy] others are MDs [medical doctors]. I'm not a person that believes that standardization for entry level is an absolute requirement."

In discussing the AACN leadership's timeline for achieving transformation, two respondents stated it would take longer than 2015 to implement the DNP program as the AACN has determined. One person added, "I am not sure if they can replace the number of master's programs with DNP programs" and added "I understand the DNP attrition rate is considerable." Another respondent, a post-master's DNP-prepared APN, conveyed concern that there are inadequate numbers of APNs to serve as faculty members. This individual also stated that people ask "what is the DNP?" and expressed surprise at the number of APNs who do not know about the DNP. One person stated that universities should wait until the APN professional groups provided support to the DNP entry to APN practice, as occurred with the pharmacy professional group that supported the move to the PharmD as sole entry level to pharmacy practice.

Regarding financial impact of eliminating the master's degree programs, five interviewees stated they did not know of any such an analysis. Two respondents discussed the fact that not all universities that now offer master's degrees are authorized to create doctoral programs and would also certainly experience a negative financial effect by eliminating the master's program. In addition, four individuals stated there would be a negative impact on universities by closing master's programs. One person stated if universities closed master's degree programs there would be reduced access to APN education and resulting fewer APNs, touching on a potential third-order effect concerning access to care. Another individual stated that universities are driven by student enrollment and if there is sufficient interest in DNP programs there would be no financial impact, however, if potential students cannot or do not wish to invest four years in an advanced practice nursing program there would be considerable unintended outcomes. Finally, two respondents, both faculty members in APN programs, stated their universities did not have plans to phase out the master's programs.

Professional Literature: Closing Master's Degree Programs

Nursing literature addressing the questions, "Will there be confusion if master's degree programs still exist? Should those programs be phased out now? Has there been a financial analysis performed of the impact on universities by eliminating the master's program?" (ANA, 2005, n.p.) reflects many of the concerns of the individuals interviewed for this work.

Dracup and Bryan-Brown (2005) emphasize that the BSN, the MSN and the PhD have become the preferred degrees for each level of nursing and are recognized internationally. These authors acknowledge that the master's degree has become the requirement for APNs as well as nurses entering teaching and administrative roles and suggest that the DNP will actually increase confusion regarding entry to advanced nursing practice. Brown (2005), an ND-prepared APN, posits that the DNP might confuse the nursing profession as well as the public and encourages academia to define the degree and the role before the degree is "adopted as a model for a clinical doctorate in both 'direct' and 'indirect' patient care" (p. 466). Having recognized that educators initiated the DNP as entry level for APNs, Dracup and Bryan-Brown:

> hope that the discipline will move slowly, encouraging input from the public, other types of healthcare professionals, and state accrediting boards before the DNP is adopted in university schools of nursing. We also hope that if universities decide the professional doctorate is important for nursing, that they will build the DNP as a post-master's degree. Maintaining an MS degree in nursing would allow nurses the flexibility to select a doctoral program that meets their career goals. (p. 280)

Conversely, from the perspective of the AACN's task force for the DNP, Lenz (2005) states that perhaps a single education entry level to advanced practice could enhance degree clarity and it was the:

> firm belief [of the task force] that the doctorate is the appropriate degree to reflect the extent and level of difficulty and sophistication of preparation required for specialized, advanced practice in today's health care system...the shift to the doctorate as the preferred preparation for advanced nursing practice will be difficult, requiring a transition period of approximately ten years...the goal is to move to the doctorate as the sole advanced practice degree. (n.p.)

Meleis and Dracup (2005) indicate that leaders in nursing education presume that master's degree APN programs will be closed. Others acknowledge that not all nursing schools currently offering master's degree APN programs are authorized to offer doctoral education and that not all master's programs for APNs are products of nursing schools (Avery & Howe, 2007; Cartwright & Reed, 2005; Fulton & Lyon, 2005). Dracup and Bryan-Brown (2005) expressed concern that master's degree programs currently preparing APNs will be forced to close, decreasing the number of health care providers available, thus reducing access to and quality of care in the larger health care system. In providing policy and planning strategies for the nursing academe, Cartwright and Reed (2005) advise the nursing profession that "for schools already preparing advanced practice nurses at the master's level, there are real downsides to a negative decision on the DNP. After 2015, preparation at the master's level will cease" (n.p.).

Third-Order Effects

Organizational Documents: Cost to Nursing

Within a system of systems approach, the third-order effects are difficult to discern as they emerge. In part, this is due to the greater lag time between first-order effects in initiation of transformation or the adoption of the innovation. It is also the result of the greater complexity of evaluating transformational outcomes within the more diverse constituent system of systems encountered. In this regard, the following questions were explored:

> What is the cost of the DNP in regards to the economics of the profession?
>
> What research demonstrates that nursing service can bear the additional cost associated with hiring someone with a DNP? If such evidence is missing, will AACN or another organization conduct such an analysis? Why or why not?
>
> Has there been a cost benefit analysis of how the DNP will affect cost of care provided by DNP prepared advanced practice nurses? (ANA, 2005, n.p.)

Concerning the cost of the DNP regarding the economics of the profession, the AACN acknowledged opportunity costs to the individual and proposed varied approaches to allow the APN to pursue the DNP. To this end, the AACN recommended multiple entry points into programs, which would ensure that APNs "who wished to obtain the doctoral degree would be provided the opportunity to earn a practice doctorate" (AACN, 2004a, p. 13). Additionally, the AACN recommends that in assisting students transitioning from master's degree to DNP, that "faculty must assess each candidate's previous educational program to determine the unique learning experiences required to meet the end-of-program competencies of the DNP" (AACN 2006a, p. 10).

In the DNP Roadmap, the AACN (2006a) acknowledged the establishment of the DNP program as resource intensive and provided essentials to guide curricula as well as administrative guidance for the DNP. The AACN recognized the increased resources involved in the transition of entry-level education for APNs, for the student as well as the profession:

> This impact should be taken into account as plans are made for the transition period to ensure a feasible and sustainable shift in educational preparation for advanced practice nurses. The Task Force believes that the benefits of such a move will outweigh the costs but recognizes that the transition plan will need to take into account the timing of costs and benefits. (AACN, 2004a, p. 13)

The AACN also addressed the possibility of a reduction of potential PhD students. The AACN states that the DNP would not affect enrollment in research doctoral programs, but create an opportunity for nurses who wish to earn a doctorate and remain clinical. "The two types of programs, research and practice-focused, would attract students with very different goals and interests" (p. 8).

Looking deeper into the greater system of systems and with regard to research demonstrating that nursing services can bear additional costs associated with hiring someone with a DNP, the AACN states only that the "earning potential will be directly related to the clinician's ability to make significant contributions to the mission or strategic goals of the employing organization" (AACN, 2006a, p. 17). The organization does not directly assess effects on nursing services, nor does the AACN address a cost benefit analysis of how the DNP will affect the cost of care provided by the DNP-prepared advanced practice nurse.

In response, the National League for Nursing expressed concerns which subsequently affect the economics of the profession in terms of third-order outcomes:

> In the midst of a very serious shortage of nurse faculty during a period of diminished resources, the DNP may have a negative effect on the current pool of students in other doctoral programs in nursing and nursing education and reduce the number of nurses whose research focus adds to knowledge development in nursing. (An unintended consequence of the practice doctorate in pharmacy is that it significantly decreased the numbers of PhD-prepared members of the discipline.)

> University nursing faculty struggle daily with an environment that requires substantial acquisition of resources and, in particular, funding through research. A decrease in doctorally prepared faculty could negatively affect the ability of deans and their faculty to maintain the research productivity that has become a standard for survival. (NLN, 2007, n.p.)

The NLN did not address nursing services or health care costs associated with DNP-prepared advanced practice nurses.

However, the economic impact of the DNP on the profession, nursing services and health care provided by DNP-prepared advanced practice nurses is expressed by the American College of Nurse–Midwives (2007):

> Data are lacking regarding the potential impact of the DNP on the applicant pool and on the cost to the health care system...In a time of critical shortage of midwives and other women's health care providers, the requirement of an additional degree decreases their availability in the workforce. (n.p.)

In addition, the National Association of Clinical Nurse Specialists (2005) articulated concerns on the effects of the DNP on the nursing profession in economic and global terms. First, the NACNS states that the AACN position on the DNP creates a possibility of further dividing the nursing profession, which has a history of a lack of cohesion. Next, the NACNS White Paper discusses the potential for the DNP to compete against the PhD for scarce resources, as occurred in the pharmacy discipline, adversely influencing the number of PhD-prepared CNSs by reducing the number of nurse scientists contributing to the "evidence base for nursing practice" (p. 2). Finally, the NACNS states that it is unknown if salaries of the DNP-prepared CNS will offset the opportunity costs and from "a health care employer perspective, it is not known if DNP-prepared advanced practice nurses will be affordable to employers and third party reimbursers" (p. 3).

Economic considerations of the DNP on the nursing profession, employers and health care are not addressed by the Nurse Practitioner Roundtable; however some member organizations have expressed concerns. The American Academy of Nurse Practitioners states, "Issues related to parity, providing reasonable methods for currently prepared NPs to obtain the DNP if desired and prevention of discrimination in reimbursement, must be addressed" (AANP, 2007, n.p.). The National Association of Nurse Practitioners in Women's' Health (2007) states:

> An economic impact study detailing market need for such credentialing has not been done. It is not known whether this credential will increase utilization of nurse practitioners or whether it will create barriers to hiring nurse practitioners, especially in public sector positions. There is no evidence that salaries will rise to reflect the advanced credentials and increased debt from a longer education. (n.p.)

The American Organization of Nurse Executives adds its perspective on the economic impact of the DNP and expressed concerns of potential unintended effects of the DNP as entry into advanced practice nursing:

> AONE Professional Practice Policy Committee's review focused on the long range plan of AACN that all nursing master's degrees, with the exception of the clinical nurse leader (CNL) will migrate to a DNP curriculum track. Therefore, eliminating any option of seeking advanced nursing specialty degrees, including nursing administration, nursing systems management or nursing leadership, at the master's level. The committee felt that many nurse managers, directors and even those nurses at the executive level will not seek a DNP for reasons of expense, time commitment and the cost/benefit of such a degree. With limited choices, many nurses, whether choosing an advanced practice focus or an aggregate/systems/organizational focus, may seek advanced degrees at the master's level in other domains such as public health, business or the social sciences.
>
> The committee's review further identified the lack of an analysis detailing the need for and the efficacy of a practice doctorate across all aspects of the care continuum. Also, the financial impact of rising salary expectations has not been fully studied. The committee concluded that the concerns and questions related to patient outcomes, salary compensation and the financial impact on organizations have not been fully identified, explored nor answered. (n.p.)

Interviews: Cost to Nursing

Participants were asked the following questions with regard to the cost of the DNP to the profession of nursing:

> What is the cost of the DNP in regards to the economics of the profession?
>
> What research demonstrates that nursing service can bear the additional cost associated with hiring someone with a DNP? If such evidence is missing, will AACN or another organization conduct such an analysis? Why or why not?
>
> Has there been a cost benefit analysis of how the DNP will affect cost of care provided by DNP prepared advanced practice nurses? (ANA, 2005, n.p.)

During this collection of data, five of the eight people interviewed addressed the increased opportunity cost, understood as increased time in school, tuition costs, and time out of the workforce, with no expected increase of APN salary. Three participants stated the opportunity cost would outweigh the benefits, adding "Who can take a four-year break to return to school?" Two added comments that the increased opportunity cost creates the potential for a decrease in the number of APN education programs as well as creates a barrier to enrolling in programs, thus constricting the supply of new APNs in practice. One person considered earning the PhD, but chose the DNP due to the opportunity cost of a five year or longer commitment to school.

In reflecting on this topic, one interviewee opined that the DNP is not economically feasible for prospective students or programs for two reasons. First, students need to continue working while attending school to support themselves or families and often take courses out of order as planned in the curriculum. This financial requirement disallows the probability that students may matriculate through the program as a cohort, creating an inefficient model of programmed instruction. Another participant stated there was a gap in evidence regarding the cost of the DNP and its value added, that the value of the DNP is simply not known at this time. This individual also added that nursing historically has not well articulated the value of nursing. Two interviewees responded that the opportunity costs may be balanced with increased status and could help nursing if "we get a critical foothold and a stronger voice." Another stated that the public would "foot the bill" on the increased costs if students are recipients of federal and state educational assistance.

Regarding the increased cost to nursing service, one participant responded there is a ceiling on salaries of non-physician providers. If an APN's pay was perceived as excessive, that APN would likely be replaced with a physician. One person stated APNs will not receive physician pay, another implied a reduction in pay might be experienced in the coming years due to changes in the health care system. Two participants also stated that nursing service would not be able to justify an increased salary for a DNP-prepared individual unless that person could produce evidence of "value added." Moreover, the DNP must demonstrate improved patient outcomes, and would receive increased compensation only if nursing could "prove there was a real benefit to the organization." Another respondent stated that the DNP does not address the most pressing needs of a director of nursing, offering a skill set that would add value to a nursing role. This participant added that in most cases, the DNP advanced practice nurse works for the medical staff, not the director of nursing.

In considering this initiative in terms of leadership responsibilities, another interviewee stated that it was "incumbent upon the AACN to conduct analyses to learn if the DNP would cost a hospital more than a master's prepared APN." This interviewee added that the DNP-prepared provider would not offer a different level of service or a different product than the master's-prepared APN. One respondent stated they did not believe "the AACN will conduct any analysis, I don't think that's a priority for them... they've already decided that this is a degree that we need and they're basically telling us what needs to be included in it."

Responding to the question regarding a cost benefit analysis of how the DNP will affect cost of care provided by DNP-prepared advanced practice nurses, one person answered that the cost of care is not dependent on the educational credentials of a provider but on the services provided. This interviewee added that the salaries of other practice doctorates did not increase based on their educational level, including physical and occupational therapists. Another responded that there would be no change in salary because there is no change in service, adding the DNP would be a "hard sell" to master's-prepared APNs, unless the APN planned to teach.

One APN participant stated that third-party payers may negotiate reimbursement if a provider "demonstrated better outcomes" and if no improvement in outcomes can be documented, then reimbursement would not change. Additionally, this person added "just because you decided you needed another degree doesn't mean they should pay for it." This person considered the DNP increased cost without increased benefits to the APN or to nursing in general. On a similar tact, one APN respondent explained the potential for reduced involvement in health care:

> When you look at the nurse anesthetist profession, I think there should be very careful consideration given to the controversy between anesthesiologists and nurse anesthetist—what this may raise—and will that controversy lead to the anesthesiologist supporting more heavily the PA programs in anesthesia that would then drive down the nurse anesthetist. For example, if I'm a group owner and I'm an anesthesiologist, I may just decide that—know what, I don't want to deal with nurse anesthetists any longer, I'm going to just hire anesthesia assistants for my group. That negatively affects our profession and ultimately negatively affects nursing practice.

Professional Literature: Cost to Nursing

Questions germane to exploring the topic of economic impact on the profession of nursing include:

> What is the cost of the DNP in regards to the economics of the profession?

> What research demonstrates that nursing service can bear the additional cost associated with hiring someone with a DNP? If such evidence is missing, will AACN or another organization conduct such an analysis? Why or why not?

> Has there been a cost benefit analysis of how the DNP will affect cost of care provided by DNP prepared advanced practice nurses? (ANA, 2005, n.p.)

Professional nursing literature presents a discourse on economic costs to the profession from several perspectives. First is the recognition that in the move to the PharmD, fewer pharmacists chose to earn the PhD (Fulton & Lyon, 2005). Dracup et al. (2005) suggest the number of nurses seeking PhDs in nursing will decline. Economically, fewer PhD-prepared nurses on faculty translates into fewer principle investigators, resulting in a loss of funded research opportunities. The effects of fewer nurses with PhDs would decrease the scholarly status of nurses within the university, eroding the hard-won equality the profession has taken many decades to achieve. More importantly, Meleis et al. (2005) contend that if nursing faculties are comprised of primarily DNP-prepared faculty, that nursing will "take secondary roles in the advancement of science" (p. 179). Moreover, the need for nurse researchers is expanding to meet the health care needs of the nation. Should the number of PhD-prepared nurses decline, the profession will be less well represented on important national initiatives such as the National Institutes of Health Roadmap Plan.

Conversely, Lenz (2005) and Sperhac and Clinton (2004) predict that the DNP will increase the credibility and enhance the image of nursing. Apold (2008) suggests that by increasing the level of education and enhancing the image of nursing, the profession may attract more people, which would help to alleviate the nursing shortage. Loomis, Willard and Cohen (2007) support that "status and parity with other health professionals may be a beginning to foster equality at the academic level" (n.p.).

Meleis and Dracup (2005) suggest that the timing of the introduction of the DNP can cost the nursing profession credibility. Focusing on a new degree for the purpose of parity with other professions gives the impression that the nursing profession is self-serving and non-responsive to the needs of the nation. The authors describe the critical nursing shortage issue which threatens the safety of patients and the retention of nurses, further compounding the problem. Meleis and Dracup state the discussion on the development of the DNP within schools of nursing consumes much time, reducing limited resources for the work of producing nurses.

Dracup et al. (2005) express the expectation of increased salaries for DNP graduates based on increased education costs, but warn that our society is addressing how to decrease health care costs. To contain costs, the authors discuss the lowering of reimbursements to physicians, the hiring of nurse practitioners, and the hiring of less educated personnel. Dracup et al. illustrate this concept with health administrators hiring one doctorally prepared individual to lead a team of "untrained helpers" (p. 180), specifically teams consisting of one PharmD-prepared pharmacist leading a team of pharmacy technicians or one orthopedic surgeon assisted by orthopedic technicians. The authors "worry that the DNP will lead patients to receive nursing care from a few select nurses and an army of unlicensed personnel" (p. 180). Fulton and Lyon (2005) express concern that the intended role of the DNP would become physician substitutes, further reducing nursing resources.

Sperhac and Clinton (2004) state that the educational degree alone will not guarantee increased salaries for DNP-prepared pediatric nurse practitioners (PNP), although it is possible that the skill set will enable the PNPs to demonstrate their increased worth by improving patient outcomes. They express optimism that "with improved patient outcomes and decreased health care costs, it would be expected that compensation for providers would be increased" (p. 296). In addition, Fulton and Lyon (2005) reveal:

> There is no data to suggest that post-graduation salaries for advanced *practice* nurses with a DNP will offset the increased educational costs. From a health care employer perspective, it is not known if DNP-prepared advanced *practice* nurses will be affordable to employers and third party reimbursers. (n.p.)

Avery and Howe (2007) explain that published reports confirm excellent patient outcomes of certified nurse midwives and certified midwives, regardless of their varying credentials. The authors state that the increased didactic and clinical experience may increase the DNP graduates' influence on policymaking in local to international areas but express apprehension about unanticipated effects of salary increases for DNP-prepared CNMs:

> Theoretical benefits are offset by concerns that creating a higher-priced graduate could contribute to the escalating costs of health care. It is also possible that the demand for higher salaries could price these graduates out of the market. As salaries of advanced practice nurses and CNMs/ CMs approach those of their physician colleagues, institutions may view the physicians' broader scope as worth a modest cost differential. (p. 18)

Moving the discussion deeper into the healthcare system, Chase and Pruitt (2006) explore the potential for increased health care costs as a critical issue:

> With increasing preparation costs, the number of NPs will decrease, yielding fewer primary care providers. A resultant demand for increased salary from graduates of longer, more expensive programs will contribute to the upward spiral of health care costs. Much of the nursing profession's success with federal support and training funds is partly a result of role preparation as cost-effective care providers. As a disruptive innovation,

NPs have provided efficient, costeffective alternatives to health care delivery. Increasing the cost and complexity of APRN preparation does not, by itself, improve the health care system. (p. 160)

Organizational Documents: Regulation and Certification

Perhaps one of the most challenging areas for discerning third-order effects lies within the regulatory bodies that impinge on the AACN's leadership initiative to transform advanced practice nursing. Research questions addressed in this regard include, "How would state nurse practice acts and regulatory language need to change upon implementation of the DNP? What will be the role of credentialing bodies? Will those entities need to create certification mechanisms and new specialty exams for DNPs?" (ANA, 2005, n.p.).

The American Association of Colleges of Nursing outlines measures to ensure the DNP-prepared advanced practice nurse is entitled by law to enter clinical practice. Each category of advanced practice nurses, ARNP, CRNA, CNM and CNS requires a specific APN license in addition to the registered nurse license in order to practice. To achieve licensure, many states require certification by a nationally recognized agency, such as the American Nurses Credentialing Center or the credentialing divisions of the AANA and the ACNM. The AACN (2004a) addresses regulation and credentialing issues in its position paper:

> It also is recognized that a change in the educational requirements for APN practice could impact certification and regulation. Stakeholders representing certifying and regulatory bodies, however, have indicated that the specific impact and need for change in these arenas cannot be identified at this point in the transition phase. These individuals further indicate that, as outcome-based competencies are identified and programs evolve, certification and regulatory changes will follow. (p. 14)

Two years later in the DNP Roadmap document, the AACN (2006a) described the disparity among states requiring certification for APN practice: CNS-29, CNM-44, CRNA-48, and NP-38. The AACN added that "a national, consensus-based model for the recognition of APN roles and specialties is being developed through the APN Consensus process" (p. 22). It is expected that this group will address licensure for DNP graduates.

In the DNP Roadmap document, the AACN (2006a) acknowledges the role of the Centers for Medicare and Medicaid Systems (CMS) in establishing educational expectations for nurse providers. In 1998, CMS authorized reimbursement for advanced practice nurses, and included language requiring the APNs to have a master's degree by January 2000 (Code of Federal Regulations, 1998). The AACN describes this action as "quasi-regulatory" (p. 24) because it mandated the master's degree as educational preparation for reimbursement for services of APNs. This document recommends that the AACN takes responsibility for preparing DNP graduates for certification, working to change language in state nurse practice acts and CMS/federal regulations from master's degree to graduate education, and working toward a uniformed approach to regulation of APNs.

Other nursing organizations addressing certification and regulation in position statements on the DNP include the ACNM, NPWH and NACNS. The American College of Nurse-Midwives (2007) states, "The American Midwifery Certification Board (AMCB) is responsible for developing and administering the national certification examination. AMCB is a member of the National Organization for Certifying Agencies (NOCA) and is accredited by the National Commission for Certifying Agencies (NCCA)" (n.p.). The document further emphasizes, "Because the educational standards for midwifery education, accreditation and certification have been and continue to be carefully updated, monitored and maintained, the practice of nurse midwives has well-documented evidence regarding its safety and positive outcomes for women and newborns" (n.p.). The National Association of Nurse Practitioners in Women's Health expresses concern that requirement of the DNP may alter regulation of currently licensed master's-prepared nurse practitioners:

> No plan has been presented to ensure uncomplicated and equitable grand-fathering of currently practicing NPs across state lines. Moving forward without such a plan may limit women's access to care as practicing NPs may be forced to discontinue practice when moving across state lines. (n. p)

In addition, the National Association of Clinical Nurse Specialists expresses concerns about changing nurse practice acts:

- The regulation of the practice of Clinical Nurse Specialists, as well as other advanced practice nurses, differs from state to state, and scope of practice will be affected differently depending on the state's nurse practice act.
- Nurse Practice Acts will need to be opened and modified in order to change language to incorporate doctoral competencies and scope of practice. Opening Acts may invite the attention of stakeholders who wish to modify existing components of the acts as well as to block the changes required.
- Variability within state level regulations exists with respect to using the title "doctor" when providing patient care.
- Certification mechanisms (new exams or portfolio) to satisfy state boards of nursing may need to be developed.

Ongoing/Implementation Concerns

- Issues related to grandfathering (a regulatory term) currently certified CNSs **must** be resolved. It is imperative that this issue be examined and that CNSs along with other advanced practice nurses who are prepared at the master's degree level be given authoritative assurance that they can continue to practice without additional graduate course preparation. (p. 4)

Interviews: Regulation and Certification

In exploring the certification and regulation of APNs, interviewees were asked, "How would state nurse practice acts and regulatory language need to change upon implementation of the DNP? What will be the role of credentialing bodies? Will those entities need to create certification mechanisms and new specialty exams for DNPs?" (ANA, 2005, n.p.).

Respondents provided three general discussion points when asked how state nurse practice acts and regulatory language would need to change in order to implement the DNP. Two respondents stated there would be no change in the scope of practice for DNP-prepared APNs, and the nurse practice acts would not require modifying; one added "I do not think we should replicate another profession's body of work." Three participants responded that the need to open the practice acts would depend upon APN scope of practice changes incidental to the introduction of the DNP. One added that changes would be required if the master's degree "went away." The three remaining participants stated changes would be required, but did not elaborate on the nature of these expected adjustments. One interviewee added that certification would soon be required for licensure and one related changes in one state's nurse practice act driven by a slight name change of an accrediting body for APNs.

Additional comments from the respondents included that nursing should regulate nurses, and that the National Council of State Boards of Nursing (NCSBN) is working to create uniform requirements to ensure that every APN obtains certification for licensure. Three respondents stated that nurse practice acts must add grandfathering clauses to guarantee that current APNs with other than DNP preparation could continue to be licensed to practice. Of the eight individuals interviewed, two discussed the possibility that stakeholders could change state practice acts by reducing the scope of practice of APNs, when opened to include DNP considerations. Lastly two participants addressed the fact that not all APNs are regulated by boards of nursing. One respondent also suggested creating boards of anesthesia and midwifery in every state to avoid undue influence of nursing.

Regarding the role of credentialing bodies, all respondents agreed that APNs should be certified by a nationally recognized agency in order to gain licensure. One person emphasized that one-half of all APNs are nurse practitioners and reiterated work in progress by the NCSBN to create a central certifying examination for APNs analogous to the National Council Licensure Examination (NCLEX) for registered nurses. When asked if this proposal would recognize that both the AANA and the ACNM provided certification for CRNAs and CNMs, the interviewee replied that the NCSBN "did not answer to the profession, they answered to the public."

Additionally, one participant stated that the American Association of Nurse Anesthetists provided both accreditation for educational programs and certification for CRNAs. This APN stressed the need for coordination between accreditation and credentialing to ensure that all educational programs teach required material. The respondent stated CRNA practice would not change and a new certifying exam would not be required.

Professional Literature: Regulation and Certification

Data gleaned from nursing literature sought to explore the questions, "How would state nurse practice acts and regulatory language need to change upon implementation of the DNP? What will be the role of credentialing bodies? Will those entities need to create certification mechanisms and new specialty exams for DNPs?" (ANA, 2005, n.p.). Several authors discuss effects of the DNP on the regulation of APNs and potential subsequent effects on APN practice. Topping the list, APNs are regulated by Boards of Nursing, Boards of Midwifery, Boards of Anesthesia, and by Joint Boards of Nursing and Medicine (Avery & Howe, 2007). Fulton and Lyon (2005) point out that practice acts are different in each state and each legal document will need to address the changes in practice for the DNP. If regulatory boards establish the DNP as a requirement to practice, even if currently licensed APNs are protected by *grandfather clauses*, APNs may not be allowed to acquire licensure in states other than that in which they are currently licensed. With reference to APN practice beyond 2015, Clinton and Sperhac (2004) state that if APNs "would move to another state, the DNP standard may be mandated. Therefore, it is essential to attend to announcements from the appropriate state board of nursing and the relevant professional organizations" (p. 150).

Along with Dracup et al. (2005), Fulton and Lyon (2005) express concern that the opening of state practice acts "may invite the attention of stakeholders who wish to modify existing components of the acts as well as to block the changes required...states vary with regard to regulations involving the use of the title "*doctor*" in clinical settings" (n.p.). Some physicians have voiced opposition to DNP nurse providers using the title *doctor*, stating nurses would misrepresent themselves to patients (AMA, 2006a). Additionally, two resolutions were introduced to control the scope of practice for all non-physician providers (AMA, 2005; AMA, 2006b). Most recently, physicians opposed APNs working independently and the American Medical Association Resolution 214 recommended that all APNs work under the direct supervision of physicians (AMA, 2008).

With regard to certification, Marion et al. (2003) recognize that there has not been a mechanism established to accredit DNP programs or certify DNP graduates. Proposals have been presented to create one accrediting and certifying body for APNs and others recommending current accrediting and certifying organizations change policies to address the DNP. Marion et al. recognize the need for both accreditation and certification for DNP-prepared APNs and add that the Institute of Medicine "has made clear the importance of addressing continuing competence as well as other critical competencies among healthcare providers through licensure, accreditation, and certification" (n.p.)

DISCUSSION: INTERPRETATION OF DATA WITHIN EFFECTS-BASED REASONING FRAMEWORK

Effects-based reasoning (EBR) demonstrates the exponential sequencing of outcomes from one specific action. The United States military employs effects-based objectives (EBO) to understand the "direct, indirect, intended, and unintended consequences" (Mann, et al., 2002, p. 9) of political and military actions. Smith describes effects-based operations as a "series of stimulus and response interactions" (Smith, 2002, p. 113). The use of this construct illustrates actions and chains of interactions in the planning, execution, and evaluation of a single event. This research utilized EBR as a framework to identify actual and potential effects of the introduction of the Doctor of Nursing Practice as the sole educational preparation for advanced practice nurses by the American Association of Colleges of Nursing into a system of systems.

The introduction of the DNP initiative by the AACN is primarily an example of transformational leadership, as by definition, this organization "explicitly communicates a vision, inspires followers to share and work toward fruition of the vision, and provides resources for developing the personal potential of the follower" (Smith et al., 2004, p. 80). The endorsement of the DNP communicated the vision that educational preparation for all APNs will move to the DNP level by 2015. Members of the AACN demonstrated the magnitude of their inspiration as they initiated DNP programs in nursing schools. AACN's DNP Roadmap document provides guidance for the development and implementation of the DNP initiative.

The American Nurses Association, a landmark organization representing the entire nursing profession, posed questions and concerns about the DNP that provided the research tool for collecting data. Data from organizational documents, interviews, and professional nursing literature were gathered and organized into first-, second- and third-order effects. These data identified the direct and indirect outcomes resulting from the AACN endorsement of the DNP, the trigger event. Effects-based outcomes of the DNP initiative are illustrated as each group of questions is analyzed.

Effects-Based Outcomes

First-order effects include the immediate, direct results of a specific action (Mann et al, 2002). In this case study research, the introduction of the DNP as sole educational preparation for APNs represents the trigger action. Second-order effects stem from first order effects, or outcomes, after the introduction of at least one variable. From this point, third-order outcomes are evident as a result of the introduction of additional variables, creating a series of response interactions (Smith, 2002) resulting from the introduction of the DNP initiative. In each level of effects, subsequent potential outcomes are extrapolated, creating a multi-linear model of actual and potential outcomes.

The immediate results of the AACN's introduction of the DNP initiative define first-order effects. Schools of nursing and professional organizations could choose to accept the paradigm change defined by establishing the DNP as sole educational preparation for advanced practice nurses, reject this change, or defer action on the initiative. Data examined issues contemplated prior to accepting, rejecting or deferring decision to adopt the DNP. Schools of nursing and professional organizations considered whether empirical evidence existed supporting the need for the DNP and if a gap between clinical practice and educational preparation was demonstrated. Organizational documents, interviews and literature failed to produce empirical evidence promoting the DNP as sole entry-level education for APNs. Also, data did not support the necessity of replacing the master's degree with the DNP as the singular APN educational preparation.

Data revealed that the movement to create the DNP as the sole educational requirement for APNs was initiated by educators seeking to provide an equitable degree for the number of credit hours required to educate APNs. This became increasingly more important as faculty and nurse practitioners identified additional desired content areas in their courses of study. Finally, the AACN sought to achieve educational and credential parity for APNs with health care providers with similar responsibilities, such as doctors of medicine and pharmacy.

Effects-Based Outcomes: Schools of Nursing Accept DNP Initiative

First-order effects consist of the acceptance, rejection or deferring decision on the DNP as the singular educational preparation for advanced practice nurses. The DNP program list posted on the AACN website, updated August 2008, lists 78 DNP programs accepting students and "more than 140 additional nursing schools are considering starting DNP programs nationwide" (AACN, 2008, n.p.). This is an outcome of the first order, the direct effect of the AACN's endorsement of the DNP. Extrapolating these figures, one can project that by 2015 there will be at least 218 DNP programs matriculating students. Should APN education cease to be offered at the master's level as Cartwright and Reed (2005) state, a significant second-order outcome would be that the 351 master's degree programs (NACNS, 2005) would no longer graduate APNs. This would create a loss of 133 programs graduating APNs, or an approximate 38% decrease in APN production. One subsequent third-order outcome would be the reduced access to health care provided by APNs. From the data available, the researcher could not distinguish between schools currently offering master's degree APN programs that have rejected the DNP initiative and those that have deferred making the decision whether to support or reject the DNP initiative.

SCHOOL OF NURSING SYSTEM Once the DNP is accepted as the appropriate educational preparation for APNs, schools of nursing must assign appropriate faculty members to design and teach curricula, a second-order effect. Data produced several options to meet this requirement. Schools could utilize: current faculty with research doctorate degrees; doctorally prepared faculty from different disciplines, both research and practice doctorates; newly graduated DNP prepared faculty; and current clinical faculty including master's-prepared APNs.

Each option presents separate variables influencing third-order outcomes. Should current faculty members be assigned to design new DNP programs, the possibility exists to further decrease the number of available nursing faculty to teach. Such action could limit enrollment, reducing the number of advanced practice nurses or more significantly, pre-licensure nursing students, which will produce a clear third-order effect in the larger health care system. It is possible that faculty selected from other disciplines to teach DNP students promotes the potential for more collegial communication within the health care team and supports initiatives by the Institute of Medicine (third-order outcome). However, some data suggest that if APNs are primarily taught by those outside the discipline of nursing, the resulting outcomes may include the loss of nursing qualities in the APN role, APNs prepared to function as physician substitutes, not nurse practitioners, or APNs taking on roles in health care which would no longer resemble nursing. The data mainly support that doctorally prepared faculty are required to teach in DNP programs, so considering master's-prepared APNs as faculty was not a viable option. In addition, should current master's-prepared APN faculty find themselves no longer qualified to teach in the new DNP programs, disenfranchisement, another third-order outcome, may occur.

Once schools of nursing accept the DNP initiative, they must also consider the financial costs required to create DNP programs. Although a cost benefit analysis has not been identified in this research, the data support that the initiation of the transition from master's degree to DNP is resource intensive. Variables presented in addressing this area include the reassignment of faculty within schools of nursing from teaching master's level to DNP and taking into account that selected faculty members must possess doctoral degrees to teach in DNP programs. The AACN recommended creating robust faculty APN practices to provide funding for faculty salaries as well as partnering between schools of nursing and community APNs to provide clinical instruction for DNP students. Another option would be to hire additional faculty, however, with the current nursing faculty shortage, schools may find difficulty in hiring qualified persons available for faculty appointment or experience bidding wars for those qualified. Relative to the discussion of leadership in a culture of change, these variables represent second- and third-order outcomes that are not within the control of the AACN. The AACN endorsed the DNP initiative and represents an example of a leadership's area of influence not matching the area of concern.

This research identified additional considerations for the nursing profession. Possibly the most detrimental third-order outcome associated with the cost of implementing the AACN vision turns on the potential to find constrained resources for nursing education drawn to the DNP initiative and away from efforts to correct the nursing shortage at the pre-licensure level. Another negative third-order effect centers on the potential new nurse researchers deciding to pursue the DNP degree rather than a PhD, the lure of a shorter and less expensive route to a doctoral degree being key in this situation. Cascading effects resulting from this outcome may include fewer PhD-prepared nurses on faculty, less nursing theory development, less respect to nursing schools in universities, and fewer dollars awarded in grant money for the university since fewer faculty members would be eligible to become principal investigators.

UNIVERSITY SYSTEM This research addressed tenure and equity of DNP-prepared faculty within the university setting. The existence of DNP-prepared faculty constitutes a second-order effect of the AACN's transformation initiative into the greater university system. The triangulated data offered several third-order outcomes sequential to the second-order outcome of DNP-prepared faculty members. All data indicated that tenure falls within the purview of individual universities and tenure status grants faculty members certain recognition and privileges within universities. Variables considered the Carnegie classifications of institutions of higher education, research expectations defined by individual universities, and the mission of the university where DNPs may hold faculty appointments. In institutions where research drives tenure, DNP-prepared APNs may not be prepared to conduct research at levels required to earn tenure, resulting in loss of employment, a third-order effect, or being reassigned to clinical track contracts. Data suggested that scholarly effort is often defined differently among universities. Some institutions tend to weigh the teaching mission higher than scholarly production; in this case, the university would more likely offer tenure to the DNP-prepared faculty. In addition, a smaller portion of the data posited that in the future, tenure will be granted based on redefined scholarly considerations or that tenure will hold less importance, with a possibility of being omitted from higher education. At this time, the data reflects a high degree of uncertainty on the issue of DNPs and tenure.

STUDENT AND ADVANCED PRACTICE NURSE CONSIDERATIONS From the student perspective, all data indicated increased opportunity cost, recognizing three second-order effects of the proposed change from master's level education to DNP preparation of the APN. Specific second-order outcomes identified were increased time in school, increased time out of the workforce, and increased financial liability. Variables identified regarding opportunity costs included career plans of the potential APN, available lead time to enter the workforce as an APN, desire to become a nurse provider rather than a medical provider, financial support, and current financial status, including educational debt.

The data currently available precludes any extrapolation that the benefit of the DNP, compared to the master's preparation, will equal or exceed the cost to an individual considering APN education. Possible third-order effects related to opportunity costs stemming from DNP education include a steady number of APN graduates accepting the increased opportunity costs, with no expectation of a direct financial return or APN graduates expecting salaries commensurate to the cost of their educational investment. Data posited that the increased opportunity cost will be a barrier to some individuals pursuing the DNP, resulting in another third-order effect, that of a reduced pool of APN applicants. Subsequent to this outcome exists the probability of the unintended consequence of reduced access to APN care in the larger health care system.

Regarding cost benefit of DNPs in health care, the data reveals that salaries will not be based on the academic degree obtained, but on the role, experience, contributions, and position of the nurse provider. The available data does not specify how the DNP will demonstrate value added in the workplace, since there is no research finding that DNPs will function clinically at a level different from the master's-prepared APNs. However, should salaries of DNP-prepared APNs be considered excessive, potential unintended, third-order outcomes include dissolution of job titles and replacement by less expensive providers such as physician assistants and anesthesia assistants. Conversely, APNs may be replaced by slightly more expensive providers such as physicians, who may be considered more cost effective due to their greater scopes of practice. Data illustrated that unlike the PharmD, Doctor of Physical Therapy, and Doctor of Occupational Therapy, the roles of NPs, CRNAs and CNMs can be filled by physicians and/or physician assistants and anesthesia assistants. Once again, the DNP initiative encounters much uncertainty in the domain of third-order outcomes.

CERTIFYING AND REGULATORY SYSTEMS Changes in certification of APNs constitute third-order outcomes, subsequent to the implementation of the DNP initiative and graduating DNP-prepared advanced practice nurses. At this time there is one agency providing certification for nurse anesthetists and one for nurse midwives. Several organizations provide certification for nurse practitioners and clinical nurse specialists. Currently the requirement for APN certification varies from state to state and among APN specialties. A potential third-order outcome of the DNP initiative could include certification for all APNs and a subsequent increase in the credibility by ensuring a constant level of quality. However, another third-order effect has been described as establishing a universal licensing examination comparable to the National Council Licensure Examination that nurses take for initial licensure. This carries potential unintended subsequent effects, since it can dismiss accomplishments and contributions of those currently providing certification and promote dissonance in the nursing profession.

An additional third-order effect requires changes in nurse practice acts and other regulatory documents to secure licensure for DNP-prepared advanced practice nurses. Because nurse practice acts are not uniform or nationally regulated, each state would need to accommodate DNP educational preparation for APNs. Currently, regulation of APNs includes legislated scopes of practice created by boards of nursing, boards of anesthesia or midwifery, and joint regulation with boards of medicine and nursing, anesthesia, or midwifery. A positive outcome could result in uniform requirements, allowing APNs to gain license to practice more easily when changing states of residency. However, when state practice acts are altered, there exists the risk that scopes of practice could be restricted, launching a cascade of effects for APNs currently practicing in the clinical setting. For example, should a state medical society lobby successfully in support of AMA Resolution 214 (AMA, 2008), nurse providers may cease to practice independently, and require the direct supervision of physicians. Should this third-order effect occur, in one or more states, the equity sought by DNP education would become a patchwork of gains and losses resulting in further barriers to health care.

Effects-Based Outcomes: Schools of Nursing Reject or Defer Decision on the DNP Initiative

According to the AACN (2008), 78 schools of nursing have begun accepting students and 140 additional schools are "considering" (n.p.) implementing DNP programs. Out of the 351 APN programs in existence (NACNS, 2005), 133 programs have either rejected or deferred the decision to support the DNP initiative. From available data, this research cannot accurately discern if a school has rejected or simply deferred a decision on the DNP initiative. Moreover, it is not possible with any degree of accuracy to predict the future behavior of these 133 remaining programs.

A stark vision of the future is presented by Cartwright and Reed (2005), who state that master's degree programs will simply cease to exist by 2015. Conversely, the data does not indicate that acceptance of the DNP initiative is mandated or that extant master's degree APN programs will lose accreditation. Further, there is no data indicating that state boards of nursing will cease to grant licenses to master's-prepared APNs. However, the accrediting agency for many of the nursing schools currently offering advanced practice nurse programs is the Commission on Collegiate Nursing Education (CCNE), the accrediting arm of the AACN. Some data suggests that this fact, coupled with the presumption that master's programs must be replaced with DNP programs, will influence first-order outcomes for schools of nursing deferring the decision to accept the DNP initiative. Those schools of nursing deferring decision on the DNP initiative produce a lag time in the emergence of second-order effects surrounding APN education, and in essence, limit the AACN's ability to achieve the intended first-order effect, the transformation of APN education.

Schools of nursing now accredited by the CCNE may choose to seek accreditation by the National League for Nursing Accrediting Commission (NLNAC) and maintain master's-prepared APN programs, a second-order outcome. Should accredited master's degree APN programs continue to exist, this option provides a career trajectory common in nursing. As a result, the master's-prepared APN could enter the workforce as a clinician, become proficient in that role, then return to school for the desired nursing doctoral degree, DNP or PhD, depending on the individual career goals of the advanced practice nurse. However, an unintended third-order outcome from the production of APNs from two educational levels may be experienced as amplified disenfranchisement, comparable to that perceived among nurses who received pre-licensure education from three levels of education. Subsequent effects include further fragmentation of the nursing profession.

The closure of master's degree APN programs represents a case-specific second-order outcome. The data revealed that some colleges currently offering master's degrees are not authorized to offer doctoral education and some nursing school faculties cannot support an additional doctoral degree. Should current APN master's programs close, cascading effects could include loss of revenue to the institution and possible closure of both master's and baccalaureate nursing programs. This would more likely occur in institutions not chartered to provide doctoral level education. Also, should a current master's degree program coexist with a faculty practice comprised of master's-prepared APNs, subsequent outcomes could include closure of both entities, further removing employment opportunities for APNs and reducing access to APN care.

Additional consideration whether to accept or reject the DNP initiative included perceptions of universities and the public. Data did not support that there would be confusion if the current master's degree model of APN education remains in existence. However, some data suggested that the DNP has and will continue to be a source of confusion for the public and potential disenfranchisement within the nursing profession.

Case-specific variables will influence the first-order outcomes of schools that have deferred decision on the DNP as the sole level of education for entry into advanced nursing practice. For example, the issue of available faculty to teach in a proposed DNP program may compel a school to accept the DNP initiative. Conversely, schools of nursing not affiliated with medical centers and not currently offering a research doctorate may lack necessary resources to create a DNP program. Should a majority of nursing schools reject or delay the decision to implement the DNP initiative, the AACN may be compelled to abandon its vision of the DNP as the sole educational route to APN or reconsider its timeframe rather than the projected 2015 date for fruition. It is also possible that leadership of the AACN will act more vigorously to achieve transformation as 2015 approaches.

Effects-Based Outcomes: Professional Nursing Organizations Accept, Reject, or Defer Decision on the DNP Initiative

The decisions made by professional nursing organizations to support, not to support or to remain neutral regarding the DNP initiative represent first-order effects of the introduction of the DNP by the AACN. The National Association of Pediatric Nurse Practitioners supports the DNP without qualification. On the other hand, the National Organization of Nurse Practitioner Faculties, a partner in the development of the practice doctorate, describes the DNP initiative as an evolutionary process and does not agree that a deadline can be applied to the transformation.

The American Organization of Nurse Executives does not support the DNP as the sole entry-level educational requirement and has articulated a number of potential unintended consequences in its position statement on the DNP. The AONE position statement suggests that nurses may seek graduate education in health care disciplines outside nursing, if appropriate or desired master's degrees within the profession are no longer offered. Outcomes beyond this second-order effect may include a perceived disenfranchisement by nurse executives as well as a shift in loyalty to other disciplines within health professions other than nursing. Although a working knowledge of other disciplines may be helpful from a health care team approach, subsequent effects include a diminished nursing influence in strategic planning regarding patient care. A subsequent third-order effect may create a generation of nurse executives possessing only undergraduate-level nursing education, in charge of leading nurses in direct care settings.

In addition to nurse executives, the American College of Nurse-Midwives does not support the DNP as the only educational preparation for entry into midwifery practice, a first-order outcome. Stemming from this rejection is a potential second-order outcome, involving philosophical dissonance within schools of nursing offering a nurse midwifery track, that have replaced master's-degree preparation with the DNP. Since there is precedence for schools of midwifery not to be affiliated with nursing schools, a third-order effect could become a complete separation of midwifery education from nursing. Should midwifery education become separate from other APN education, a subsequent outcome would be the loss of midwifery faculty to teach specialties such as women's health or family nurse practitioners. Another possible second-order effect may be the development of the Doctor of Midwifery Practice, sought within or outside schools of nursing. Yet an additional set of cascading effects could have potential midwifery students opting for medical school (second-order effect), resulting in fewer midwives and a loss of midwifery options for childbirth in the United States, a third-order outcome.

The creation of the Nurse Practitioner Roundtable (NPR), bringing together individual nurse practitioner organizations to comprise its membership, represents a collective second-order effect. Although the individual organizations of the NPR varied in terms of accepting, rejecting, or deferring the decision on the DNP initiative, the resulting third-order outcome was the publication of a unified statement in support of the DNP as an evolutionary transformation in APN education. In addition, this organization supports certification for all advanced practice nurses and use of the title *doctor* for the DNP-prepared nurse provider.

Summary

The AACN endorsed its vision of the Doctor of Nursing Practice Degree as the sole educational preparation for advanced practice nurses by 2015. Transformational leaders, such as the AACN with its DNP initiative, are presented with second-order and third-order effects within their circle of concern but not within their circle of direct influence. The DNP initiative, as a catalyst for change within the health care system of systems, introduced several exponential sequences of outcomes that the AACN cannot control or bring to fruition. This research identified first-, second- and third-order effects or outcomes resulting from the DNP initiative. Data collected from organizational documents, interviews and professional literature identified direct, indirect, intended, and unintended effects, which can now be addressed to better control outcomes as they influence the nursing profession.

CHAPTER V: SUMMARY AND IMPLICATIONS

Scholars describe leadership as a dynamic process of influencing groups toward goal achievement, where leaders and followers interact within specific circumstances (Hughes et al., 1993; Roach & Behling, 1984). Gardner (1993) stresses that leadership must be based on shared values with followers and that trust is fundamental in the leader–follower relationship. O'Toole (1995) asserts that leadership responsibilities include creating and maintaining order while directing change in turbulent environments. Pullan (2001) adds that although change can be led, variables and outcomes cannot be controlled and leadership must create coherence during this dynamic event. Pascale et al. (2000) state change within a system does not occur along a linear path because unforeseen variables will be introduced into the change process. The process of change may approach chaos; the challenge to leadership is to guide the system toward the desired outcome. In essence, effects-based reasoning seeks to highlight the variables associated with change so that leadership may effectively produce intended and mitigate unintended outcomes. In this case study, the outcome is a transformational change in nursing education.

In October 2004, the American Association of Colleges of Nursing introduced a paradigm change by its endorsement of the Doctor of Nursing Practice degree as the singular educational preparation for advanced practice nurses by the year 2015. Transformational leadership best describes the AACN regarding its introduction of this initiative into a system of systems. According to Smith (2004), transformational leadership effectively communicates a vision, inspires followers to pursue fruition of the vision, and provides resources to the followership for development. The AACN published its position statement illustrating its vision and developed the DNP Roadmap Report to provide guidance for implementing the degree. Inspiring members to action, this transformational leadership resulted in the establishment of 78 DNP programs in less than four years after the endorsement and an additional 140 programs in developmental stages.

The introduction of the DNP initiative by the AACN provides the focus for understanding a leadership process within effects-based methodology. Effects-based outcomes and effects-based reasoning will be discussed in terms of the AACN initiative as well as a method to be employed in the planning, implementation and evaluation of change from a leadership perspective. In addition, the implications and recommendations based on this case study are discussed.

Summary of Research

This research explored the leadership process of one organization's introduction of change into a system of systems. Specifically, this research identified outcomes or effects created by the introduction of the Doctor of Nursing Practice degree by the AACN as the sole educational degree for entry into advanced practice nursing. Employing a qualitative case study design, data were mined from the published documents of professional nursing organizations, interviews were conducted with a maximum variation sample of nursing leaders and advanced practice nurses, and relevant professional literature provided additional data for analysis. The triangulation of the data provided internal validity for this case study.

First-order outcomes resulted directly from the *trigger* action of the endorsement of the DNP initiative, absent any influence from variables. First-order effects included acceptance of the DNP as the preferred educational preparation for advanced practice nurses, rejection of this proposed change, or the deferral of decision on the DNP. Subsequent to the response of first-order outcomes, second-order effects occurred after the introduction of variables by the affected systems. The resulting variables included faculty, student and university concerns as well as variables introduced by professional organizations after their acceptance, rejection or deferral of the AACN initiative. A greater number of third-order effects were identified, however, with less certainty due to the exponential opportunity for the introduction of variables within the larger health care system.

Major findings included the establishment of 78 DNP programs and 140 additional schools considering DNP programs (AACN, 2008, n.p.), which constitute first-order outcomes. Significantly, 351 programs currently graduate advanced practice nurses (NACNS, 2005) and even if all 140 potential programs enrolled students by 2015, there would still be 133 fewer programs producing APNs, a second-order outcome, should master's programs no longer exist. From this point in time, the third-order outcome would be reduced access to APN care. However, the data revealed that most DNP programs admitted post-master's-prepared APNs and did not indicate if DNP and master's degree APN programs coexisted or if the master's programs had been eliminated at the institution. Third-order outcomes then become either a steady production of APNs from both master's and DNP programs or simply a reduction in the number of graduating APNs. This branching is an example of where effects-based reasoning could guide leaders to establish conditions to prevent unintended outcomes.

Several sequences of effects were identified that carry the potential for unintended effects within the profession of nursing. One begins with the first-order outcome of accepting the DNP followed by the second-order effect establishing a new and perhaps an additional doctoral program. Recognizing this process as resource intensive, this research identified a second-order effect, that of transferring resources away from master's and possibly prelicensure nursing programs. Third-order outcomes include a decrease in the number of faculty available for teaching as they are shifted to establish and instruct DNP curricula, forcing reduced enrollment and resulting in the reduction of advanced practice or prelicensure graduates.

Another set of second-order outcomes initiated by the universal acceptance of the DNP as the sole educational entry requirement for advanced practice nursing results in a reduction of students pursuing the PhD and a subsequent loss of nurse scientists. Consequences of the loss of nurse scientists include loss of academic respect for the profession of nursing, loss of principal investigators eligible for major grants, and loss of the development of nursing theory. Although some PhD programs admit BSN graduates, most PhD and other nursing doctorate programs are designed to accept master's-prepared nurses. Conversely, the DNP is an attractive terminal degree because most post-master's DNP programs can be accomplished in one or two years, greatly reducing the opportunity costs compared to the PhD in Nursing, which averages over eight years to completion (Berlin & Sechrist, 2002). The difference in opportunity costs alone, in terms of time in school, time out of the workforce and financial investment, would encourage many to seek the practice doctorate rather than the research doctorate. This would then lead to a troubling third-order effect of reduced nursing scholars. Again, effects-based reasoning reveals potential unintended outcomes that can be addressed by leaders.

Proponents of the AACN initiative posit that DNP-prepared individuals will help relieve the nursing faculty shortage. Although the DNP would require additional education for success in the university setting, data remained inconclusive regarding possibility of tenure and career success of the DNP-prepared faculty member. Should master's programs preparing APNs be eliminated, all

APNs will enter advanced practice nursing with the DNP degree. It is unknown if the DNP-prepared APN will have an interest or the opportunity to return to school to pursue a post-DNP research doctorate. Indeed, both post-master's and post-baccalaureate DNP programs for APNs translate into the third-order outcome of fewer PhD-prepared APNs educated to conduct research and teach the next generation of advanced practice nurses.

The researcher is unable to distinguish from the available data schools that rejected the DNP and schools that deferred decision to accept or reject. In this case, both first-order outcomes spark separate chains of stimulus and response interactions. In terms of rejecting the DNP as the appropriate level of educational preparation for APNs, schools may continue to offer master's degree APN programs or close them. In support of this second-degree outcome, schools may seek accreditation from the Commission on Collegiate Nursing Education, the accrediting body of the AACN, seek accreditation from the National League for Nursing Accrediting Commission, or possibly create a new organization for accreditation. In addition, remaining master's programs offer potential APNs educational options that may be more accommodating to student needs and ability to bear the opportunity cost of advanced practice education. However, the existence of two levels of educational preparation may result in professional dissonance among APNs as is currently experienced among nurses prepared at the associate degree, diploma, and baccalaureate levels, another third-order outcome.

Following the Diffusions of Innovations framework used by the AACN to introduce the DNP, schools that defer the decision to accept or reject the DNP are labeled as late adopters. This research cannot predict if those schools will eventually accept or reject the DNP innovation. In an evidence-based framework, deferring the decision creates a lag time, which in turn influences the AACN's effectiveness in producing its desired outcome of DNP for all APNs by 2015. It is useful to note that the Nursing Doctorate (ND) provides one example of a protracted response time resulting in second-order effects that prevented the achievement of the ultimate goal of establishing the nursing practice doctorate. Introduced in 1979, there were four programs matriculating students when the DNP was endorsed as the appropriate practice doctorate for nursing (AACN, 2004a). The lag time produced by late adopters may compel the AACN to reconsider the goal or the timeline for achievement of its vision.

Implications

Having identified first-, second-, and third-order effects, implications of this study include considerations with regard to the introduction of the Doctor of Nursing Practice degree as well as the usefulness of Effects-Based Reasoning as a leadership tool. Thus far, this research identified outcomes resulting from the introduction of the DNP, which created many chains of stimulus and response interactions. From this analysis, leaders in the nursing profession have the opportunity to act to direct and set conditions so that the subsequent cascading effects achieve desirable outcomes and avoid unintended and negative outcomes.

Implications Regarding the Introduction of the DNP

The overarching goal of the AACN's endorsement of the DNP was the transition from the master's degree to the DNP as the singular educational preparation of advanced practice nurses. Within four years of the publication of its position, the AACN guided the establishment of 78 programs enrolling students and 140 others in stages of development. As was encouraged in the DNP Roadmap Report, some universities successfully partnered with others to provide faculty and academic requirements to achieve the transition. Because research supports that baccalaureate nurses improve patient outcomes, one of the more exciting implications would be to apply the AACN model for collegial partnership to transition associate and diploma programs to baccalaureate-level prelicensure nursing education.

The DNP initiative also introduced an alternate educational progression for the nursing profession. Unlike research regarding baccalaureate-prepared nurses, it is currently unknown if the DNP-prepared APN will produce patient outcomes that are different from master's-prepared APNs. Since many APNs who have earned the DNP entered advanced practice nursing with a master's degree, it is unknown if the role of the DNP-prepared APN will differ from that of a master's-prepared APN. At this time, data is insufficient to evaluate a difference in outcomes of care provided by the master's- and the DNP-prepared APN. Preparing nurse providers at the doctoral level incurs greater economic cost for all concerned, which is a second-order outcome. This increase in cost will be paid by the practitioner, the system in which the APN works, or the person seeking health care from the APN, the third-order effect. In today's health care system where evidence-based practice is expected, implications require that the DNP degree must demonstrate value added, evidenced by improved outcomes of the advanced practice nurse.

Although 78 programs currently matriculate students and 140 additional programs are planned, if master's programs are eliminated, second-order variables may produce a significant reduction in the number of educational programs graduating APNs. Identifying this second-order effect before master's programs are eliminated allows nursing leadership to act on this information.

The nursing profession has the opportunity to exercise influence, based on second-order effects to allow two levels of education for APNs, acting to avoid the third-order outcome of decreased access to health care.

Additionally, one professional organization identified second- and third-order effects should the master's degree in nursing no longer offer specialization. This group posited that nurses would seek master's degrees outside nursing, an unintended second-order effect, if appropriate graduate education at the master's level would no longer be offered in nursing administration. Resulting consequences would reduce the nursing influence in health care agencies and in the health care system, constituting an unintended third-order effect. Illustrating these second-order effects allows nursing leadership to guide the educational system to a desired outcome.

Research identified an unintended second-order effect as potential nursing researchers may choose to pursue a DNP, resulting in the loss of nurse scientists. Compared to the research doctorate, the practice doctorate offers a terminal degree at a fraction of the opportunity costs of the PhD. Implications derived from this effects-based outcome include evaluating the career path to nursing researcher and working to create a more inviting course of study to achieving a nursing research doctorate. This is especially important when considering that time to completion approaches 20% longer than other scientific research doctorates (Berlin & Sechrist, 2002). Another implication is to explore the demographics of those entering DNP programs especially with regard to age and career goals and closely examine the influence of lesser opportunity costs of DNP education. Because a generational interest in the DNP was identified in the data, further research on generational implications may be insightful for achieving this transformational goal.

One goal of establishing the DNP as entry-level education for APNs was to create parity among health care professionals, to raise the academic status of nurse providers to that of other health care providers. From an academic perspective, a practice doctorate demonstrating academic equity would accomplish this. However, there is inadequate available data to support or refute that the roles of nurse provider, pharmacist, physical therapist and occupational therapist are currently perceived inequitably by the health care team or the American public.

The question remains if nurse practitioners with practice doctorates will achieve equity with physicians. Actions of the medical society imply otherwise. This research revealed four resolutions made by the American Medical Association since the introduction of the DNP; one proposed the prevention of nurse practitioners using the title *doctor* and three advocated physician control of the scope of practice of advanced practice nurses and other non-physician providers (AMA, 2005; AMA, 2006a; AMA, 2006b, AMA, 2008). Based on these second-order effects, implications for leaders include the need for the nursing professionals to work with physicians to build interprofessional trust in order to produce a health care environment where all legitimate health care providers are recognized and respected, an important third-order outcome. It is vital to the future of advanced practice nursing that actions of the AMA do not lead to restriction of the scope of practice for nurse providers or the dissolution of current partnerships between nurse providers and physicians.

Subsequent outcomes identified include decreased communication among health care professionals leading to decreased safety and quality of health care, which counters goals established by the Institute of Medicine. Although APNs may practice differently than physicians and physician extenders, it is important to understand that the roles of nurse providers can be filled by others, specifically, physicians, physician assistants, and anesthesia assistants. With replacement of nurse providers identified as a potential third-order outcome, leaders have the opportunity to set the conditions to avoid this and create an environment where patient-centered care can be provided by an effective health care team, which includes advanced practice nurses.

Leadership Implications for Use of Effects-Based Methodology

This research introduced a concept used by military leaders, effects-based methodology, to examine the leadership process of the AACN's introduction of a paradigm change into a system of systems. Among the reasons for using this approach, Mann et al. (2002) highlighted the importance of identifying military requirements for involving "interservice, interagency and international coordination" (p. 9) in the planning of actions to produce intended objectives and avoid unintended consequences. Moreover, this approach is used to compare possible courses of actions designed to set conditions or produce effects to achieve an objective. Considering the complexities and challenges of leading change described by scholars in the fields of leadership and transformation, effects-based reasoning allows leadership to predict stimulus and response interaction chains that achieve goals. This methodology illustrated the immediate effects of the AACN's *trigger* action and identified outcomes resulting from variables introduced into the process by members of the larger health care system.

Effects-based reasoning provides a framework for critical thinking permitting the leader to evaluate a course of action prior to its implementation. Leadership was defined for this study as the "process of influencing the activities of an organized group toward goal achievement" (Roach & Behling, 1984, p. 46). Effects-based reasoning assists leaders to identify effects and variables that hold potential for altering the direction of the intended change process. By creating conditions for change and building coalitions prior to initiating change as well as evaluating potential variables and outcomes at different levels of effects, the leader may more effectively produce the desired results of the trigger action and lead an organization toward achieving its goal. In this regard, the course of action chosen by the AACN leadership to introduce change into a complex system of systems can be examined in detail.

Limitations

This qualitative study proposed to develop a greater understanding of the leadership process of the American Association of Colleges of Nursing endorsement of the Doctor of Nursing Practice as the sole educational entry into advanced practice nursing. Applying effects-based methodology and approaching research from a systems perspective, this research identified outcomes, both intended and unintended. Selected questions posed by the American Nurses Association created the tool for collecting data from organizational documents, study participants, and relevant professional literature, but could not evaluate all outcomes resulting from the DNP initiative.

Organizational documents included the AACN Position Statement on the Practice Doctorate in Nursing, the DNP Roadmap Task Force Report, and position statements published by nursing organizations. Although a maximum variation sample was selected, comprised of nursing leaders and advanced practice nurses, the relatively small number of participants does not allow extrapolation of ideas into the general population in the nursing profession. Professional literature on the DNP and other practice doctorates continues to be published; therefore literature contributing to this analysis cannot be considered conclusive. Finally, variables continue to be introduced into the health care system and chains of stimulus and response interactions continue to develop, as second and third orders of effects from the endorsement of the DNP.

Recommendations

Based on outcomes identified in this case study, further research is recommended to determine demographics and career aspirations of DNP students, roles that DNP-prepared advanced practice nurses fill, pay range, and patient outcomes. For example, it is possible that the generational interest identified in the data is driven by a simple realization that eight or more years to a nursing research doctorate is too long to consider. From this information, the Diffusion of Innovations should be more effective in convincing the late adopters to decide whether to accept or reject the practice doctorate education for APNs. A cost benefit analysis will further assist in the support of this educational transformation. To justify the resource intensive transformation, research must support that the DNP provides value added in the four roles of the APN, the ARNP, CNM, CNS, and the CRNA.

Further research on the baccalaureate as entry level to professional nursing should be conducted. An historical research endeavor, taking into consideration the 1965 status of nursing in universities compared to the present day, may reveal reasons the transition was unsuccessful and identify different methods to pursue this proposal. A further recommendation includes an exploration of an intercollegiate model for transitioning the entry level of nursing practice to the baccalaureate degree by the American Nurses Association along with the National League for Nursing and the American Association of Colleges of Nursing, employing effects-based reasoning.

Nursing researchers must continue to create theory to ensure the future of nursing. In conjunction with the Council of Graduate Schools, nursing research may reveal innovations to reduce the average time required to complete nursing research doctorates, resulting in increased recruitment and retention of students pursuing research doctorates in nursing. Directors of nursing research doctoral programs should study alternate methods for admission and matriculation of students, alternate tracks for pursuing research interests, and provide increased support for doctoral candidates to ensure completion of courses of study.

In addition, all nursing organizations must work toward the common goal of patient-centered, quality health care. The American public needs additional education on the abilities and legitimacy of nurse providers. Advanced practice nursing organizations should work together to prevent medical organizations from successfully lobbying to interfere with advanced practice nurses' scope of practice.

Moreover, the American Association of Colleges of Nursing has made substantial progress in realizing their vision to change the entry-level education for advanced practice nursing to the practice doctorate level. Research may reveal how a small number of individuals can make such a significant change in a system of systems. Using a systems framework and effects-based methodology, nursing leadership may identify variables throughout the health care system which may lead to overall goal attainment.

Conclusion

In fewer than four years after endorsing its vision, the American Association of Colleges of Nursing has influenced the nursing education system to produce 78 programs currently enrolling students earning the Doctor of Nursing Practice Degree, with an additional 140 programs in varying stages of development. This is no small feat in terms of transformation leadership. However, the nursing profession has not presented evidence that the DNP will produce an improvement in the safety and quality of care provided by advanced practice nurses. Moreover, data are lacking to support that the benefits of this degree justify the increased costs incurred.

Nursing professionals have expressed concern that the DNP represents a temporary solution to the faculty shortage, which will ultimately come at the expense of nursing science. Specifically, the DNP, whether acquired for the purpose of entering APN practice or sought because of its attractive opportunity cost compared to the PhD, will divert some nurses from pursuing research doctorate degrees. This third-order outcome threatens the academic status for which the nursing profession has diligently worked for decades as well as endangers the future of nursing science.

From a practice perspective, master's-prepared advanced practice nurses may be concerned that their ability to continue practice and earn incomes are threatened by physicians attempting to control APN scope of practice motivated by the AACN's endorsement of the DNP. Other APNs may worry that the Center for Medicare and Medicaid Services will repeat actions of 1998, requiring APNs to return to school and earn a DNP in order to continue eligibility for third-party payment. Nurses with aspirations to become advanced practice nurses may abandon this path to professional development because the opportunity costs have become too great.

From data collected and analyzed in this case study, the primary impetus for the development of the DNP was to achieve educational parity in terms of credit hours required to produce advanced practice nurses. Master's degree programs preparing nurses for advanced practice often require many more credit hours than other master's degrees. Educational leaders may have chosen to limit the addition of courses not directly supporting the APN scope of practice to address this issue. The solution chosen by the AACN leadership was the establishment of the DNP as entry-level education for APNs by 2015, launching a myriad of cascading effects. These effects are described by leadership scholars as outcomes that cannot easily be controlled or directed by the leaders involved. The most troubling third-order outcomes identified in this work include greater dissonance within the nursing profession, discord among health care providers risking the replacement of nurse providers with physicians or non-physician providers, the potential decrease of nursing researchers with subsequent loss of academic status and nursing science, and the loss of focus and resources to address the nursing shortage.

This research supports the conclusion that evidence-based reasoning is a useful methodology in assisting leadership to create conditions and identify variables that may become catalysts or barriers in achieving change. The American Association of Colleges of Nursing introduced change into a system of systems, which generated many variables, producing numerous chains of stimulus and response interactions influencing the establishment of the DNP. Systems where the AACN exerts the greatest influence include the schools and colleges of nursing. Although within its area of concern, the AACN does not assert direct influence in most of the other systems which comprise the health care system. At this juncture of the change process introduced by the AACN, the application of effects-based reasoning may assist nursing leadership to identify and guide variables to create coherence during this dynamic process and lead the profession toward a desirable outcome.

REFERENCES

American Academy of Nurse Practitioners. (n.d.) *Qualifications of candidates.* Retrieved October 5, 2005 from http://www.aanp.org/Certification/Certification +Application.htm

American Academy of Nurse Practitioners. (2005). *American Academy of Nurse Practitioners discussion paper of DNP.* Retrieved September 22, 2006 from http://www.aanp.org/NR/rdonlyres/eohypbva5ab2yefiszlbl3nttmi3czv2lojklfechu-5w3lecyuy6gmnn6ykpzv6xhjmropsmeo2wou3ebo6qhdsafgf/Doctor+of+Nursing +Practice+_DNP_+Discussion+Paper.pdf

American Academy of Nurse Practitioners. (2006a). *Documentation of quality of nurse practitioner practice.* Retrieved October 4, 2006 from http://www.aanp.org/ NR/rdonlyres/ezmxdxkxur67qi67zg3sicvgqmspdy762keglxoqlndmutu7iifgbcs6v656 ktczfzyxbbsvise3n7ni4fauusv4npxe/AANP+Doc+Quality+of+NP+Practice.pdf

American Academy of Nurse Practitioners. (2006b). *American Academy of Nurse Practitioners fact sheet.* Retrieved September 22, 2006 from http://www.aanp .org/NR/rdonlyres/eic6ud5lllxzevpfhioihtduah5zbgw6wxdyyuksiarbsla5mlq2slt jagqpggzck32rxumeevldjyoozyqg3ytd3ac/2006+Fact+Sheet+9-26-06.pdf

American Academy of Nurse Practitioners. (2007a). *AAPN information.* Retrieved July 3, 2008 from http://www.aanp.org/AANPCMS2/AboutAANP/AANP +Information

American Academy of Nurse Practitioners. (2007b). *Discussion paper: Doctor of Nursing Practice.* Retrieved July 3, 2008 from http://www.aanp.org/NR/ rdonlyres/9DC9390F-145D-4768-995C-1C1FD12AC77C/0/DiscussionPaperDoctor _of_NursingPrac.pdf

American Academy of Nurse Practitioners. (2007c). *American Academy of Nurse Practitioners: Quality of nurse practitioner practice.* Retrieved July 3, 2008 from http://www.aanp.org/NR/rdonlyres/34E7FF57-E071-4014-B554-FF02B82FF2F2/ 0/Quality_of_NP_Prac112907.pdf

American Association of Colleges of Nursing. (2004a). *AACN position statement on the practice doctorate in nursing* [Electronic Version]. Washington, DC: Author.

American Association of Colleges of Nursing. (2004b). *Mission*. Retrieved June 30, 2007 from http://www.aacn.nche.edu/ContactUs/strtplan_mission.htm

American Association of Colleges of Nursing. (2005). *Press release: Commission on Collegiate Nursing Education moves to consider for accreditation only practice doctorates with the DNP degree title*. Retrieved June 30, 2007 from http://www.aacn.nche.edu/Media/NewsReleases/2005/CCNEDNP.htm

American Association of Colleges of Nursing. (2006a). *DNP roadmap task force report: October 20, 2006* [Electronic Version]. Washington, DC: Author.

American Association of Colleges of Nursing (2006b). *The essentials of doctoral education for advanced practice nurses*. October 2006 [Electronic Version]. Washington, DC: Author.

American Association of Colleges of Nursing. (2007a). *AACN member schools*. Retrieved July 1, 2007 from http://www.aacn.nche.edu/Memberservices/membdir.htm

American Association of Colleges of Nursing (2007b). *Doctor of nursing practice (DNP) programs*. Retrieved July 1, 2007 from http://www.aacn.nche.edu/DNP/DNPProgramList.htm

American Association of Colleges of Nursing (2007c). *Institutions offering doctoral programs in nursing and degrees conferred (N=132) Fall 2007*. Retrieved August 6, 2008 from http://www.aacn.nche.edu/IDS/pdf/DOC.pdf

American Association of Colleges of Nursing (2008). *Doctor of nursing practice (DNP) programs*. Retrieved August 6, 2008 from http://www.aacn.nche.edu/DNP/DNPProgramList.htm

American Association of Nurse Anesthetists (2006a). *Council on Accreditation of Nurse Anesthesia educational programs/schools*. Retrieved October 5, 2006 from http://www.aana.com/credentialing.aspx?ucNavMenu_TSMenuTargetID=105&ucNavMenuTSMenuTargetType=4&ucNavMenu_TSMenuID=6&id=118&

American Association of Nurse Anesthetists. (2006b). *Interim position statement on the DNP as entry into advanced practice of nurse anesthetists*. Retrieved September 22, 2006 from http://www.aana.com/uploadedFiles/Professional_Development/Nurse_Anesthesia_Education/Educational_Resources/DTF_Report/interim_pos_stmt.pdf

American Association of Nurse Anesthetists. (2006c). *The Doctorate in Nursing Practice (DNP): Background, current status and future activities*. Retrieved September 22, 2006 from http://www.aana.com/professionaldevelopment.aspx?ucNavMenu_TSMenuTargetID=131&ucNavMenu_TSMenuTargetType=4&ucNavMenu_TSMenuID=6&id=1742&

American Association of Nurse Anesthetists. (2007). *AANA position on doctoral education of nurse anesthetists: Adopted, July 2, 2007*. Retrieved September 30, 2007 from http://www.aana.com/uploadedFiles/Members/Membership/Resources/dtf_posstatemt0707.pdf

American Association of Nurse Anesthetists. (2008). *National Council on Certification and Recertification of Nurse Anesthetists*. Retrieved July 3, 2008 from http://www.aana.com/Credentialing.aspx?ucNavMenu_TSMenuTargetID =111&ucNavM enu_TSMenuTargetType=4&ucNavMenu_TSMenuID=6&id=13

American College of Nurse-Midwives. (2004). *Position statement: Definition of a certified nurse-midwife: Definition of midwifery practice*. Retrieved October 16, 2006 from http://www.midwife.org/siteFiles/position/Def_of_Mid _Prac,_CNM,_CM_05.pdf?CFID=1350590&CFTOKEN=73843576

American College of Nurse-Midwives. (2005). *ACNM Division of Accreditation statement on midwifery education*. Retrieved October 16, 2006 from http://www.acnm.org/siteFiles/DNPstatementedited.doc

American College of Nurse-Midwives. (2006, March). *Position statement: Mandatory degree requirements for entry into midwifery practice*. Retrieved September 22, 2006 from http://www.midwife.org/siteFiles/position/Mandatory _Degree_Requirements_3.06.pdf?CFID=1350590&CFTOKEN=73843576

American College of Nurse-Midwives. (2007, June). *Position statement: Midwifery practice and the Doctor of Nursing Practice (DNP)*. Retrieved October 12, 2007 from http://www.midwife.org/siteFiles/position/Midwifery_Ed_and_DNP_6_07.pdf

American College of Nurse Practitioners. (n. d.a). *ACNP position paper on nurse education*. Retrieved March 6, 2008 from http://www.acnpweb.org/files/public/ Position_Statement_NP_Education.pdf

American College of Nurse Practitioners. (n. d.b). *The American College of Nurse Practitioners Membership*. Retrieved July 3, 2008 from http://www.acnpweb.org/ i4a/pages/index.cfm?pageid=3295

American Medical Association. (2005). *American Medical Association House of Delegates Resolution: 814*. Retrieved June 21, 2008 from http://www.aaom.info/ ama814.pdf

American Medical Association. (2006a). *American Medical Association House of Delegates Resolution: 211*. Retrieved September 24, 2006 from http://www.ama-assn.org/ama1/pub/upload/mm/471/211a06.doc

American Medical Association. (2006b). *American Medical Association House of Delegates Resolution: 904*. Retrieved June, 21, 2008 from http://www.acnpweb .org/files/public/AMA_Resolution_904_11_06.pdf

American Medical Association. (2008). *American Medical Association House of Delegates Resolution: 214*. Retrieved June, 21, 2008 from http://www.ama-assn .org/ama1/pub/upload/mm/471/214.doc

American Nurses Association. (1965). American Nurses' Association first position on education for nursing. *American Journal of Nursing, 65*, 106–111.

American Nurses Association. (2005). *Handout: Questions/concerns to be addressed regarding the Doctorate of Nursing Practice*. Retrieved May 8, 2007 from http://nursingworld.org/gova/state/april19call/dnphandout.pdf

American Nurses Association. (2006). Nursing facts: *Advanced practice nursing: A new age in health care.* Retrieved October 16, 2006 from http://nursingworld.org/readroom/fsadvprc.htm

American Organization of Nurse Executives (2007). *AONE position statement: Doctorate of Nursing Practice.* Retrieved November 29, 2007 from http://www.aone.org/aone/docs/PositionStatement060607.doc

Apold, S. (2008). The Doctor of Nursing Practice: Looking back, moving forward. *Journal for Nurse Practitioners, 4*, (n. p.). Retrieved April 30, 2008 from http://www.medscape.com/viewarticle/571070

Avery, M. D. & Howe, C. (2007). The DNP and entry into midwifery practice: An analysis. *Journal of Midwifery & Women's Health, 53*, 14–22.

Bennis, W. (1994). *On becoming a leader.* Reading, MA: Addison-Wesley Publishing Company.

Berlin, L. E., & Sechrist, K. R. (2002). The shortage of doctorally prepared nursing faculty: A dire situation [electronic version]. *Nursing Outlook, 50*, 50–56.

Berlin, L. E., Wilsey, S. J., & Bednash, G. D. (2005). *2004–2005 Enrollment and graduations in baccalaureate and graduate programs in nursing.* Washington, DC: American Association of Colleges of Nursing.

Berman, A., Snyder, S., Kozier, B., & Erb, G. (2008). *Kozier & Erb's fundamentals of nursing: Concepts, process, and practice* (8th ed.). Upper Saddle River: Prentice Hall.

Brown, M. A., Draye, M. A., Zimmer, P. A., Magyary, D., Woods, S. L., Whitney, J., et al. (2006). Developing a practice doctorate in nursing: University of Washington perspectives and experience [electronic version]. *Nursing Outlook, 54*, 130–138.

Burke, A. M. (2004). The history of nursing. *Bert Rogers Schools of Continuing Education.* Retrieved December 1, 2007 from http://www.bertrodgers.com/_healthcare/pdf_healthcare/History%20of%20Nursing.pdf

Busch, J. A. & Busch, G. M. (1992). *Sociocybernetics: A perspective for living in complexity.* Jeffersonville, IN: Social Systems Press.

Capra, F. (1996). *The web of life.* New York: Anchor.

Carr, K. C. (2005). The Doctor of Nursing Practice degree: Is this the right degree at the right time for nursing and is it right for midwifery? *Quickening, 36*(6), 3–7.

Cartwright, C., & Reed, C. (2005). Policy and planning perspectives for the doctorate in nursing practice: An educational perspective. *Online Journal of Issues in Nursing, 10*, (n.p.). Retrieved September 15, 2006 from www.nursingworld.org/ojin/topic28/tpc28_6.htm

Chase, S. K., & Pruitt, R. H. (2006). The practice doctorate: Innovation or disruption? [Electronic Version]. *Journal of Nursing Education, 45*, 155-162.

Cheal, N. E. (1999). *Medicine and nursing: Professions bound by gender, pre-scribed by society. An analysis of the Goldmark Report.* Retrieved November 29, 2007, from CINAHL Plus with Full Text database.

Christopher, P. (2004). *The ethics of war & peace: An introduction to legal and moral issues.* (3rd ed.). Upper Saddle River: Pearson Prentice Hall.

Clinton, P. & Sperhac, A. M. (2006). National agenda for advanced practice nursing: The practice doctorate [Electronic Version]. *Journal of Professional Nursing, 22,* 7–14.

Code of Federal Regulations (1998). *42 CFR 410.75 for nurse practitioners.* Washington, DC: Federal Register. Retrieved September 24, 2007 from http://www.access.gpo.gov/nara/cfr/waisidx_99/42cfr410_99.html

Courtney, M., Galvin, K., Patterson, C., & Shortridge-Baggett, L. M. (2005). Emergent forms of doctoral education in nursing. In S. Ketefian & H. P. McKenna (Eds.), *Doctoral education in nursing: International perspectives.* (pp. 163–184). London: Routledge.

Creswell, J. W. (2005). *Educational research: Planning, conducting, and evaluating quantitative and qualitative research.* Upper Saddle River: Pearson Education, Inc.

DeValero, Y. F. (2001). Departmental factors affecting time-to degree and completion rates of doctoral students at one land-grant research institution [Electronic Version]. *The Journal of Higher Education, 72,* 341–367.

Dracup, K., Cronewell, L., Meleis, A. I., & Benner, P. E. (2005). Reflections of the Doctorate of Nursing Practice [Electronic Version]. *Nursing Outlook, 53,* 177–182.

Draye, M. A., Acker, M. & Zimmer, P. A. (2006). The practice doctorate in nursing: Approaches to transform nurse practitioner education and practice [Electronic Version]. *Nursing Outlook, 54,* 123–129.

Eisenhauer, L. & Bleich, M. (2006). The clinical doctorate: Whoa or go? *Nursing Education. 45,* 3–4.

Fairholm, G. W. (1994). *Leadership and the culture of trust.* Westport, CT: Praeger Publishers.

Fontaine, D., Stotts, N., Saxe, J., & Scott, M. (2007). *To DNP or not: One school's decision-making process.* Paper presented at the First National Conference on the Doctor of Nursing Practice: Meanings and Models, Annapolis, MD.

Freebody, P. (2003). *Qualitative Research in education: Interaction and practice.* London: Sage Publications.

Fulton, J. S. & Lyon, B. L. (2005). The need for some sense making: Doctor of Nursing Practice. *Online Journal of Issues in Nursing.* September 1, 2005. Retrieved October 15, 2006 from http://aumnicat.aum.edu:2229/ehost/detail?vid=29&hid=1 01&sid=ba1a2dd5-793b-4a50-9098-42a7f2977317%40sessionmgr4

Gardner, John W. (1993). *On leadership.* New York: Free Press.

Gardenier, E. F. (1991). *The transformation from the hospital school to the community junior college: A step towards the professionalization of nursing (1873–1965).* Retrieved December 6, 2007 from ProQuest Database.

Hathaway, D., Jacob, S., Stegbauer, C., Thompson C., & Graff, C. (2006). The practice doctorate: Perspectives of early adopters [Electronic Version]. *Journal of Nursing Education, 45,* 487–496.

Hughes, R. L., Ginnett, R. C. & Curphy, G. J. (1993). *Leadership: Enhancing the lessons of experience.* Burr Ridge, IL: Richard. D. Irwin, Inc.

Institute of Medicine. (1999). *To err is human: Building a safer health system.* Washington, DC: National Academies Press.

Institute of Medicine. (2001). *Crossing the quality chasm.* Washington, DC: National Academies Press.

Institute of Medicine. (2003). *Health professions education: A bridge to quality.* Washington, DC: National Academies Press.

Jacobs, L. A., DiMattio, J. K., Bishop, T. L., & Fields, S. D. (1998). The baccalaureate degree in nursing as an entry-level requirement for professional nursing practice. *Journal of Professional Nursing, 14,* 225–233.

Klein, T. (2007). Are nurses with a Doctor of Nursing Practice degree called "Doctor"? *Medscape Nurses.* October 11, 2007. Retrieved November 30, 2007 from http://www.medscape.com/viewarticle/563176

Kotter, J. P. (1996). *Leading change.* Boston: Harvard Business School Press.

Lenz, E.R. (2005). The practice doctorate in nursing: An idea whose time has come. *Online Journal of Issues in Nursing. 10* (3), (n. p.). Retrieved September 15, 2005 from http://www.nursingworld.org/MainMenuCategories/ANAMarketplace/ANAPeriodicals/OJIN/TableofContents/Volume102005/Number3/tpc28_116025.aspx

Loomis J. A., Willard, B., Cohen, J. (2007). Difficult professional choices: Deciding between the PhD and the DNP in nursing. *Online Journal of Nursing, 12,* (n.p.). Retrieved March 2, 2008 from http://www.nursingworld.org/MainMenuCategories/ANAMarketplace/ANAPeriodicals/OJIN/TableofContents/Volume122007/No1Jan07/ArticlePreviousTopics/tpc28_816033.aspx

Mann, E. C., Endersby, G., & Searle, T. R. (2002). *Thinking effects: Effects-based methodology for joint operations.* Maxwell Air Force Base, AL: Air University Press.

Maraldo, P. J., Fagin, C., & Keenan, T. (1988). Nursing and private philanthropy [Electronic Version]. *Health Affairs, 7,* 130–136.

Marion, L., Viens, D., O'Sullivan, A. L., Crabtree, K., Fontana, S. & Price, M. M. (2003). The practice doctorate in nursing: Future or fringe? *Topics in Advanced Practice Nursing eJournal, 3,* 1–7. Retrieved September 15, 2005 from http://www.medscape.com/viewarticle/453247

McKenna, H. (2005). Doctoral education: Some treasonable thoughts [Electronic Version]. *International Journal of Nursing Studies, 42*, 245–246.

Merriam, S. B. (1988). *Case study research in education: A qualitative approach.* San Francisco: Jossey-Bass Publishers.

National Association of Clinical Nurse Specialists. (n.d.a). *FAQS.* Retrieved October 15, 2006 from http://www.nacns.org/faqs.shtml

National Association of Clinical Nurse Specialists. (n.d.b). *NACNS mission.* Retrieved July 5, 2008 from http://www.nacns.org/mission.shtml

National Association of Clinical Nurse Specialists. (2005). *NACNS white paper on the nursing practice doctorate.* Retrieved July 4, 2007 from http://www.nacns .org/nacns_dnpwhitepaper2.pdf

National Association of Nurse Practitioners in Women's Health. (2007). *NPWH position statement: The DNP and practice in women's health care.* Retrieved June 28, 2008 from http://www.npwh.org/files/public/DNP.pdf

National Association of Pediatric Nurse Practitioners. (2004). *About NAPNAP.* Retrieved July 4, 2008 from http://www.napnap.org/index.cfm?page=9

National Association of Pediatric Nurse Practitioners. (2008). *NAPNAP position statement on the Doctorate of Nursing Practice (DNP).* Retrieved June 28, 2008 from http://www.napnap.org/userfiles/File/NAPNAP_DNP_PS_final.pdf

National Conference of Gerontological Nurse Practitioners. (n.d.). *About NCGNP.* Retrieved July 4, 2008 from http://www.ncgnp.org/displaycommon.cfm?an=17

National League for Nursing. (2005). *Position statement: Transforming nursing education.* Retrieved March 6, 2008 from http://www.nln.org/aboutnln/ PositionStatements/transforming052005.pdf

National League for Nursing (2007). *Reflection and dialogue: Doctor of nursing practice (DNP).* Retrieved May 8, 2007 from http://www.nln.org/aboutnln/ reflection_dialogue/refl_dial_1.htm

National Organization of Nurse Practitioner Faculties. (2006). *Statement on the doctorate in nursing: Response to recommendations on clinical hours and degree title.* Retrieved June 28, 2008 from http://www.nonpf.com/NONPF2005/ PracticeDoctorateResourceCenter/PDstatement1006.htm

Nelson, M. A. (2002). Education for professional nursing practice: Looking backward into the future. *Online Journal of Issues in Nursing.* May 31, 2002. Retrieved September 20, 2006 from http://www.nursingworld.org/ojin/topic18/tpc18_3.htm

Nurse Practitioner Roundtable. (2008, June). *Nurse practitioner DNP education, certification and titling: A unified statement.* Retrieved July 2, 2007 from http://www.acnpweb.org/files/public/DNP_GROUP_LETTER_6-08_w_copyright.pdf

O'Toole, J. (1995). *Leading change: Overcoming the ideology of comfort and the tyranny of custom.* San Francisco: Jossey-Bass Publishers.

Pascale, R. Millemann, M., & Gioja, L. (2000). *Surfing the edge of chaos*. New York: Crown Business Publishing.

Phillips, S. (2006). 18th annual legislative update: A comprehensive look at the legislative issues affecting advanced practice nurses. *The Nurse Practitioner, 31*, 6–398.

Phillips, S. (2007). 19th annual legislative update: A comprehensive look at the legislative issues affecting advanced practice nurses. *The Nurse Practitioner, 32*, 14–16.

Pullan, M. (2001). *Leading in a culture of change*. San Francisco: Jossey-Bass Publishers.

Roach, C., F. Jr. & Behling, O. (1984). Functionalism: Basis for an alternate approach to the study of leadership. In J. G. Hunt, D. M. Hosking, C. A. Schriesheim, & R. Stewart (Eds.), *Leaders and managers: International perspectives on managerial behavior and leadership*. Elmsford, NY: Pergamon.

Rogers, E. M. (2003). *Diffusion of innovations*. (5th ed.). New York: Free Press.

Smith, B. N., Montagno, R. V. & Kuzmenko, T. N. (2004). Transformational and servant leadership: Content and contextual comparisons. *Journal of Leadership and Organizational Studies, 10*(4), 80–91.

Smith, E. A. (2002). *Effects based operations: Applying network centric warfare in peace, crisis, and war*. Washington, DC: CCRP Publication Series.

Sperhac, A. M., & Clinton, P. (2004). Facts and fallacies: The practice doctorate. *Journal of Pediatric Health Care, 18*, 292–296.

Stake, R. E. (1995). *The art of case study research*. Thousand Oaks, CA: Sage Publications.

Upvall, M. J., & Ptachcinski, R. J. (2007). The journey to the DNP program and beyond: What can we learn from pharmacy? *Journal of Professional Nursing, 23*, 316–321.

U. S. Department of Health and Human Services, Health Resources and Services Administration, Bureau of Health Professions. (2004) *The registered nurse population: National sample survey of registered nurses March 2004: Preliminary findings* [Electronic version]. Washington, DC: U.S. Department of Health and Human Services.

Varney, H. (1997). *Varney's midwifery*. (3rd ed.). Sudbury: Jones and Bartlett Publishers.

Waldspurger-Robb, W. J. (2005). PhD, DNSc, ND: The ABCs of nursing doctoral degrees. *Dimensions of Critical Care Nursing, 24*(2), 89–96.

Appendix C

"Untidy": The Pre-War Policy Process for Post-War Iraq

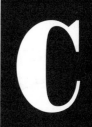

Review the following research project in its entirety. Analyze it to find implementation of each of the steps of the research process.

QUESTIONS TO GUIDE YOUR ANALYSIS

1 What is the research problem? What is the population being studied?

2 Was a hypothesis used or a research question? Was the author's choice appropriate for the type of study implemented? Give your rationale for your answer. Write additional hypotheses or research questions that could have been utilized.

3 Can a theoretical or conceptual framework be identified? If it is not clearly stated, is it implied at some point in the document? Was it an appropriate choice for this project?

4 Was the literature review thorough enough for the topic? Give your rationale for your answer.

5 Was informed consent or an institutional review board utilized in this research project? Was the author's choice to utilize an IRB or not appropriate? Give your rationale for your answer.

6 What type of research design was utilized for this project? How could this project have been implemented differently with a different type of research design?

7 What type of sampling was used in this research project? How could this project have been implemented with a different type of sampling utilized?

8 What type of data collection method was used? Was it the most appropriate one for this study? Give your rationale for your answer.

9 What type of statistical analysis was used with this study? Are there other statistics that could have been utilized but were not selected? Does this study have implications for the population being studied?

10 If you were to replicate this research project, what would you decide to do differently?

"Untidy": Tracing the Pre-War Policy Process for Post-War Iraq[1]

Sylvia B. Gage

CHAPTER 1: INTRODUCTION

Two years have passed since the U.S. military initiated ground operations in Operation Iraqi Freedom and declared Iraq's liberation from the Saddam Hussein regime. Contrary to predictions by U.S. Department of Defense officials, an insurgency in Iraq threatens Iraqi and regional security. Plans for post-war reconstruction and stability operations in Iraq, a policy outcome of the U.S. national security interagency process, have not accomplished the transition from war to peace. It is important to analyze the policy process for development of post-war operations to determine what went wrong and provide lessons learned for future operations.

Common criticisms of U.S. post-war policy in Iraq are allegations of poor intelligence leading to flawed policy, and failure of the Department of Defense to provide sufficient forces for policy implementation. Although both of these criticisms may be credible, the use of information in the policy process and design of a policy implementation plan are part of the overall policy process and need to be explored, as such. This research argues that institutional differences between the Department of State and the Department of Defense in their missions, structures, problem definitions, agenda setting, and use of information impeded the development of effective post-war policy.

The differences between these departments are constitutionally designed to strengthen U.S. foreign policy by providing discourse to the policy process and alternative instruments of national power, diplomacy and military force. It is the National Security Council (NSC) that is responsible for bringing the departments together to develop interagency policy in a collaborative process. A secondary criticism of U.S. post-war policy on Iraq is that the NSC failed to adequately synthesize interagency discourse to support the policy process.

This research is a qualitative descriptive analysis of the interagency policy process, as applied to a specific case: the policy outcome for reconstruction and stability operations in Iraq at the conclusion of Operation Iraqi Freedom. Unclassified U.S. Government documents and publications provided initial evidence of the national security interagency policy process as it worked in this specific case. To ensure an accurate view of formal roles and interactions in the evolution of policy development, official documents were used as

---

[1] Courtesy of Dr. Sylvia B. Gage.

evidence in the initial analysis. Public statements and analysis by stakeholders, academicians, and international relations practitioners provided supporting analyses and hindsight vision to the policy process.

This introductory chapter begins with a discussion of the evolution of post-war policy in Iraq. It continues with a description of the implementation plan developed by civilian Department of Defense personnel. When available, the "going in" assumptions of the planners are noted. Policy outcomes are described with regard to reconstruction and humanitarian assistance, as well as security and stability operations. The final section of this chapter describes the current insurgency, as it is an unintended consequence of the policy process.

Chapter 1 describes the policy process, including outcomes and unintended consequences for post-war planning of Operation Iraqi Freedom. This description provides the dependent variable for this research, or the thing we hope to explain. Chapter 2 provides a descriptive analysis of the independent variables covered in this research and begins with a discussion of the existing framework for the national security policy process.

Chapter 2 outlines the statutory structure of the formal policy process, including an examination of the changing structure of the national security policy process post Goldwater-Nichols, the evolution of civil-military affairs and the balance between diplomacy and military instruments of power. The role of the president is also discussed, as it contributes to an understanding of the informal policy process within the National Security Council, and may help explain one argument of this research, that the National Security Council failed to synthesize interagency discourse to support the policy process.

Chapter 2 also describes the institutional frameworks with which key stakeholders, the Department of State and the Department of Defense, approach the policy process, as this research argues that it is the differences between those institutional frameworks that impeded development of a successful post-war policy in Iraq.

Chapter 3 provides a brief description of the framework for analysis of the post-war policy process. It discusses how we might compare the policy process as it is statutorily defined to the actual policy process for post-war planning in Operation Iraqi Freedom. It will also provide a structure for how we might systematically apply the differences between the institutional frameworks of the Department of State and the Department of Defense to the post-war policy process. Finally, Chapter 3 includes a discussion of why the post-war policy process in Iraq is a useful case for analysis.

Chapter 4 includes an analysis of the policy process and its outcomes from Chapter 1, as affected by the variables outlined in Chapter 2. Chapter 5 provides a summary of the findings, notes limitations of the research, and recommends further study to clarify key concepts.

Evolution of Iraq's Post-War Policy

Planning for a regime change in Iraq did not begin as a build-up to Operation Iraqi Freedom, but resulted from the history of U.S. military actions in Iraq over the past 20 years. The United States has varied interests in the region. Apart from ensuring regional stability, and countering the proliferation of weapons, it is in the best interest of the United States to guarantee the stable flow of oil from the region. The Persian Gulf War in 1990–1991 drove the Hussein regime from the Kuwait oil fields, but stopped short of regime change. Operations Desert Fox and Desert Thunder in the late 1990's were initiated by the United States to degrade or destroy Saddam Hussein's ability to manufacture weapons of mass destruction, as well as his ability to pose a threat to his neighbors. Although Saddam Hussein did not escalate military action during the late 1990's, contingency plans were developed at that time to stabilize Iraq should a regime change become a U.S. foreign policy objective.

These military plans, developed primarily by General Anthony Zinni, were available for policy analysis and implementation in the build up to Operation Iraqi Freedom.[2] The Zinni plan could best be likened to heart surgery, in that he envisioned surgical removal of the Saddam Hussein regime and quick insertion of a temporary government, as a place-holder, until the Iraqi people could form new institutions. Zinni's concept was to use existing ministries and security forces to maintain stability during the transition.[3]

The U.S. Department of Defense notes that the planning for post-war Iraq began as an interagency policy process involving officials from the Departments of Defense, State, Justice, Treasure, Energy, and Commerce; the United States Agency for International Development (USAID), the Central Intelligence Agency and staff members of the National Security Council and the Office of Management and Budget. Although the order to go to war had not been given, and in fact would not be given until March 2003, interagency working groups began in July 2002 to coordinate post-war policy with regard to defining criteria to measure Iraq's transition to sovereignty, determining military requirements and diplomatic strategy, preparing for humanitarian and reconstruction assistance and developing policy recommendations for the National Security Council.[4]

Civilian officials on these interagency teams developed post-war plans for health, education, water and sanitation, electricity, shelter, transportation, governance and rule of law, agriculture and rural development,

[2] Michael E. O'Hanlon, "Iraq Without a Plan," *Policy Review*, No. 128, (Stanford University, The Hoover Institution, December 2004 and January 2005).

[3] Michael E. O'Hanlon, "Iraq Without a Plan," *Policy Review*, No. 128, (Stanford University, The Hoover Institution, December 2004 and January 2005).

[4] http://www.defenselink.mil/policy/isa/nesa/postwar_iraq.html.

telecommunications, economic and financial policy. Meanwhile, military officers at Central Command produced an extensive (300-page) operational order for the transition from war to peace, focusing on seven operational lines: unity of effort, security, rule of law, civil administration, governance, humanitarian assistance, and resettlement.[5]

In October 2002, a civilian policy planning group, "The Directorate of Special Plans," was formed at the Department of Defense to coordinate the interagency effort and produce policy options for decision makers.[6] It was specifically not named the "Iraq Planning Group" so as not to inflame ongoing diplomatic efforts. This group originated in the Office of Near East and South Asia (NESA) Affairs, under the Assistant Secretary of Defense for International Security Affairs. It was renamed the NESA/NG (Northern Gulf) in 2003.

On January 20, 2003, President Bush signed a directive creating the Office of Reconstruction and Humanitarian Assistance (ORHA) within the Department of Defense. Jay Garner, who would later deploy to preside over the initial postwar reconstruction work in Iraq, built the office from the ground up. ORHA took plans prepared in the interagency process and developed execution plans. These plans were "rehearsed" less than a month later at the National Defense University to check for surprises or unintended consequences of policy implementation.[7]

The purpose of ORHA was to organize interagency efforts to work in coordination with "Phase IV" operations should the U.S. invade Iraq and topple the Saddam Hussein regime. Military campaigns consist of four series of operations, or phases. Phase I is to deter if possible, and if not, to engage the enemy. Phase II is to deploy troops to seize the initiative, Phase III is to win decisively, and Phase IV is to transition from war to peace. These operations are sequenced, but overlap is anticipated, particularly between Phase III and Phase IV. This is because as troops win decisively, they continue to pursue new territory. While they pursue Phase III operations in new territory, Phase IV operations to support the transition from war to peace should occur in the area just taken by military force.[8] At the completion of major conflict, Phase IV includes the redeployment of forces and support of stability and reconstruction operations including humanitarian and peacekeeping operations.

The Under Secretary for Defense Policy announced the following Iraq Post-War policy objectives in February 2003:

---

[5] http://www.defenselink.mil/policy/isa/nesa/postwar_iraq.html.

[6] http://www.defenselink.mil/policy/isa/nesa/postwar_iraq.html.

[7] United States Department of Defense, Background Briefing on Reconstruction and Humanitarian Assistance in Post-War Iraq. March 11, 2003. Available at http://www.defenselink.mil/news/Mar2003/t03122003_t031bgd.html.

[8] Joint Pub 3-0, Doctrine for Joint Operations (Washington, D.C.: Joint Chiefs of Staff, 10 September 2001) p. III-21.

- First, continue to demonstrate to the Iraqi people and the world that the United States and its coalition partners aspire to liberate the Iraqis and not to occupy or control them or their economic resources.
- Second, eliminate Iraq's chemical and biological weapons, its nuclear program, the related delivery systems, and the related research and production facilities.
- Third, eliminate Iraq's terrorist infrastructure. A key element of U.S. strategy in the global war on terrorism is exploiting the information about terrorist networks that the coalition acquires through our military and law enforcement actions.
- Fourth, safeguard Iraq's territorial unity.
- Fifth, reconstruct the economic and political systems, putting Iraq on a path to become a prosperous and free country. The U.S. and its coalition partners share with many Iraqis the hope that their country will enjoy the rule of law and other institutions of democracy under a broad-based government that represents the various parts of Iraqi society.[9]

These objectives were offered with a commitment by the United States to stay as long as necessary to achieve these objectives, and a commitment to leave Iraq once institutional structures allow the Iraqi people to govern their own country and provide for their people. Testimony regarding these policy objectives specifically addressed and encouraged participation from foreign governments, non-governmental organizations and international organizations.[10]

The mixing of strategic and operational objectives for post-war policy is evident. The first objective clearly falls within the context of the national security strategy, foreign policy or international affairs. As such, it fits in the domain of the U.S. National Security Council or the U.S. Department of State. Only as an information operation, an attempt to shape the perception of the enemy, would this be included as a military objective. The second, third and forth objectives are clearly operational objectives of the Department of Defense and the appropriate military commands, or at best, part of the strategic concept of U.S. Central Command's Crisis Action Plan. The final objective is again a strategic objective, the narrative of which is almost verbatim from the U.S. National Security Strategy.[11] The objectives demonstrate integration of concepts developed by the U.S. Department of Defense and the U.S. Department of State, but lack a descriptor of accountability for policy implementation.

---

[9] Douglas Feith, Under Secretary of Defense for Policy, Testimony before the Senate Foreign Relations Committee, February 11, 2003.

[10] Douglas Feith, Under Secretary of Defense for Policy, Testimony before the Senate Foreign Relations Committee, February 11, 2003.

[11] The White House, *The National Security Strategy of the United States of America*, September 17, 2002. Particular attention should be paid to Section VI, Ignite a New Era of Global Economic Growth through Free Markets and Free Trade.

The Implementation Plan

Baghdad fell on April 9, 2003. General Tommy Franks, the Commander of Coalition Forces, declared dissolution of the Ba'ath Party and liberation of Iraq from the Saddam Hussein regime on May 10, 2003. General Franks temporarily headed the CPA until a civilian administrator could be positioned in Iraq. Ambassador L. Paul Bremer, selected prior to initiation of military action, assumed the position of Civilian Administrator of the Coalition Provisional Authority, on May 13, 2003. On May 16, 2003, the order establishing the Coalition Provisional Authority (CPA) was signed by Bremer and as civilian administrator, he became responsible for overseeing all civilian U.S. personnel in Iraq, including those working in the Office of Reconstruction and Humanitarian Affairs (ORHA). However, the CPA reported to the U.S. President through the U.S. Department of Defense.

Implementation of Iraq policy objectives would be supported by coalition military forces as part of Phase IV military operations, but carried out by the newly created CPA. The CPA was to act as a temporary government of Iraq, during the development of new government institutions. As such, the plan was for the Coalition Provisional Authority to remain in control of Iraq until an Iraq Interim Government could be formed. A background briefing provided by a senior defense official in March 2003 implied the Deputies and Principals of the U.S. National Security Council were developing the plan for development of a new Iraq government.[12]

Testimony to the House Committee on International Relations in May 2003, by the Under Secretary for Defense Policy, indicated that although plans had not been fully crystallized, the Iraqi Interim Government would be a representative and inclusive body in which Iraqis would feel free to participate in economic and political reconstruction. It was envisioned that the most important function of the Iraqi Interim Government would be to replace itself through design of new government institutions that would be representative of the Iraqi people. These institutions would include a constitution and rule of law, and means of political participation such as development of political parties and fair and free elections.[13]

The implementation plan allowed existing Iraqi government ministries to be kept in place until the United States decided to either disestablish that ministry or turn it back over to the Iraqis. Additionally, the Iraqi regular army would be kept on the payroll to aid clean-up and reconstruction efforts, as

---

[12] United States Department of Defense, Background Briefing on Reconstruction and Humanitarian Assistance in Post-War Iraq. March 11, 2003. Available at http://www.defenselink.mil/news/Mar2003/t03122003_t031bgd.html.

[13] Douglas Feith, Under Secretary of Defense for Policy, Testimony before the Committee on International Relations U.S. House of Representatives, May 15, 2003.

would over two million employees of the various ministries for critical services such as healthcare, education, food programs, law enforcement, and the courts system.[14] Although government institutions would remain in place, the plan called for "De-Ba'athification," or the removal of all Ba'athist leaders from positions of authority in government institutions.

The implementation plan did not clearly distinguish between civilian and military roles and called for a senior civilian administrator to head the post-war effort.[15] It is unclear why the U.S. Department of Defense was given the lead in planning and implementation of post-war policy. In previous wars, the role of the military was peacekeeping, that is, providing a safe and secure environment in which nation building can occur. In this case, the responsibility of nation building, or transitioning Iraq into a viable, self-sustaining country, friendly to the United States, was tasked to Department of Defense personnel of the Office of Reconstruction and Humanitarian Assistance (ORHA).

The ORHA was to coordinate efforts with the military Civil Affairs brigades, part of the Coalition Forces Land Component Command (CFLCC). ORHA pre-positioned civilian Disaster Response Teams from USAID in Kuwait to be the first responders for reconstruction efforts. Additional resources were anticipated to arrive from the United Nations, the International Committee of the Red Cross, and other non-governmental and international organizations.[16] "Free Iraqis," those who hade been in exile in the United States, Britain, or other free countries would be hired by the ORHA for a short term of 90 to 120 days to help with reconstruction efforts and would "explain" to the people in Iraq, how to live in a democracy.[17]

Pre-War Assumptions on Post-War Challenges

Prior to the initiation of hostilities by the United States in Iraq, the Congressional Research Service of the Library of Congress, as well as the ORHA, noted the potential for tremendous humanitarian issues in post-war Iraq.[18] Primary

---

[14] United States Department of Defense, Background Briefing on Reconstruction and Humanitarian Assistance in Post-War Iraq. March 11, 2003. Available at http://www.defenselink.mil/news/Mar2003/t03122003_t031bgd.html.

[15] Douglas Feith, Under Secretary of Defense for Policy, Testimony before the Committee on International Relations U.S. House of Representatives, May 15, 2003.

[16] United States Department of Defense, Background Briefing on Reconstruction and Humanitarian Assistance in Post-War Iraq. March 11, 2003. Available at http://www.defenselink.mil/news/Mar2003/t03122003_t031bgd.html.

[17] United States Department of Defense, Background Briefing on Reconstruction and Humanitarian Assistance in Post-War Iraq. March 11, 2003. Available at http://www.defenselink.mil/news/Mar2003/t03122003_t031bgd.html.

[18] Rhoda Margesson and Johanna Bockman, "Potential Humanitarian Issues in Post-War Iraq: An Overview for Congress," Congressional Research Service, The Library of Congress, March 18, 2003.

concerns included contamination of water supplies, food shortages, basic health concerns, refugees and preparation for entry of aid organizations. The Department of Defense ORHA, in conjunction with the Department of State and USAID, was tasked with developing an operational concept for humanitarian assistance and the delivery of aid to avert a humanitarian crisis.

The ORHA also was concerned about the development of a new political culture, democratic government institutions, and rule of law, as noted in the policy objectives. Ethnic and religious fragmentation between Sunnis, Shias, and Kurds was of concern, but not deemed to present insurmountable challenges. It was also believed that the concept of "Nationalism" would bring Iraqis together regardless of their differences. Nationalism might be defined as being an Iraqi first, or an Arab first, thus subjugating small group interests to the greater good.[19] It was envisioned that Iraq was a fairly sophisticated country that would be able, with a helping hand, to run itself fairly efficiently.[20] It was also assumed that Iraqis would welcome the return of somewhere between 80 and 150 expatriates to serve in leadership positions. Their purpose would be to assist in the reconstruction effort until local Iraqis could be developed to assume a greater role in their new government.[21]

With regard to security and stability in Iraq, the ORHA assumed that coalition forces would provide secure conditions for reconstruction and humanitarian efforts, as well as development of new government institutions. The Iraqi regular army would be trained in law enforcement functions and would assist coalition troops in patrolling Iraq. Iraqis, with the assistance of international advisors, would maintain security. Other security issues, notably the security of Iraq's oil production facilities, the location and elimination of weapons of mass destruction (WMD) and the destruction of terrorist infrastructure, would be the responsibility of coalition forces and their civilian agencies with related expertise.[22] Securing Iraq was thought to be a short-term effort, once coalition forces were in country.[23] The assumption was that once Iraqis believed that the Saddam Hussein Regime was over, they would diligently work with the United States to build their new government. The Iraqi expatriate community,

---

[19] Douglas Feith, Under Secretary of Defense for Policy, Testimony before the Committee on International Relations U.S. House of Representatives, May 15, 2003.

[20] United States Department of Defense, Background Briefing on Reconstruction and Humanitarian Assistance in Post-War Iraq. March 11, 2003. Available at http://www.defenselink.mil/news/Mar2003/t03122003_t031bgd.html.

[21] Douglas Feith, Under Secretary of Defense for Policy, Testimony before the Committee on International Relations U.S. House of Representatives, May 15, 2003.

[22] Douglas Feith, Under Secretary of Defense for Policy, Testimony before the Committee on International Relations U.S. House of Representatives, May 15, 2003.

[23] United States Department of Defense, Background Briefing on Reconstruction and Humanitarian Assistance in Post-War Iraq. March 11, 2003. Available at http://www.defenselink.mil/news/Mar2003/t03122003_t031bgd.html.

a major source of information in the Department of Defense post-war policy process, supported this view.[24] The Office of Reconstruction and Humanitarian Assistance (ORHA) assumed that financing for the reconstruction and stability operations in Iraq would be accomplished through existing congressional appropriations, financial support from coalition partners, contributions from international organizations, and revitalization of Iraq's oil production capability. One large expense would be payment of wages to approximately two million Iraqis, for their work to keep government services flowing during the transition.

Post-War ORHA Realities

When U.S. forces entered Iraq, it became obvious that reconstruction efforts would be more challenging than anticipated. This was partially because the infrastructure of Iraq was in far more deteriorated condition than anticipated. This was particularly true with regard to availability and functioning of public utilities and the nation's oil production capability. Since the worldwide oil crisis of 1973, Iraq's economy has been primarily based on oil production rather than agriculture. Although coalition forces prevented the destruction of most oil fields during the war, the condition of the equipment prevented immediate and effective management of production. In fact, soon after the war Iraq experienced tremendous shortages of gasoline and propane, and it became necessary to supplement Iraq's production capability by importing these products.[25]

The funding requirements for Iraq's reconstruction remain unknown, just as the length of time the U.S. will remain in Iraq is to be determined. It was believed prior to the war that oil revenues would contribute a large portion of the funds necessary for rebuilding. Additionally, the U.S. government froze approximately $1.7 billion in Iraqi assets in the United States prior to the war. During the combat phase of Operation Iraqi Freedom, another $700 million in cash was seized by the United States and is available to provide assistance to the Iraqi people. As of May 2003, public pledges from the international community totaled over $1.2 billion to be used in the food, health, agriculture, and security sectors. Congress had also appropriated $2.5 billion for reconstruction efforts.[26]

---

[24] Douglas Feith, Under Secretary of Defense for Policy, Testimony before the Committee on International Relations U.S. House of Representatives, May 15, 2003.

[25] Chip Cummins, "Export, Storage Troubles Snarl Iraq's Oil Industry," *The Wall Street Journal*, May 7, 2003.

[26] Douglas Feith, Under Secretary of Defense for Policy, Testimony before the Committee on International Relations U.S. House of Representatives, May 15, 2003.

Security and Stability Realities

U.S. post-war policy as it relates to post-war stability and security is a focal point for this research. Stability and security, or the lack thereof, affect the ability of coalition forces to achieve policy objective one, "demonstrate to the Iraqi people and the world that the United States and its coalition partners aspire to liberate the Iraqis and not to occupy or control them or their economic resources," and policy objective five, "…reconstruct the economic and political systems, putting Iraq on a path to become a prosperous and free country. The U.S. and its coalition partners share with many Iraqis the hope that their country will enjoy the rule of law and other institutions of democracy under a broad-based government that represents the various parts of Iraqi society."[27]

Even though basic security and stability provide the environment in which democratic institutions can grow, very little is mentioned in the literature regarding pre-war planning for post-war stability. This may be due to the prevailing assumption that Iraqis would welcome coalition forces as liberators. Failure to address security and stability operations in policy discussions is troubling at best, and will be further discussed in Chapter 4.

One description of this policy deficit is portrayed by Colonel Christopher C. Conlin, a marine who experienced first-hand the immediate consequences of the policy failure. Conlin described the situation in Baghdad in April 2003 once coalition forces had won the city: "We were now the single center of authority." Conlin noted he was surprised at the immediacy with which he became responsible for the day-to-day events of Iraqis. He was inundated with requests from locals, for everything from electricity to medical care. The former "secret police" had melted into the crowds and in the uncontrollable aftermath, looting was rampant. Conlin indicates that he and his men struggled with how to be "the government" and with no contingency plan, made up the rules as they went along. His mission was to run a city of approximately five million, with a battalion of men who were unprepared to govern and had very little information on which to make decisions.[28]

Conlin's experience of being "the government" lasted less than two weeks, after which the responsibility was handed over to several U.S. Army units. He observes, "There did not seem to be a unity of purpose throughout the theater in defining a cohesive political end state fully supported in all phases of the operation."[29] Conlin's observations include a need to provide civil solutions to civil power vacuums and merge high-intensity combat operations with

---

[27] Douglas Feith, Under Secretary of Defense for Policy, Testimony before the Committee on International Relations U.S. House of Representatives May 15, 2003.

[28] Christopher C. Conlin, "What Do You Do for an Encore?" *Marine Corps Gazette*, September 2004.

[29] Christopher C. Conlin, "What Do You Do for an Encore?" *Marine Corps Gazette*, September 2004.

nonmilitary solutions. He notes there was not an identifiable plan to address the transition from war to peace in Iraq.[30]

The Insurgency—A Policy Outcome

It is too early to know if the Iraq insurgency was avoidable, but it must be explored as an outcome of the policy process, if for no other reason than it prevents the achievement of policy objectives in Iraq. It did not cause the failure of coalition policy, but rather resulted from the failure of the policy process to adequately address security and stability operations.

Insurgency is a strategy, employing the use of subversion and armed conflict to fight an existing civil authority or to liberate a country from outside occupiers. At a minimum, the following conditions must exist for an insurgency to be effective:

1. Preconditions—frustration, conspiratorial history, culture
2. Effective strategy for force protection, augmentation and erosion of the enemy's will as well as the strength and legitimacy of his regime
3. Effective ideology that explains discontent and offers a remedy
4. Effective leadership[31]

Preconditions in Iraq

Iraq is an oddly shaped nation state with an ethnically and culturally diverse population of which approximately half are 19 years of age or younger. There is a strong Iraqi identity regardless of ethnic and religious cleavages. The beginnings of Iraq as a nation state came with occupation by the British (1920–1932) to serve their own strategic economic interests. Economic gains from the oil-based economy during the 1970's were squandered by the Hussein regime in costly wars against Iraq's neighbors. Additionally, during the 1990's economic development was stifled by economic sanctions imposed by western powers to punish the regime for its actions. Iraqis have reason to feel exploited, not only by Western powers, but by their own government. As an independent state, Iraq also has an internal history of political violence. As the United States continues to provide the Interim Iraqi Government with "security support" and advice on building democratic institutions, one can not help but wonder if Iraq has traveled full circle back to the "provisional government" maintained during the post–World War I, British occupation.

---

[30] Christopher C. Conlin, "What Do You Do for an Encore?" *Marine Corps Gazette*, September 2004.

[31] Steven Metz and Raymond Millen, "Insurgency and Counterinsurgency in the 21st Century: Reconceptualizing Threat and Response," (Strategic Studies Institute monograph, November 2004) 2.

Effective Strategy

The Iraqi insurgency began almost immediately as U.S. military forces entered Iraqi towns. Imbedded media representatives first reported fire from Iraqi guerrilla fighters on day three of the war.[32] The welcoming parades predicted by Pentagon analysts did not occur. Two years later it is safe to say that Iraqi insurgents have demonstrated their capability to sustain the insurgency. The insurgents include a variety of religious and ethnic sects. Their numbers have increased and now include foreign fighters. They represent a wide range of religious, political and economic interests, some of which pertain to an internal struggle for power within Iraq and some of which pertain to resistance against an outside power.

The tactics of Iraq insurgents run the gamut from passive resistance by surrounding buildings and blocking traffic, to brutal torture and beheadings. No matter how repulsive, the tactics are not new and have been seen in prior insurgent movements across the world. For example, beheadings occurred during the Korean War. Military scholars generally refer to such tactics as part of the "strategic environment," and note that use of these tactics most commonly reflects the availability of resources and access to conventional weapons. However, another important consideration in modern insurgencies has been the continuous news cycle that drives public opinion. The tactics used by insurgents seem to be selected not only by the availability of resources, but the impact of the use of such tactics on public opinion and political will.[33]

Effective Leadership/Who Are the Insurgents?

Even by the most generous estimates, the actual number of insurgents represents less than one half of one percent of the Iraqi population.[34] The actual number of insurgent groups is unknown, but they may be categorized by their interests into four broad groups: Sunnis who are Saddam loyalists and remnants of the secular Ba'ath Party; Sunni religious elements previously quelled by the secular Hussein regime: Shi'a Muslims indigenous to Iraq, some of whom are supported by Iran and led by clerics such as Muqtada al-Sadr; and

---

[32] Lt. Gen. John Abizaid, CENTCOM Operation Iraqi Freedom Briefing. March 23, 2003. Available at http://www.globalsecurity.org/wmd/library/news/iraq/2003/iraq-030323-centcom02.htm.

[33] Ivan Eland, "'Turning Point' in the War in Iraq: But Which Way Is It Turning?" November 19, 2003. Available at http://www.independent.org/tii/antiwar/e111903.html.

[34] Unnamed source, reports insurgents number between eight to twelve thousand individuals who represent various interests and ideologies. Reported in *New York Times*, October 22, 2004. Available at http://www.msnbc.com/id/6304304/. Michael Ware reports in "The Enemy with Many Faces," *Time*, September 24, 2004 that total insurgents including those providing food shelter and logistic support may number over 100,000.

international Jihad warriors, such as Abu Mousab al-Zarqawi.[35] These groups may share interests and cooperate in the insurgency. However, enmity between certain Sunni and Shi'a elements may also escalate the insurgency.

Effective Ideology/Why Are They Acting?

The United States has struggled in the post–Cold War era to replace George Kennan's "containment" policy with a policy of economic, social and political engagement, known as "globalization." Because America values political and economic liberalism, peaceful relationships with and between nations, and respect for human dignity, these standards underpinned our foreign policy development and engagement in this new arena.

An argument can be made that economic globalization is merely a shiny new package for the delivery of democratic values, as it requires the development of economic and political institutions. It also has the potential to create a strong middle class in countries with struggling economies, and democracies require a strong middle class.[36] In fact, some researchers have isolated economic growth as a key causal variable to the emergence and stability of new democratic regimes.[37]

Although globalization was an acceptable foreign policy strategy during the 1990's, the unintended consequences of its implementation have had far-reaching and dangerous effects. These include perception of the United States as a self-serving hegemonic crusader and a growing resistance from those who do not share the same enthusiasm for economic and political liberalism.

The emphasis on political liberalism, modernization, and the development of western-styled democratic institutions is not acceptable to a large number of countries in the Middle East. Political scientist Robert Clark has written extensively on the effects of development and modernization in the non-Western world. He notes three potentials for political instability brought on by modernization. First, he theorizes that democratization has the potential to dislodge

---

[35] Roshan Muhammed Salid, "Al-Zarqawi: America's new bogeyman," *Al Jazeera*, July 1, 2004. Salid refers to al-Zarqawi as a 38-year-old Jordanian who previously fought the Soviet forces in Afghanistan and was sentenced to death in Jordan for plotting attacks on Israeli and American tourists. He fled to Afghanistan to fight with Usama bin Ladin against the U.S.-led invasion in 2001 and later sought refuge in Iraq after being injured in Afghanistan. Salid reports Al-Zarqawi is "probably a pretty significant figure," but he is being used by the United States to discredit the resistance by internal Iraqi insurgents. In a later article, November 18, 2004, *Al Jazeera* reports "U.S. exaggerated foreign fighters in Iraq," and quotes U.S. Ground Commander General George Casey's report that of the 1000 men captured in Falluja last week, only 15 were foreign fighters.

[36] Robert A. Dahl, *On Democracy*, (New Haven: Yale University Press, 1998), 166–9.

[37] Ross E. Burkhart and Michael S. Lewis-Beck, "Comparative Democracy" *American Political Science Review*, (88: 1994), 903–910.

traditional elites, creating friction between the former elites and the new regime. Second, he notes that secularism may weaken traditional cultural values and lead to a weaker society. Finally, he notes that economic development may increase the economic and socio-cultural cleavages, as not all individuals will receive equal benefit or growth at the same rate.[38]

The first two potentials are frequently cited as reasons why Western democracy will not work in the Middle East. Even so, in a December 2002 speech at the Heritage Foundation, U.S. Secretary of State Colin Powell introduced an initiative referred to as the "U.S.–Middle East Partnership," to promote Western democracy and support for economic, political, and educational reform in the Middle East. Three months later, the United States invaded Iraq, displaced the traditional Sunni elites and called for a secular democratic government. In a predictable conflict, the United States' presence in Iraq is now portrayed by Arab media outlets as an occupation, in which the U.S. interests are focused on oil reserves and economic expansionism, rather than helping the people of Iraq and the broader Middle East.[39]

An additional concern in the Middle East is the fit of the Shari'ah, (referred to as Islamic democracy, but actually Islamic law), with Western style democratic institutions and constitutionalism. The Shari'ah is a standard to which all law must adhere. If a law is inconsistent, or in conflict with Islamic law, it is considered null and void. Stanley N. Katz, of the Princeton University Program of Law and Public Affairs, provides a recent analysis of this issue. He concludes that although it may be difficult to merge the concept of constitutionalism with Shari'ah, we just do not know yet if it can be done. He notes that constitutionalism is a long contested process whereby a commitment is made to the structure of political power that balances state power with individual rights. It is not something that one country can provide to another or invoke on another. This process may be particularly difficult in Iraq, because of the distinct ethnic and religious cleavages of the population.[40]

To summarize, the U.S. policy of globalization during the 1990's became synonymous with democratic values of economic and political liberalism. This policy was aligned with U.S. interests, but in some cases created an even larger gap between the world's "haves" and "have-nots." As nations struggled to build democratic institutions in order to receive aid and assistance from international entities such as the International Monetary Fund and the World Bank, their illiberal governments exploited financial support. This tarnished

---

[38] Robert P. Clark, Jr., *Development and Instability, Political Change in the Non-Western World*, (Hindale, Illinois: The Dryden Press, 1974). 10.

[39] http://www.usembassy-israel.org.il/publish/peace/peace1.htm.

[40] Stanley N. Katz, "Gun Barrel Democracy? Democratic Constitutionalism Following Military Occupation: Reflections on the U.S. Experience," *Princeton Working Papers, No. 04-010*. Available online at Social Science Research Network Electronic Library.

the United States' image abroad and set the stage for claims that the United States' foreign policy is merely interested in economic expansionism and control of energy resources in the Middle East. That, combined with a forced shift in political power, an uncertainty regarding the role of Islamic law in the new rules of the game, and fear of the effects of secularism on traditional cultural values, has produced an anti-democracy sentiment in Iraq.

Few interviews have been conducted with the insurgents to confirm their motivations. However, statements by these groups suggest differing motives. The Saddam loyalists and remnants of the Ba'ath Party have two primary motives. First, they express opposition to an invading force instituting a new form of government. Although always secular, the government of Iraq has for the past 70 years been based on power obtained through internal political violence rather than democratic institutions. Not only is the outside occupier forcing a change in Iraqi leadership and the form of government, it is changing the rules of power.

Second, in Saddam Hussein's regime, there were many government administrators who served as subject matter experts. They did not necessarily involve themselves in the brutality of the regime, but as career bureaucrats they administered day-to-day government operations. The group also included military and police personnel. At the completion of major military operations, these individuals were removed from their positions because they were identified as Ba'athists. Contrary to the initial policy plan, this created a group of highly trained, unemployed, and angry military and security personnel, as well as former bureaucrats with the logistics knowledge of materials, weapons, personnel, and funds, to support the insurgency.

Apart from the Sunni insurgents affiliated with the former Ba'ath regime, another group of Sunni insurgents seem focused on Islamic ideology. Their motivation varies from group to group. Wahhabi insurgents are primarily driven by religious beliefs that are antagonistic to western freedoms. They want to protect Iraq from what is perceived as western influences and immoralities. Sheikh Harith Sulayman al-Dhari, a Sunni leader, former professor of Islamic Law at Baghdad University and chairman of the Association of Muslim Scholars, is thought to have provided financial and organizational assistance to the religious Sunni insurgency.[41] However, al-Dhari has also condemned the atrocities by other, more violent, insurgent groups.

Shi'a insurgents are also defending their country from outside occupiers. Again two primary motives seem plausible. First, during Ba'ath rule of over 40 years, Shi'a Muslims, who represented over sixty percent of the Iraqi population, were denied a role in government. In fact, Saddam Hussein ordered the execution of many of their leaders to prevent opposition to the regime. Framed

---

[41] http://news.bbc.co.uk/1hi/world/middle_east/3770065.stm.

in the cultural context of political violence and winner take all, removal of the predominantly Sunni regime has not elevated the Shi'a to what they hoped would be their new place in the power structure of Iraq. Indeed, there is a lack of consensus among Shi'a citizens regarding whether they are better off today than before the arrival of U.S. troops.

Second, during the 1970's Iranian clerics attempted to further the Islamic movement by supporting a Shi'a resistance in Iraq. The Iraqi Ba'ath Party crushed this move. Some of the Shi'a leaders were executed and many fled to Iran. These Shi'a are returning from Iran with hopes of driving out the occupiers and establishing an Islamic state in Iraq. They are fighting against the development of a secular government. Grand Ayatollah Ali al-Sistani, a political moderate, is the spiritual leader of the Shi'a Islamic movement and is not directly involved in the insurgency.[42] Early on, Moqtada al Sadr emerged as a figurehead for the Shi'a insurgency. He formed the Mehdi Army to protect Shi'a religious institutions in Najaf and was thought to have a relatively large following of approximately 3000. His participation in the insurgency has moderated of late, and his group has expressed a desire to participate in the political process. Al-Sistani is credited with influencing al-Sadr's decision.

International Jihad warriors have altogether different motivations for launching an insurgency in Iraq. Although they are not necessarily attempting to liberate their own country, it could be argued through a discussion of the concepts of "One Islamic Nation," or "Arab Nationalism," or even "Pan Arabism," that they have a vested interest in liberating a politically fragmented and economically depleted Iraq from outside occupation. Two primary motives seem to drive this group of insurgents. The first is the desire to drive western powers, and particularly the United States, out of Arab lands. The second is to force the United States to abandon its support of Israel with regard to the Israeli-Palestinian conflict. These insurgents are reported by the U.S. government to be led by Abu Musab al-Zarqawi. Zarqawi, a Jordanian, and possibly of Palestinian descent, is an experienced warrior. He previously fought along side Usama bin Laden to expel the Soviets from Afghanistan.

Strategy and Objectives, Again

As previously defined, the Iraq insurgency is a strategy used by several groups with varied interests to liberate Iraq from outside occupation. These groups may act individually or in cooperation with one another, using tactics that are based on the availability of resources. The insurgents do not use conventional weapons or necessarily push for a military victory, but focus on the philosophy

---

[42] Sharon Otterman, "Grand Ayatollah Ali al-Sistani," Middle East Information Center. January 16, 2004. Available at http://middleeastinfo.org/article3861.html.

of the conflict to discredit the occupation and push for public will to resist the occupying force. The insurgents have two effective objectives in this regard: the first is external, and involves the destruction of the will of the occupiers to remain. The second is internal, and involves calling into question the legitimacy of the occupiers and their recommendations for a new government.

Violent tactics have been used to destroy the will of outside occupiers. Initially low levels of violence, approximately 30 to 50 attacks daily, were carried out primarily by Saddam loyalists. These attacks produced an attrition mentality. Military planners counted the attacks, consisting of drive-by shootings, suicide bombings, mortar attacks, and placement of improvised explosive devises to destroy coalition vehicles and personnel, as a means of measuring the progress of post-war stability operations. This is not unlike the use of a body count for tracking progress in the Vietnam Conflict. These tactics are designed to wear down an occupying force, which eventually decides that the political costs are not worth the benefits of remaining. Another example of violence perpetrated to influence political will was the bombing of trains in Madrid, Spain. This tactic successfully influenced the presidential elections in Spain and ultimately the withdrawal of Spanish troops from Iraq.

Although significant, and costly in terms of human life, these random attacks are not as defining as the beheading of civilian contractors. The escalation of violence by the international jihad warriors shocked the Western world and significantly reduced the number of companies willing to send employees to Iraq. Additionally, the brutality of these acts has caused some to question the legitimacy of the occupation and the logic of attempting to build a democracy in Iraq. The strategic purpose of this violence is not to win the war or overcome major weapons systems but to destroy the will of the "enemy" to fight. In this case, it is not directed as much at the will of the armed forces, as U.S. domestic political will and the will of the international coalition.

The second objective of insurgents has been to call into question the legitimacy of the occupiers and their recommended government. The tactical pursuit of this objective has varied greatly depending on the group involved in the implementation. One constant among the groups, however, has been the use of the Arab press to show the horrors of war perpetrated by the occupying force. The photographs of mangled and burned Iraqi bodies are widely shown around the world, with the exception of the United States, where they are available only on Internet links. This information campaign, as a tactic, has been quite effective in discrediting those who claim to be helping Iraqis. Additionally, although small in number, there are citizens in Iraq who remember the British occupation and know that life did not improve significantly after the British departure. To them, the concept of outside occupation and the legitimacy of the resulting government will have to be proven.

The Shi'a insurgents initially attacked the legitimacy of the occupation with political rhetoric and weekly uprisings at the conclusion of Friday prayers. Gradually, the level of violence incorporated in their tactics escalated and culminated with the capture and execution of several military personnel. Moderate Shi'a religious leaders seem to have effectively intervened to quell the violence. These insurgents appear to have modified their tactics. They recently laid down their weapons and expressed an interest in pursuing their rightful place in the emerging political process. As reported by Michael Ware, in his recent article, "The Enemy with Many Faces,"

> Sources inside the insurgency say al-Zarqawi's willingness to sanction terrorist attacks against all civilians has created splits among the various rebel groups. As a result, nationalist insurgent groups are attempting to create their own leadership and forge ties with moderate Islamists. Their goal is to create a political party that can contest and win elections, held after U.S. withdrawal.[43]

One other tactic used to call into question the legitimacy of the new government has been to execute Iraqi citizens who choose to participate in the process of institution building. Although many view this as an intimidation technique, it also signals a weakness of the government, in that it is unable to protect its personnel. The executions have not been limited to government officials, but police officers and security forces of the new Iraqi army as well.

Summary

The post-war policy process was primarily managed by the U.S. Department of Defense. Five policy objectives were announced by DOD, of which two related to security and stability operations, and the other three to more operational concepts of eliminating weapons of mass destruction, destroying terrorist infrastructure and safeguarding Iraq's territorial sovereignty. Implementation of post-war policy was the responsibility of civilian DOD personnel.

The plan relied on certain assumptions: that there would be huge needs for humanitarian assistance, that Iraqis would stick together to run their country, that securing Iraq would be a short-term requirement, and that financing reconstruction efforts would be accomplished through existing allocations, as well as support from the international community.

The post-war realities were that reconstruction efforts were far more challenging than anticipated because the existing infrastructure was in far worse

---

[43] Michael Ware, "The Enemy With Many Faces," *Time*, September 27, 2004.

condition than originally thought. Additionally, the oil production infrastructure was in such a state of disrepair as to prevent production in a capacity that would help finance reconstruction efforts.

Plans for security and stability operations in Iraq did not exist, or were not communicated to the military forces. Chaos ensued as coalition forces struggled to become "the government." As frustration mounted among some Iraqis who anticipated a better way of life without Saddam Hussein, and in others who had been stripped of power and employment, a chaotic situation evolved into an insurgency.

At the conclusion of major conflict, all the necessary conditions were in place for the Iraq insurgency to be effective as a strategy to liberate Iraq from foreign occupation. The culture of political violence, the history of prior occupation and the frustration from unfulfilled promises of a better life offered by coalition forces, set the stage for insurgent leaders to use ideology and discontent to motivate their followers.

The insurgents have used well-reasoned tactics to disrupt the development of new government institutions and call into question the legitimacy of coalition forces. Department of Defense policy objective one, demonstrating to the Iraqi people that the coalition is not there to occupy or exploit their resources, and Department of Defense policy objective five, reconstructing the economic and political systems in hopes that Iraq will enjoy the rule of law and other institutions of democracy, are unachievable in the current environment.

Why did this happen? What went wrong? How did we fail in our assumptions? How did we arrive so unprepared? These are all valid questions, and an analysis of the post-war planning process for Operation Iraqi Freedom is critical to provide an explanation, as well as lessons learned, regarding the policy process for the transition from war to peace.

Given the post–Cold War trend of using the U.S. military in "other than war operations,"[44] it is important to examine the policy process for the new mission. Of particular importance are the institutional differences between the Department of State and the Department of Defense and the workings of the mechanism to synthesize these differences into effective policy, the National Security Council. This researcher examines the Iraq case in a descriptive qualitative analysis that tests two hypotheses:

1. Institutional differences between the Department of State and the Department of Defense in their missions, structures, core values, culture, use of information, and training impeded the development of effective post-war policy.
2. The National Security Council failed to synthesize interagency discourse to support the policy process.

---

[44]Dana Priest, *The Mission*, (New York: W.W. Norton & Company, 2003). See Priest's discussion of "The Rise of the American Military," 41–57.

Criticism of the post-war policy process has also been directed at the "neo-conservative" ideology of certain members of the George W. Bush Administration. Although this may also be a valid observation, it is not a clearly defined argument. Pursuing it would invite methodological concerns with regard to how one might measure ideology and its impact on the decision-making process. Evidence of ideology, as appropriate to the discussion, is included in the description of institutional differences and the bureaucratic decision-making process. It is not isolated as a separate variable.

This chapter has described in detail what this research hopes to explain—the post-war policy process including the results of the policy implementation plan. The next chapter provides a descriptive analysis of the independent variables argued in this research. It begins with a discussion of the existing framework for the national security policy process and outlines the statutory structure of the formal policy process. It examines the changing structure of the national security policy process post–Goldwater-Nichols, the evolution of civil-military affairs and the balance between diplomacy and military instruments of power. The role of the President is discussed, as it may help explain one argument of this research, that the National Security Council failed to synthesize interagency discourse to support the policy process.

Finally, the next chapter describes the institutional frameworks and organizational cultures that key stakeholders, the Department of State and the Department of Defense, bring to the policy process. This research argues that differences in these institutional frameworks and organizational cultures impeded the development of a successful post-war policy in Iraq.

GLOSSARY

AOR	Combatant Commander's Area of Responsibility
CAP	Crisis Action Plan (prepared by combatant commander)
CENTCOM	Central Command
CIA	Central Intelligence Agency
CFLCC	Coalition Forces Land Component Command
CJTF	Coalition Joint Task Force
COM	Chief of Mission
CPA	Coalition Provisional Authority
DOD	United States Department of Defense
DOS	United States Department of State
IIG	Iraqi Interim Government
NDS	National Defense Strategy
NMS	National Military Strategy
NSA	National Security Advisor to the President

NSC　National Security Council
　　　　NSC Principle's Committee:
　　　　Vice-President
　　　　Secretary of Defense
　　　　Secretary of State
NSS　National Security Strategy
ORHA　Office of Reconstruction and Humanitarian Assistance
OIF　Operation Iraqi Freedom
Phase IV　Transition by military commander from war to peace operations
TSC　Theater Security Cooperation
USAID　United States Agency for International Development
WMD　Weapons of Mass Destruction

CHRONOLOGY

1920–1932	British occupation of Iraq
1990s	Plans for Iraq regime change developed by combatant commanders as part of ongoing U.S. military actions in the region
July 2002	Interagency working groups began coordinating post-war policy
October 2002	The Directorate of Special Plans formed at DOD to produce policy options for decision makers
January 20, 2003	President George W. Bush creates the Office of Reconstruction and Humanitarian Assistance (OHRA) within the DOD
February 2003	Post-war stability operations and reconstruction plan is rehearsed at National Defense University
March 20, 2003	President George W. Bush orders the initiation of military action known as Operation Iraqi Freedom
March 23, 2003	Lt. General John Abizaid notes Iraqi resistance from "irregular" Iraqi forces
April 09, 2003	Baghdad falls, looting of Iraq government buildings begins
April 11, 2003	First humanitarian assistance flight arrives in Baghdad
April 22, 2003	Acknowledgment by CENTCOM that security was a problem, that this was not the enemy the U.S. wargamed against and that even though humanitarian assistance was ongoing to provide food, water, and utilities, the military was still in Phase III
May 01, 2003	President Bush announces end of major combat in Iraq

May 10, 2003	Dissolution of Ba'ath Party claimed by General Tommy Franks
May 13, 2003	Ambassador L. Paul Bremer became Civilian Administrator of the Coalition Provisional Authority
May 13, 2003	Lt. General David McKiernan states 150,000 troops not enough to maintain security while conducting ongoing combat operations
May 15, 2003	Testimony by DOD to House Committee on International Relations regarding Iraq post-war policy objectives
May 15, 2003	Admission that the security situation in Baghdad was poor; Saddam's release of criminals blamed
May 16, 2003	Order by Ambassador L. Paul Bremer, to establish the Coalition Provisional Authority
June 12, 2003	Ambassador Bremer announces first part of plan (return of basic services) is completed. Second part will focus on economic activity.
June 18, 2003	Secretary Rumsfeld claims success with humanitarian assistance and security concerns are ongoing
June 30, 2003	Secretary Rumsfeld announces launch of Operation Sidewinder to round up remnants of the Saddam Hussein regime as well as foreign terrorists and common criminals. He refuses to term the current situation an "insurgency" or a "quagmire," stating that would cast the war on terror with a Vietnam analogy
July 13, 2003	Inaugural session of the Iraq Governing Council (members appointed by the Coalition Provisional Authority)
March 08, 2004	Iraq Governing Council and Coalition Provisional Authority sign transitional law (Rule of Law)
June 28, 2004	Coalition Provisional Authority transfers power to Iraqi Interim Government
June 28, 2004	U.S. Department of State takes the lead in Iraq
January 30, 2005	Elections for an Iraq National Assembly

CHAPTER 2: THE POLICY PROCESS: STAKEHOLDERS AND ROLES

Chapter 1 examined the process of policy development for post-war planning in Operation Iraqi Freedom. It provided a description of the policy process, the implementation plan, and the policy outcomes. This chapter sets the stage for analysis of the post-war policy process by providing an examination of the independent variables argued in this research. Graham Allison and Philip

Zelikow's discussion of the governmental politics paradigm in *Essence of Decision* is used as a rough guide to help organize the discussion. Using their original logic, policy decisions are the result of political games that can be organized around the concept of who plays, what they bring to the game, their impact and the rules of the game. The policy process is viewed as a political outcome of interagency activity.[45]

This chapter begins with a contextual overview of the framework for national security policy development, including an examination of the changing structure of the national security policy process after passage of Goldwater-Nichols, the evolution of civil-military relations, and the balance between diplomatic and military instruments of power. This helps to explain the rules of the national security decision-making process.

Continuing, the discussion turns to a description of the institutional differences between two primary stakeholders in the national security policy process, the U.S. Department of State (DOS) and the U.S. Department of Defense (DOD). These differences are critical to one argument of this research, that the institutional differences between those departments impeded development of post-war policy in Iraq. The role of the President is also discussed, as it contributes to an understanding of the policy process within the National Security Council, and may help explain the other argument presented in this research, that the National Security Council failed to synthesize interagency discourse to support the policy process.

The Existing Framework for the National Security Policy Process

The national security policy process has been shaped by several events. Pivotal influences have been the National Security Act of 1947, the Defense Reorganization Act of 1986, (also referred to as the Goldwater-Nichols Act), the end of the Cold War, the terrorist acts of September 11, 2001 and the responsive National Security Strategy of 2002. This section provides an overview of how the existing national security policy framework has been shaped by these events.

The National Security Act and the National Security Council

Authority and accountability for the development of national security policy in general, and post-war planning for Operation Iraqi Freedom specifically, fit within the roles and responsibilities of the National Security Council (NSC). Established by the National Security Act of 1947, the NSC's primary function is

---

[45] Graham Allison and Philip Zelikow, *Essence of Decision: Explaining the Cuban Missile Crisis*, 2nd ed. (New York: Addison-Wesley Educational Publishers, Inc., 1999), 294–313.

to "advise and serve the President in all matters of defense and foreign policy."[46] The statutory members of the NSC are the President, the Vice-President, the Secretary of State and the Secretary of Defense. Some presidential administrations have also included the Secretary of Treasury as a member of the National Security Council. The National Security Advisor serves as the primary administrator of the NSC decision-making process and is the official point of discourse between the Secretary of State and the Secretary of Defense in negotiating foreign and military policy.[47] The NSC Principals Committee is comprised of the statutory members of the NSC, excluding the President. It was formalized to provide a means of resolving issues at the cabinet level, if they did not require presidential approval. Success depends on the ability of these stakeholders to integrate instruments of national power (economic, diplomatic and military) to support the national security strategy.

The relative power of the NSC as a decision-making body, and the National Security Advisor, as honest broker of information and policy preferences, has varied within presidential administrations, but it remains the premiere advisory council on national security matters.[48] The Chairman of the Joint Chiefs of Staff and the Director of Central Intelligence serve as advisors to the NSC and the President.[49] Although structure (how units are arranged) and process (how units interact) are not necessarily the same, this author depicts the structural arrangement of these relationships in Figure C-1.

The national security decision-making process is very similar to the "Stages Approach" to policy development.[50] Stages of the policy process include initial recognition of a problem, placing the problem on the policy agenda, development of policy goals, searching for information to support policy options, selection of an option, policy implementation and evaluation of policy effectiveness.

Ideally, interagency teams within the NSC framework negotiate the national security policy process. Practitioners may be on rotational assignments to the National Security Council from their home organizations within the executive branch, or they may be permanent staff employees of the National Security Council. Either way, they participate in working groups to coordinate the policy process and provide information to decision makers at all levels of the policy process.

In theory, executive branch agencies and departments are represented in any interagency working group if their agency or department would be affected by development or implementation of the subject policy. As noted by Gabriel

---

[46] U.S. Code, Title 50, *National Security Act of 1947*, Section 101.

[47] U.S. Code, Title 50, *National Security Act of 1947*, Section 101.

[48] www.whitehouse.gov/nsc/history.html.

[49] www.whitehouse.gov/nsc/history.html.

[50] Wayne Parsons, *Public Policy*, (Northampton, MA: Edward Elgar Publishing, Inc., 2001) See Parson's synopsis of Carol and Johnson's (1990) discussion of the policy decision-making process. 357–358.

FIGURE C-1 Structure of the National Security Council.

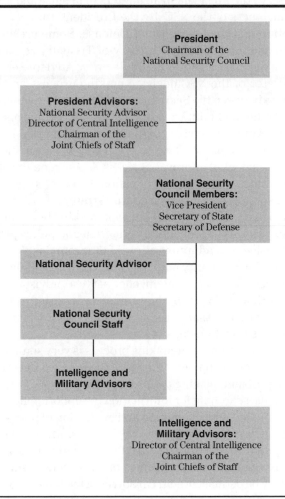

Marcella, an Instructor of Strategy in the Department of National Security and Strategy at the Army War College, in his review, "National Security and the Interagency Process," there is a functional interdependency. The resources, personnel and expertise of each organization must be merged to produce effective policy because no issue can be resolved by one agency acting alone.[51] This discourse is critical to policy development, as the most common reasoning

---

[51] Gabriel Marcella, "National Security and the Interagency Process: Forward Into the 21st Century," *Organizing for National Security*, Carlisle Barracks: Strategic Studies Institute, November, 2000.

flaws are drawing conclusions from inadequate information and overlooking plausible alternatives.

Just as Charles Lindblom theorized that there is no "best answer" to any problem and that the decision-making process is just as important as the decisions made, the interagency working group struggles to form collaborative policy recommendations. Lindblom criticized the basis of the "rational-comprehensive" method of decision making—goals, objectives, criteria, and measurement—or the scientific model, arguing that policy development is a slow deliberative process of reaching agreement or consensus between those involved in and affected by the policy process.[52]

Theoretically, the NSC staff represents both constructs of policy making, in that the staff "works" issues, determining how they should be framed and which ones should be placed on the agenda for higher level consideration. Development of policy options and analysis of policy feasibility are also conducted by the interagency staff at the NSC.

Goldwater-Nichols and the National Security Strategy

The Defense Reorganization Act of 1986, also known as "Goldwater-Nichols," increased accountability in the national security decision-making process by requiring the President to submit an annual report to Congress detailing the National Security Strategy (NSS).[53] The NSS provides an overview of threat analysis and reflects the strategic plan to protect U.S. national interests. Compared with the stages model of policy development, the NSS broadly defines strategic problems, provides international notification of the national security agenda, lists the national security goals and objectives, and in some cases, suggests the implementation process and delivery mix.

Although officially named the Department of Defense Reorganization Act of 1986, the requirement in Goldwater-Nichols for publication of the President's National Security Strategy guides the activities of other executive branch departments and agencies that develop, administer, and/or support foreign policy and defense activities. The effects of Goldwater-Nichols on national policy extend to the Department of State and the Intelligence Community, as they also prepare policy statements and plans to support the President's National Security Strategy.

The Department of State's Strategic Plan presents how the Department and the U.S. Agency for International Development (USAID) will implement U.S. foreign policy and development assistance within the guidance of the National

---

[52] Charles E. Lindblom, "The Science of Muddling Through," *Public Administration Review,* 1959, 78–88.

[53] U.S. Code, Title 10, *The Goldwater-Nichols Department of Defense Reorganization Act of 1986.*

Security Strategy.[54] The Intelligence Community, comprised of both civilian and military intelligence agencies and organizations, uses the guidance of the National Security Strategy to develop intelligence collection requirements and priorities, collect and process information to support national security objectives, and provide intelligence products to decision makers.[55]

The Post–Cold War Evolution of Civil-Military Relations

"Civil-military relations" define the distribution of political power in the national security decision-making process and in the implementation of national security policy. Constitutionally, the President and civilian leadership in the executive branch develop national strategic objectives and the military is funded by Congress to protect national interests and accomplish national defense.

In a top-down formation, national guidance from the National Security Strategy is converted to civilian defense concepts, then to concepts of military operation, then to testing scenarios, and finally to developing the metrics to determine size and availability of force constructs. The Department of Defense publishes the National Defense Strategy to establish the objectives that guide national defense activities and provide direction for the National Military Strategy. Leaving the civilian arena, the Chairman of the Joint Chiefs of Staff publishes the National Military Strategy detailing the strategic direction with which the Armed Forces will accomplish national defense.

Theater Security Cooperation (TSC) plans are developed by Combatant Commanders to sustain engagement with allies, friendly nations and potential coalition partners and "support the U.S. defense strategy, advance regional defense policy goals, and enable wartime operations" within their respective Areas of Responsibility (AOR's).[56] The Goldwater-Nichols Act of 1986 substantially increased the authority and financial resources of Combatant Commanders in their AOR's. In keeping with the commander's responsibility to organize, train and equip his forces, financial resources are provided to meet these goals.

Theater Security Cooperation activities include multinational military exercises, training and education events; facilitation of national security programs, humanitarian and civic assistance; arms control and treaty monitoring activities; as well as senior official visits that publicly acknowledge the cooperative

---

[54] U.S. Department of State, *FY 2004–2009 Department of State and USAID Strategic Plan,* August 20, 2003.

[55] http://www.intelligence.gov/1-relationships.shtml.

[56] Chairman of the Joint Chiefs of Staff, "Theater Security Cooperation Planning," Draft, Joint Publication 5-0, Doctrine for Planning Joint Operations, December, 2002.

relationship.[57] The funding of these activities and one on one contact with international leaders in a commander's AOR raised the profile of the military and significantly reduced the influence of the Ambassador and the effectiveness of the Department of State in conducting foreign policy. That the military commanders were now tasked with developing engagement plans to sustain support for U.S. policy abroad further blurred the demarcation of roles and responsibilities between the two executive entities.

A draft copy of the joint publication on Theater Security Cooperation Planning, released in December 2002, included the objective to "shift emphasis from broad-based theater engagement to a more focused program of bilateral and multilateral cooperation that advances U.S. strategic interests" under control of the Secretary of Defense.[58] This shift is a natural outgrowth of the increased responsibility and authority given to military commanders in their AOR's by the Goldwater-Nichols Act of 1986.

The post–Cold War era has seen a transition from a military organized, trained and equipped to fight a traditional enemy to one that must also be prepared to conduct "military operations other than war." In this new venue, the military has come face to face with the political realities of domestic politics and international affairs. As discussed above, even though the Department of State is the primary actor in the conduct of diplomacy, the military Combatant Commander is now active in what previously would be considered diplomatic missions.

September 11, 2001, and the National Security Strategy of 2002

The National Security Strategy of the United States of America, published in 2002 by the George W. Bush Administration, set the following national security policy objectives:

- Champion aspirations for human dignity
- Strengthen alliances to defeat global terrorism and work to prevent attacks against us and our friends
- Work with others to defuse regional conflicts
- Prevent our enemies from threatening us, our allies, and our friends with weapons of mass destruction
- Ignite a new era of economic growth through free markets and free trade
- Expand the circle of development by opening societies and building the infrastructure of democracy

---

[57] Chairman of the Joint Chiefs of Staff, "Theater Security Cooperation Planning," Draft, Joint Publication 5-0, Doctrine for Planning Joint Operations, December, 2002.

[58] Chairman of the Joint Chiefs of Staff, "Theater Security Cooperation Planning," Draft, Joint Publication 5-0, Doctrine for Planning Joint Operations, December, 2002.

- Develop agendas for cooperative action with the other main centers of global power
- Transform America's national security institutions to meet the challenges and opportunities of the twenty-first century[59]

In the current context, the Department of State and the Department of Defense supporting a global war on terror, the concept of "statecraft" is less defined. This may be because international relations theories and diplomatic practice are usually built within the context of nation states and instruments of power, while current security and defense concepts are built within the context of "threats," many of which are now transnational. Nonetheless, the mission has become less distinct.

"Statecraft" traditionally held that the United States used three instruments of power in the conduct of foreign policy: economic instruments of power, diplomatic instruments of power and military instruments of power. The Goldwater-Nichols Act ceded to military commanders additional funding, responsibility, and authority for the conduct of U.S. policy in their areas of responsibility. This began the blurring of authorities between the Departments of State and Defense with regard to the use of instruments of power. The post-September 11, 2001 environment of a global war on terror increased the confusion. Traditional mechanisms of policy, use of incentives, diplomatic discussions and coercion, to gain cooperation and support of nation states, remain effective. However, these policy mechanisms are not as applicable to non-state actors. It is increasingly difficult to determine how best to formulate policy in the context of a war against a tactic, rather than a nation state.

On July 10, 2003 the National Security Council issued a letter of instruction from President Bush to the Department of State's Chiefs of Mission (COM) and all other departments and agencies concerned to clarify several issues of concern. First, the COM was instructed that he held full responsibility for the coordination, supervision, and protection of all Department of Defense personnel on official duty in country, unless the personnel were otherwise assigned to a military commander. The COM was also instructed that differences that could not be resolved in the field should be reported to the Secretary of State and the Secretary of Defense for mediation. Second, the official tasking for the Chiefs of Mission was clarified as follows:

- Waging a relentless global war against terrorism, to defeat those who seek to harm us and our friends;
- Overcoming the faceless enemies of human dignity, including disease, starvation, and poverty; and
- Assisting American citizens, institutions, and businesses as they pursue their charitable and commercial interests.[60]

---

[59] The White House, *The National Security Strategy of 2002*, September 17, 2002.
[60] U.S. Department of State, "Department Notice," July 10, 2003.

Although this communiqué was issued to clarify roles and responsibilities of civilian agencies, it tasked the Department of State with waging a global war on terror; a tasking that traditionally is a military or Department of Defense mission.

One year later, on June 28, 2004 the Department of State took the lead in managing and representing U.S. interests to a sovereign Iraqi government. The Department of Defense was to continue to support a sizable force in Iraq. An Interagency Transition Planning Team, headed by Ambassador Frank Ricciardone and General Mick Kicklighter planned for how the two agencies would work together, including how their roles, missions, resources, responsibilities, and authorities would support each other.[61]

Institutional Differences Between DOS and DOD

Students of military strategy and military practitioners have long discussed the institutional and cultural differences between the Department of State and the Department of Defense. The context of these discussions generally focused on the communication gap between the two organizations and how the interagency process might be improved. The effect of institutional differences on the policy process has not received much attention in the literature.[62] Particularly in an environment in which the President clarified the role of the Chief of Mission in such a way that the Department of State and the Department of Defense share the mission to wage a global war on terror, it is important to explore the possibility that these institutional differences, once thought to strengthen the collaborative process, actually impede the development of cogent policy.

The Department of State and Department of Defense are both functionally and structurally differentiated. The organizations look different. They process information differently. They have different cultures and different core values. Until recently, they have had different missions. These differences lead to differences in the manner in which they address problem definition, agenda setting, and the use of information. These differences remain even though their missions are being redefined.

---

[61] Richard L. Armitage, Prepared Statement before the Senate Committee on Foreign Relations, May 18, 2004.

[62] Douglas A. Hartwick, "The Culture at State, the Services, and Military Operations: Bridging the Communication Gap," 1994. This student at National Defense University suggested that U.S. experiences in Panama, Grenada and Somalia demonstrate a lack of attention to civilian-military coordination until operations are nearly underway. He does not necessarily attribute this to institutional differences. Rickey Rife, author of "Defense is from Mars, State is from Venus," a research paper prepared at the Army War College, Carlisle Barracks, in 1998, provided a brief account of operational efforts in Bosnia to illustrate the need for better interagency coordination at the operational level. The primary focus of his paper was the difference in Myers Briggs "types" between the two departments.

Functional and Structural Differences

Both the Department of State and the Department of Defense develop policies in support of the United States national security objectives. The similarities end there. The Department of Defense mission is to provide military forces needed to deter war and protect the security of the United States. The Secretary of Defense is responsible for the development and execution of general defense policy.[63] The Department of Defense functions in accordance with military doctrine. This doctrine assumes a Clausewitzian "Theory of War," in that war is a means of carrying out the policy of the nation by imposing its will on others.

On the other hand, the Department of State functions to support national security objectives by building relationships with other nation states through sustained engagement. Keys to engagement are communication, understanding of other countries' cultures and interests, and immersion of State Department personnel in foreign countries. The stark difference in functions is really that of administration of policy by coercion and administration of policy by persuasion.

An overview of the structural differences of these departments illustrates these functional differences. Note the organizational charts provided in Figures C-2 and C-3.

As evident by the organizational charts, the departments are structured to reflect their functional missions. The structure of the Department of Defense is very hierarchical, with well-defined lines of authority and accountability. It is designed to provide efficiency in the movement of large groups of people and equipment around the world for the support of national defense. The Department of State is organized conceptually around issues of engagement, those of political affairs, economic affairs, arms control and international security, public affairs, and global affairs.

One criticism of the Department of State is that its structure prevents other agencies and departments from establishing a single point of contact to work interagency issues. For example, if someone at the Department of Justice wished to talk with someone at the Department of State regarding the use of African refugees to transport narcotics and procure weapons in the global war on terror, it would be unclear to the layman where to start. The possibilities might include African Affairs, Arms Control and International Security Affairs, or Global Affairs.

Perhaps the most critical difference between the two departments, with regard to national security policy, is that they do not necessarily have a shared "end state." An end state is the thread of continuity that ties strategic objectives

---

[63] Department of Defense Directive 5100.1. Originally promulgated by the National Security Act of 1947, it has been modified several times to accommodate changing legislation regarding the roles of the Department of Defense.

FIGURE C-2 Organizational structure of the U.S. Department of State.

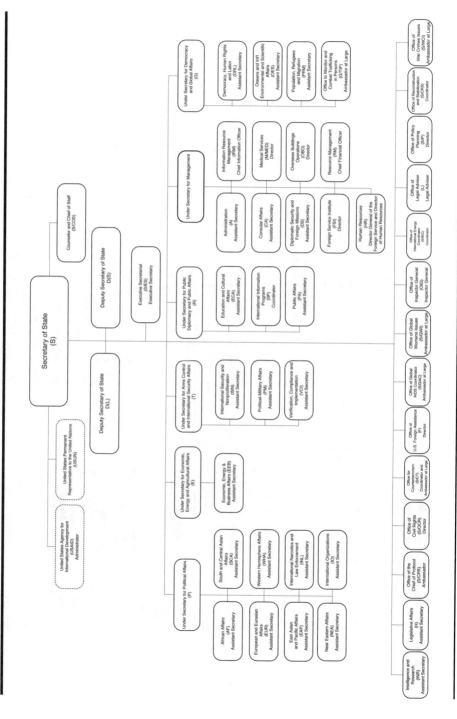
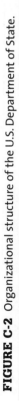

FIGURE C-3 Organizational structure of the U.S. Department of Defense.

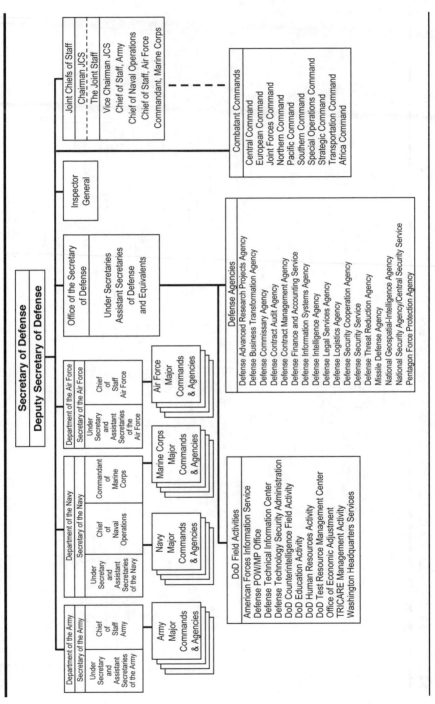

to the operational and tactical levels of administration. The end state is simply the required conditions that achieve the strategic objectives. In terms of military definitions, it is a set of conditions that when met, indicate the situation has been stabilized to allow for transition from war to peace. The process of working backward, known in the political science public policy literature as "Backward Mapping," is conceptually known in military planning as effects-based operations. This type of planning first requires a clear definition of the end state and stated policy objectives. Next, it is important to determine what successful achievement of these objectives would look like. This allows achievement of objectives to be measured or determined. Then, evaluation of alternatives provides a means of determining the best way to reach the end state, possibly choosing between coercion and diplomacy. Finally, planning includes an assessment of what resources are required to accomplish the mission. Although "effects-based" planning is considered a revolutionary concept in military affairs, it is not. Clausewitz stated, "The first, the supreme, the most far-reaching act of judgment that the statesman and commander have to make is to establish...the kind of war on which they are embarking." [64]

The Iraq post-war policy objectives included a mix of strategic and operational objectives, culminating in the reconstruction of economic and political systems that placed Iraq on a path to prosperity and freedom.[65] This is the most transparent definition of an end state available in public documents. The extent of collaboration in development of these objectives is unclear. Additionally, the Department of Defense was given the lead for policy implementation, even though the identified end state clearly falls within the traditional roles and responsibilities of the Department of State.

The Importance of Bureaucratic Culture

Organizational culture influences the decision-making process through development of standard operating procedures that are risk adverse and resistant to change, development of internalities that affect which information is valued, how it is evaluated, and how it is used in the decision-making process, and development of an emotional tie to the decision-making process and outcomes within the organization. Organizations influence political behavior and policy outcomes.

Political scientist James Q. Wilson theorized that organizations have a complex pattern of interaction or culture. As such, complex organizations have

---

[64] Carl von Clausewitz, *On War*, trans. Michael Howard and Peter Parent (Princeton, NJ: Princeton University Press, 1989), 88.

[65] Douglas J. Feith, Under Secretary of Defense for Policy, Testimony before the Committee on International Relations, U.S. House of Representatives, May 15, 2003.

developed standard operating procedures with which they respond to outside stimuli.[66] In other words, organizational culture shapes behavior. Sociologist Peter Berger, in his discussion of the social construction of reality, notes that the development of operating procedures occurs slowly over time. Based on normative information, these procedures are in keeping with habit, and people simply act in a manner that is familiar to them because alternatives do not seem feasible.[67]

In their book, *Essence of Decision: Explaining the Cuban Missile Crisis*, Graham Allison and Philip Zelikow explained the crisis decision-making process could be viewed through three "conceptual lenses," or theoretical paradigms: the rational actor approach to decision making, the organizational-behavior model of decision making and the governmental politics model of decision making.[68] This second edition publication offers updated theoretical arguments and integration of recently declassified material that was not available when Graham Allison published the first edition in 1971. In 1969, Allison published a preliminary article in which he argued that the lens of the decision maker affects what information is evaluated, what information is discarded, what the information means, and the conclusions of the decision maker. In this article, Allison theorized that alternative frames of reference produce different models for decision making and that different models produce different outcomes, even though all models initially had access to the same information.[69]

Briefly, the rational actor lens assumes that the state acts in its best interest, based on the information available to decision makers at the time of the decision. The organizational-behavior model assumes individual actors in the decision-making process have biases and preferences in policy development based on their affiliation with particular bureaucratic organizations. This model assumes that the bureaucratic decision-making process develops policy with little regard for interests, other than those internal to the organization, such as standard operating procedures and avoidance of risk. This parallels the work of Wilson, in which he theorizes large, complex bureaucratic cultures with standard operating procedures are slow to adapt to a changing environment.[70]

The impact of organizational behavior is sometimes referred to as "where you stand is determined by where you sit." An excellent example of this concept is the difference between Colin Powell the military leader, who advised against

---

[66] James Q. Wilson, *Bureaucracy: What Government Agencies Do and Why They Do It* (New York: Basic Books, 1989), 91–93.

[67] Peter L. Berger and Thomas Luckman, *The Social Construction of Reality: A Treatise in the Sociology of Knowledge* (New York, NY: Anchor Books, 1966), 54.

[68] Graham Allison and Philip Zelikow, *Essence of Decision: Explaining the Cuban Missile Crisis*, 2nd ed. (New York: Addison-Wesley Educational Publishers, Inc., 1999), 391.

[69] Graham Allison, "Conceptual Models and the Cuban Missile Crisis," American Political Science Review, Vol. 63, No.3, 689–718.

[70] James Q. Wilson, *Bureaucracy: What Government Agencies Do and Why They Do It* (New York: Basic Books, 1989), 91–93.

extended military operations without a clear end state, and Colin Powell the Secretary of State, who advocates the use of civilian and military personnel to build security and democratic institutions in post-war Iraq.

Allison and Zelikow concluded that during the Cuban Missile Crisis, each lens or model of decision making contributed something to the policy process, but that it was the governmental politics lens that best explained the impact of competing views and preferences by key decision makers in the policy development process.[71]

The vast changes in the national security decision-making process since the 1960's, as explained earlier in this chapter, limit the usefulness of the Allison and Zelikow models to explain the current decision-making process for post-war reconstruction and stability operations. However, individually, their discussion of the organizational-behavior model of decision making and their bureaucratic politics model is useful to remind us that bureaucratic organizations function with their own internal cultures (norms, values, missions and operating procedures) and that conflict between these cultures in the form of bureaucratic politics has the ability to impede the national decision-making process.

Organizational culture and standard operating procedures make it easier for bureaucracies to operate on a day to day basis. However, as noted by Richard Scott, another organizational theorist, institutionalized behaviors and thought processes sometimes inhibit innovation. He suggested that bureaucrats become so entrenched in bureaucratic norms and expectations that they are unable to respond to new challenges that require bureaucratic change.[72] This is consistent with Wilson's view that when confronted with a new situation, organizations may respond in traditional ways. This protectionist mentality may not only be counterproductive to the mission, but can create bureaucratic conflict when more than one organization is involved in a struggle to control the decision-making process.[73]

In addition to the tendency of bureaucracies to develop standard operating procedures based on internal culture and organizational environment, Herbert Simon theorized that once institutionalized, the values associated with decision making lead toward discovery of "the one best decision" and there is an emotional tie between the organization and that decision.[74] So we must ask, what are the culture and standard operating procedures of the Department of State and the Department of Defense? Do their institutional cultures and core values lead each to discover "the one best decision?" If so, are their respective decisions compatible? Do they support or impede the national policy process?

---

[71] Graham Allison and Philip Zelikow, *Essence of Decision: Explaining the Cuban Missile Crisis*, 2nd ed. (New York: Addison-Wesley Educational Publishers, Inc., 1999), 392–397.

[72] Richard Scott, *Institutions and Organizations* (Thousand Oaks: Sage Publications, 2001), 57–58.

[73] James Q. Wilson, *Bureaucracy: What Government Agencies Do and Why They Do It* (New York, NY: Basic Books, 1991), 93.

[74] Herbert A. Simon, "The Proverbs of Administration," *Public Administration Review*, Vol. 19, 1946, 79–88.

Institutional Differences — Culture and Core Values

First perhaps it is best to explore what the Department of State and Department of Defense have in common. David Sorenson, Professor of International Security Studies at the Air War College, notes that bureaucracies tend to reinforce rivalries with competing organizations. Bureaucracies also tend to minimize risk and uncertainty, sometimes leading to traditional rather than innovative responses to problem solving. Bureaucracies also tend to draw heavily from lessons learned in order to make policy recommendations, and finally, bureaucracies tend to be output oriented, rather than outcome oriented.[75] If this were true, we would expect to find conflict between these departments and the tendency for them to become entrenched in their own arguments and use of historical lessons to illustrate their positions.

The differences between the Department of State and the Department of Defense, however, go far beyond the tendencies of bureaucratic institutions to engage in conflicts of ideas. There is a tremendous difference in culture and core values. Hartwick, in 1994 noted the communication gap between these departments. Hartwick's paper, prepared at National Defense University, seemed an effort to "understand" the different perspective that the Department of State brings to military operations.

Hartwick notes four critical differences between institutions that are reflected in their missions and personnel. First, he observes that state department personnel tend to frame issues and define problems in very broad terms. This, he attributes, is done to maintain maximum flexibility in problem solving. The military, meanwhile, is not comfortable with ambiguity, preferring instead to frame issues through use of doctrine that simplifies the decision-making process.[76]

Second, Hartwick states that military professionals participate in detailed planning, as evidenced by preparation of the National Defense Strategy, followed by the National Military Strategy, followed by development of Theater Security Cooperation Plans. It is important to note that for almost any future military action, there is an existing plan for military engagement sitting on the shelf, ready to be reviewed and altered to meet the current need. Hartwick characterizes state department personnel as thinkers, rather than planners. The tendency of state department personnel is to think of the possible outcomes, while the military plans from the perspective of the most likely outcome.

A third and related difference is the tendency of state department personnel to receive "on the job training" by working issues, rather than participating in training as part of officer development. Conceptually, state department

---

[75] David Sorenson, Lecture at Air War College, August 2, 2004.

[76] Douglas A. Hartwick, "The Culture at State, the Services, and Military Operations: Bridging the Communication Gap," National Defense University Paper, April, 1994.

personnel find it a waste of time to train for an event that might not occur. Marianne Goodwin, Deputy Director of the Political Training Division of the Department of State Foreign Service Institute, recently acknowledged state department training usually occurs "just in time."[77] On the other hand, the military values training and officer development as a means of grooming leaders to be prepared for almost any eventuality or contingency plan.

A fourth critical cultural difference between the Departments of State and Defense is the value placed on individual performance. The State Department values and rewards analytical thinking and writing ability, both individualized tasks. The Defense Department values team work, leadership, and the command structure.

There are few natural points of discourse or exchange between the two Departments, structurally or functionally, and the lack of experience that both have with the other complicates the sharing of information and the ability to find the "right" person to answer even a simple question. It is possible for a request for information from the Department of Defense to the Department of State to digress to a request for a supervisor, only to find there is not a traditional supervisory relationship for a particular piece of analysis. In such cases, the frustration of Department of Defense personnel toward the "lack of command structure" at Department of State impedes the working relationship. It does not appear that either recognizes they are not good or bad, efficient or inefficient, they are different and they have few shared experiences.

Additional differences between the two organizations are noted in the literature as follows: the Department of Defense values competence, efficiency, and achievement. DOD personnel see themselves as problem solvers, ready to carry out a mission. The Department of State values competence, intellectual ability and a fluid approach that includes the integration of facts to form an understanding of the situation.

The decision-making processes of the two departments reflect these differences. The Department of Defense uses a linear, formal, problem-solving process that finds the "approved solution," while the Department of State views decision making as the opportunity to explore many possible solutions, considering all angles in an informal problem-solving process. Rife notes antagonism between these departments which he terms "polar opposites in character, in their approach to problem solving, and in worldview."[78]

It is also important to recognize that these institutional differences affect how information is solicited and used by these departments. The tendency of Department of State personnel to explore many possible solutions leads them

---

[77] Discussion at Air War College, December 13, 2004.

[78] Rickey Rife, "Defense is from Mars, State is from Venus," a research paper prepared at the Army War College, Carlisle Barracks, in 1998.

to seek much larger volumes of contextual information to integrate into the decision-making process. On the other hand, the selection of military strategy is "determined by the interaction of rational calculation, motivational biases, especially those due to institutional interests, and the cognitive and organizational need for doctrinal simplification."[79] This leads to discrepant information being ignored and new problems not being thoroughly understood, as in a struggle for cognitive consistency, information that does not fit preexisting perceptions or doctrine is rejected.[80]

Summary of Differences

The Department of State and Department of Defense are structurally and functionally different. The Department of State focuses on diplomacy and is structured around issues of engagement. The Department of Defense is structured in a manner to efficiently move personnel and equipment around the world. Culturally, these departments hold different core values and preferences as depicted in Table C-1.

They have different approaches to problem definition, agenda setting, and their use of information. Although it might be said the Departments of State and Defense do not share a mutual "end state" for strategic objectives, it might also be argued that the Department of State does not pursue an end state, but rather a continuation or evolution of relationships. The differences in their approach to policy development may be summarized as a conflict between the use of an inductive versus a deductive approach to problem solving. These differences are depicted in Table C-2.

The Duty of NSC to Arbitrate

There are two types of conflict inherent in the bureaucratic decision-making process. The first is internal conflict or discourse between members of an organization as they promote their agendas in the decision-making process. A second type of conflict arises from bureaucratic roles and barriers between organizations. It is the second type of conflict that is critical to this discussion.

In 1988, political scientist Deil S. Wright attempted to explain the role of intergovernmental relations in the decision-making process. Theorizing that conflict arises as dual organizations attempt to identify the proper sphere or jurisdiction of responsibilities, he also noted that antagonism is the natural

---

[79] Jack Snyder, "Military Bias and Offensive Strategy," *The Ideology of the Offensive: Military Decision Making and the Disasters of 1914* (Cornell Studies in Security Affairs, 1984), 26.

[80] Jack Snyder, "Military Bias and Offensive Strategy," *The Ideology of the Offensive: Military Decision Making and the Disasters of 1914* (Cornell Studies in Security Affairs, 1984), 218–219.

TABLE C-1 Organizational Differences of the Departments of State and Defense

	Department of State	Department of Defense
Mission	Foreign Diplomacy and Engagement	Defense of Homeland and Vital National Interests
Core Values	Intellect and Individual Strengths	Efficiency, Leadership and Teamwork
Structure	Functional Around Issues of Engagement	Span of Control—Bureaucratic Authority and Accountability
Culture	Think and Analyze	Plan and Operationalize
Use of Information	Inductive—From Concrete to General—Evolving	Deductive—From General to Concrete—Ending
Training	On the Job or Just in Time	Ongoing—Grooming of Leaders

result of this struggle. In this regard, it is not the decision about what is the best alternative that is at issue. The conflict revolves around the determination of who will control the decision-making process.[81]

James Q. Wilson's writings also echo that concept by noting that when confronted with a new situation, organizations may respond in traditional ways, even if less effective. This protectionist mentality may not only be counterproductive to the mission but can create bureaucratic conflict when more than one organization is involved in a struggle to control the decision-making process.[82] A former Department of Defense policy practitioner, Chris Jefferies, described bureaucratic politics within the national security decision-making process as follows:

> ... it is finally the process by which these individuals and groups exercise their influence in competition with other individuals and groups that determines the extent of their influence and thus, the policy itself. That process is bureaucratic politics.[83]

Framed in this manner, it is not surprising that bureaucratic conflicts occurred between the Department of Defense and the Department of State in the post-war planning process for Operation Iraqi Freedom.

---

[81] Deil S. Wright, *Understanding Intergovernmental Relations*, 3rd Edition (Belmont, CA: Brooks/Cole, 1988), excerpts reprinted in *Classics of Public Administration*, Jay M. Shafritz and Albert C. Hyde, editors (Orlando, FL: Harcourt Brace & Company, 1997), 578–594.

[82] James Q. Wilson, *Bureaucracy: What Government Agencies Do and Why They Do It* (New York: Basic Books, 1989), 93.

[83] Chris Jefferies, "Bureaucratic Politics in the Department of Defense: A Practitioner's Perspective." *Bureaucratic Politics and National Security*, Edited by David C. Lozak and James M. Keagle (Bolder, CO: Lynne Rienner, 1988), 109.

TABLE C-2 Differences in Approach to the Policy Process

	Department of State	Department of Defense
Approaches to the Policy Process	Diplomacy	Coercion
Problem Definition	Evolutionary and Flexible	Concrete and Doctrine Driven
Agenda Setting	Subject to Change Based on New Information	Part of the Planning Process to Organize, Train and Equip for Troop Deployment
Desired Goal/End State	Infinite—Always More to be Done	Completion of Strategic Objectives
	Changes as New Information and Possibilities Arise	The Beginning Point for Operational Planning
Policy Option Development	Fluid—Based on International Relationships	Based on Military Doctrine
	Assumes Sustained Engagement	Assumes Imposition of U.S. Will on Others and Departure
Evaluation Criteria	Effectiveness, Equity, Efficiency	Efficiency, Effectiveness, Equity
Implementation	Persuasion	Decisive Victory

The National Security Act of 1947 provided a mechanism, the National Security Council, to resolve conflicts prior to presidential action. The National Security Council is the primary point of discourse between the Secretary of State and the Secretary of Defense in negotiation of foreign and military policy. The job of the National Security Advisor (NSA) is to manage competing interests between members of the National Security Council and present a cogent set of alternatives to the President. While the Secretary of State's mission is diplomacy, the Secretary of Defense works to coerce compliance or wage war when diplomatic means are not achieving national objectives.

The Principals Committee of the National Security Council (Vice President, Secretary of State, and Secretary of Defense) defined the post-9/11 reality with regard to problem definition and national security goals and objectives. The military put forth goals to strengthen the deterrence and response systems to protect Americans at home and abroad. They planned to "build defenses beyond challenge" and participate in multilateral coalitions of convenience in defense planning and strategy.[84] The State Department put forth goals of strengthening America's image abroad and developing a strong relationship with coalitions of the willing, resulting in a foreign policy of integration. The objective of the

---

[84] The White House, "The National Security Strategy of the United States," 2002.

State Department was to lock in support of democratic values and opposition to terrorism by major powers, while building policies and institutions that locked them in even more. As noted by Deputy Secretary of State Hass, "The United States cannot compel others to become more democratic."[85]

The Iraq post-war policy objectives, announced by the Under Secretary of Defense Policy in February, and later in May 2003, included a mixture of strategic and operational objectives.[86] As noted in Table C-3, these defense policy objectives did not fall within the traditional roles of the Department of Defense. The decision to place the Office of Reconstruction and Humanitarian Assistance (ORHA) within the Department of Defense line of authority and span of control quickly became problematic to the policy implementation process. The Department of Defense did not appear to be trained or equipped to carry out this nontraditional role.

This research in part argues that the National Security Council did not effectively arbitrate the functional and cultural differences between these executive entities and that there was not synthesis of interagency discourse to support the policy process. One of the best indicators of this lack of synthesis is the all or nothing approach to policy implementation. As the Department of Defense assumed responsibility for the entire mission, the implementation of policy objectives was destined to fail. Table C-3 below shows the traditional roles that would be played in the implementation of national policy objectives by the Departments of State and Defense.

The Role of the President to Direct

Terry Moe explains that a contractual relationship exists between policy decision makers and public administrators, as well as decision makers and the public. He theorizes that citizens depend on the government to complete the tasks of making decisions, enacting laws, and administering programs for the "public good." The people elect the President, who appoints executive administrators. They also elect Congress, which provides executive oversight by its ability to control funding. There is a contractual expectation that both branches of government will act in the best interest of the country.[87]

Carl Friedrich theorized that as government broadened its scope of service and responsibility, it became increasingly difficult to secure bureaucratic accountability. Seen as a continuous process, according to Friedrich, public

---

[85] Richard N. Hass, "Defining U.S. Foreign Policy in a Post–Cold War World," U.S. Department of State, 2002.

[86] Douglas Feith, Under Secretary of Defense for Policy, Testimony before the Committee on International Relations, U.S. House of Representatives, May 15, 2003.

[87] Terry M. Moe, "The New Economics of Organization," *American Journal of Political Science*, Vol. 28 (1984), 771–772.

TABLE C-3 Traditional Departmental Roles in Policy Implementation

Traditional Roles in Policy Implementation	Department of State	Department of Defense
Policy Objectives of Department of Defense		
1. Continue to demonstrate to the Iraqi people and the world that the United States and its coalition partners aspire to liberate the Iraqis and not to occupy or control them or their economic resources.	Persuasion Diplomacy	N/A
2. Eliminate Iraq's chemical and biological weapons, its nuclear program, the related delivery systems, and the related research and production facilities.	N/A	Coercion Decisive Victory
3. Eliminate Iraq's terrorist infrastructure. A key element of U.S. strategy in the global war on terrorism is exploiting the information about terrorist networks that the coalition acquires through our military and law enforcement actions.	N/A	Coercion Decisive Victory
4. Safeguard Iraq's territorial unity.	Diplomacy	Coercion
5. Reconstruct the economic and political systems, putting Iraq on a path to become a prosperous and free country. The U.S. and its coalition partners share with many Iraqis the hope that their country will enjoy the rule of law and other institutions of democracy under a broad-based government that represents the various parts of Iraqi society.	Diplomacy	N/A

policy is inseparable from execution. He notes, policies "are decisions about what to do or not to do in given situations."[88] Although the legislative branch oversees policy development to ensure a reflection of the will of the people, it is becoming more an administrative function. He notes, "… even the most far-reaching of public policies are often formed by executive agencies under the pressure of circumstances and are merely legalized by subsequent legislation."[89]

With regard to military planning, *The Federalist Papers* demonstrate that the framers of the U.S. Constitution worked diligently to determine the appropriate role of the President and Congress in the conduct of war and foreign policy. James Madison advocated a coordination, or mix, of powers between the two branches of government, with a provision for the President to act alone in

---

[88] Carl Friedrich, "Public Policy and the Nature of Administrative Responsibility," in *Public Policy*, Carl J. Friedrich (ed.), Cambridge, MA: Harvard University Press, 1940, 3–8.

[89] Carl Friedrich, "Public Policy and the Nature of Administrative Responsibility," in *Public Policy*, Carl J. Friedrich (ed.), Cambridge, MA: Harvard University Press, 1940, 15.

a state of emergency, if the Congress was not in session.[90] The framers agreed that Congress would maintain control over "the purse," or the funding of functions of foreign policy and defense. The President would have the power to conduct war and diplomacy but not commit the nation to either. Historically, the courts have upheld these authorities and the mix of powers between the executive and legislative branches of government.

The framers clearly drew the line between the branches of government to prevent abuse of executive power. This arrangement was not the most efficient means of decision making, but the process forced deliberation, discourse, and consensus building, all basic tenants of democracy. As a result of Goldwater-Nichols, the centralization of power from the President to the Secretary of Defense, to the Combatant Commander, has placed the military clearly at the disposal of the President and diminished congressional oversight of military action.[91] The required National Security Strategy is a representation of the President's role to direct the national security policy process. It guides not only the national military strategy, but also the conduct of public diplomacy.

Summary

Chapter 1 examined the policy development process for post-war operations in Operation Iraqi Freedom. This chapter has provided contextual information on the national security decision-making process and described the two independent variables of this research: institutional differences between two primary stakeholders in the national security process, the U.S. Department of State and the U.S. Department of Defense, and the role and responsibility of the National Security Council to synthesize interagency discourse in the national security policy process. It has also explained several of the organizing concepts by which we can examine post-war policy: who plays, what they bring, and the rules of the game.

Chapter 3 will provide a brief overview of the framework for analysis of the post-war policy process. It discusses the process of searching for meaning by tracing the policy process and explains how it might be possible to compare the policy process as it is statutorily defined to the actual policy process for post-war planning in Operation Iraqi Freedom. It provides a structure for the systematic application of differences between the institutional frameworks of the Department of State and the Department of Defense to the post-war policy process. It will focus on the following questions: What evidence exists to determine if institutional differences between the Department of State and the Department of Defense impeded the post-war policy process for Operation Iraqi Freedom? What

---

[90] James Madison, The Federalist Papers, as accessed on December 15, 2004. Available at: http://www.federalistpapers.com.
[91] Dana Priest, *The Mission* (New York: W.W. Norton & Company, Inc., 2003), 92–98.

evidence exists to determine if the National Security Council failed to synthesis interagency discourse to support the policy process? How will these qualitative variables be measured and analyzed? Why is the Iraq case useful for analysis?

CHAPTER 3: METHODOLOGY

The content of research questions and their theoretical propositions should have a bearing on the selection of research methods. This research is a qualitative analysis of the policy process for reconstruction and stability operations in Iraq at the conclusion of Operation Iraqi Freedom. As such, the policy process is the unit of analysis. It is studied through an archival review of the literature regarding the post-war policy process. This researcher examines the Iraq case in an explanatory analysis to determine how institutional differences between the Departments of State and Defense may have shaped the policy development process and how these executive departments and the National Security Council interacted to result in the post-war policy outcome for Operation Iraqi Freedom.

Two hypotheses are tested:

1. Institutional differences between the Department of State and the Department of Defense in their missions, core values, structures, culture, use of information, and training impeded the development of effective post-war policy.
2. The National Security Council failed to adequately synthesize interagency discourse to support the policy process.

This chapter provides a brief description of the framework for analysis of the post-war policy process. It proposes how we are able to systematically apply the institutional differences between the Departments of State and Defense to the post-war policy process. It then discusses how we might compare the policy process as it is statutorily defined, including the role of the National Security Council to arbitrate differences, to the actual policy process for post-war planning in Operation Iraqi Freedom. This chapter also discusses the availability of evidence with which to argue the two hypotheses listed above and includes a discussion of why the post-war policy process in Iraq is a useful case for analysis.

Framework for Analysis

The framework for analysis of the interagency post-war policy process is discussed below. This framework explains why qualitative analysis utilizing process tracing is the preferred methodology for this case study research.

Chapter 1 reported the post-war policy process, its implementation and outcomes. Chapter 2 examined the organizing concepts (independent variables) for study of the policy process. A discussion of the national security decision-making process described the statutory rules of the game and the decision-making hierarchy. It provided information about the interaction channels for the policy process.

Chapter 2 also depicted institutional differences of stakeholders, as well as their differing approaches to the policy process. It included a discussion of the institutional players, what they bring to the process in terms of organizational culture and how they process information to define problems and set goals. This chapter details the process by which the researcher searched for evidence to explain how institutional differences affected stakeholder interactions during the development of post-war policy for Operation Iraqi Freedom and how those interactions were mediated and synthesized by the National Security Council.

Qualitative or Quantitative Analysis?

Peter deLeon observed that the utility of a research design should determine the appropriateness of the research methods used.[92] Quantitative and qualitative analysis produce different but complementary types of information. Qualitative analysis generally provides normative data, or an understanding of political reality, as opposed to empirical data, or the verification of knowledge of what is.[93] A debate exists between theorists advocating the use of qualitative vs. quantitative methodology in policy analysis and policy research. This debate is part of a larger historical debate between positivism and post-positivist orientations to policy analysis. The debate continues, although the issue is of appropriateness of methods and strategy, not of right and wrong.

Theorists such as Peter deLeon and Ann Chih Lin worked to bridge the conflict between those who advocated strict adherence to empirical testing, including random sampling and those who espoused the need for interpretative analysis from a non-random, directed population or purposeful selection of cases.[94] The move toward qualitative research in the 1990's grew out of a need

---

[92] Peter DeLeon, "Models of policy discourse: Insights versus prediction," *Policy Studies Journal*, Vol. 26, 1998, 147.

[93] Matthew B. Miles and A. Michael Huberman, *An Expanded Sourcebook: Qualitative Data Analysis* (Thousand Oaks, CA: Sage Publications, Inc., 1994), 1.

[94] Ann Chih Lin, "Bridging Positivist and Interpretivist Approaches to Qualitative Methods," *Policy Studies Journal*, Vol. 26 (1), 1998) 163.

to incorporate facts within a contextual basis, so that researchers might better understand phenomena that affected policy development and policy success.[95]

Although it may be important to know the available facts for post-war planning, it is the interaction between stakeholders that sheds light on the decision-making process. Qualitative research makes it possible to detail the internal organizational dynamics, in addition to the facts that are included in the policy decision-making process. It is also possible to analyze the dynamics between institutions, leaders and stakeholders during the decision-making process. As such, it is possible to detail the how and why of policy development, as well as the intent of the decision.

For example, in the George W. Bush Administration's development of policy regarding the Global War on Terror (GWOT), it was important to know not only the facts regarding terrorist groups, but the political positions of government leaders, the negotiation process that lead to development of a new National Security Strategy, and the effects of this policy on stakeholders around the world. In this regard, only so many variables could be quantified. Although quantitative methods might have produced a quick analysis inferring that the root cause of terrorism is poverty (because many terrorist groups are located in poverty stricken nation states), it took qualitative analysis to incorporate other variables such as culture, religion and values into the causation model. Additionally, the role of stakeholders in supporting the GWOT could not be quantified.

This research is an analysis of the policy decision-making process, rather than an evaluation of the merits of the policies developed. Stakeholder roles and interactions are the mechanisms through which post-war policies were developed, and they are the organizing concepts for this analysis. They help us incorporate facts within the context of the decision-making process. As noted in the previous example, these interactions are not easily quantified. For this reason, a qualitative analysis of those interactions is the best-suited methodology for this case.

An analysis of these mechanisms in the national security policy process, as it should work, and how it appears to have worked during Operation Iraqi Freedom, should yield the information necessary to explain the decision-making process that lead to development of post-war strategy in Iraq.

Case Study

Political science, as a relatively new discipline, originally borrowed traditional scientific research methods from other sciences to explain political systems, political actions, policy development, and policy success and failures. These

---

[95] Matthew B. Miles and A. Michael Huberman, *An Expanded Sourcebook: Qualitative Data Analysis* (Thousand Oaks, CA: Sage Publications, Inc., 1994), 1.

traditional scientific methods focused on causation. Sometimes it is enough to understand causation, but there are situations in which it is more important to describe the nature of the relationship between variables. Such instances are better served by a detailed analysis of cases, in which the primary purpose is to obtain descriptions of situations, events, people and their behaviors.[96] Robert Yin, a proponent of case study research, asserts that the ability of the technique to provide contextual information lends itself to questions that deal with operational links that need to be traced over time.[97]

In 1971, Lijphart suggested that a single case study, of a descriptive nature, might contribute to theory building.[98] In the last decade case study methodology has gained wider acceptance, as researchers agree it is sometimes more important to understand how and why, than to merely verify what is.[99] The design of case studies may be accomplished to explore and develop a theoretical account of an isolated event, develop theories, prove or disprove theories, or explain deviation from proven theories.

Graham Allison and Philip Zelikow's analysis of the Cuban Missile Crisis, *Essence of Decision*, is an early example of case study analysis for development of a theoretical account. Their governmental politics paradigm is generally helpful to this case analysis.[100] However, there are several crucial contextual differences between *Essence of Decision* and this research. Whereas Allison and Zelikow attempted to explain decisions regarding the use of military instruments of power during a national security crisis, this research explores the decision-making process for post-war policies. Additionally, the Cuban Missile Crisis occurred before implementation of the Goldwater-Nichols Act of 1986, which gave substantially more authority to combatant commanders and diminished the role of the Department of State. Finally, *Essence of Decision* attempted to explain an external strategic event in which one nation state opposed another nation state. Analysis of the decision-making process for post-war planning focuses internally on the bureaucratic policy process. Given these differences, the role of governmental politics and organizational behaviors remain important to the discussion and the rationality of nation state actors is less a concern.

---

[96] Michael Quinn Patton, *Utilization Focused Evaluation* (Thousand Oakes: Sage Publications, 1996). See discussion regarding use of case study analysis to provide descriptive information of the decision-making process, 265–299.

[97] Robert K. Yin, *Case Study Research: Design and Methods*, 2nd ed. (Thousand Oaks: Sage Publications, 1994), 6.

[98] Arend Lijphart, "Comparative Politics and the Comparative Method," *American Political Science Review, 65*: (3), 1971, 685.

[99] Princeton University Press, "The Role of Theory in Comparative Politics: A Symposium," *World Politics, 48*(1), 1995, 1–49.

[100] Graham Allison and Philip Zelikow, *Essence of Decision: Explaining the Cuban Missile Crisis*, 2nd ed. (New York: Addison-Wesley Educational Publishers, Inc., 1999), 294–311.

Explaining the roles of independent variables (institutional differences between the Departments of State and Defense and the role of the National Security Council to arbitrate those differences) in the policy decision-making process for post-war operations is different from pursuing cause and effect. As noted by King, Keohane and Verba, "framing a case around an explanatory question may lead to more focused and relevant description, even if the study is ultimately thwarted in its attempt to provide even a single valid causal inference."[101] Differences between executive entities and the arbitration of those differences were relevant to post-war planning. It is the interplay between the two that tells us how decisions were made and how the decision-making process actually worked.

This case study seeks to explain the decision-making process for development of post-war operations for Operation Iraqi Freedom. It does not seek to prove causation, but provide a focused and relevant description of an event. From analysis of this event, it may be possible to determine what went wrong and provide lessons learned for future operations. In that sense, a case study approach is most appropriate because it readily lends itself to theory building and a discussion of corrective action.

The post-war Iraq case is important for analysis because we know the national security policy process worked as it is statutorily designed to work when it produced the National Security Strategy in 2002. As discussed in Chapter 2, the NSS sets the tone for subsequent operational planning and policy development by executive departments. If the policy process for post-war planning did not work as it was statutorily designed to work, it is important to discover why executive departments were unable to move from the strategic level to the operational level of planning. One explanation is that the National Security Council did not adequately synthesize interagency discourse to support the policy process.

Process Tracing

The technique of process tracing is used to observe and analyze the decision process from initial conditions to final outcomes.[102] It may be used to discover causal mechanisms and understand how the independent variables influenced the dependent variable, if they did. It does not test causation in a manner that would necessarily be generalized to predict future events.

Bennett and George, in their discussion of process tracing in case study research, note that knowing how causal mechanisms work can be useful, even

---

[101] Gary King, Robert O. Keohane, and Sidney Verba. *Designing Social Inquiry: Scientific Inference in Qualitative Research* (Princeton, NJ: Princeton University Press, 1994), 45.

[102] Gary King, Robert O. Keohane, and Sidney Verba. *Designing Social Inquiry: Scientific Inference in Qualitative Research* (Princeton, NJ: Princeton University Press, 1994), 226.

if the entire causal process is not clearly understood.[103] They further note the previously referenced work of King, Keohane and Verba, stating, "Identifying causal mechanisms can sometimes give us more leverage over theory by making observations at a different level of analysis into implications of the theory."[104]

Although tracing the decision-making process may not lead to a discovery of causal effects, it can lead to theories of causality that are appropriate for further research. In this research, process tracing will be used to understand how institutional differences between the Departments of State and Defense impeded the development of an effective post-war policy, if they did. Additionally, it will look for evidence of how the National Security Council synthesized interagency discourse, if it did, to support the policy process. Further research, perhaps a triangulation of this qualitative analysis and quantitative analysis employing control variables, would be required to show causality in the national security decision-making process

Process tracing is an appropriate technique for analysis of this particular case because the analysis includes a discussion of the statutory national security decision-making process as well as the process as it worked in the post-war policy development for Operation Iraqi Freedom. Process tracing allows for a comparative view of "process verification," or how the process should work based on prior theory or rule, and "process induction," or how the causal mechanisms are actually observed to have worked.[105] Additionally, process tracing explores the evolution of the policy process by noting evidence of the causal mechanisms (stakeholder roles and interactions) along the way.

Process Verification and Process Induction

Chapter 2 established the theoretical framework for the national security decision-making process, as it is statutorily designed to work. It is a process of stakeholder discourse and consensus building. The development of the 2002 National Security Strategy, although controversial because of its policy of preemption, provides documentation that the policy process as statutorily designed worked to produce a cogent policy that integrated both diplomatic and defense missions to protect national security interests. This provides

---

[103] Andrew Bennett and Alexander L. George, "Process Tracing in Case Study Research," A paper presented at the MacArthur Foundation Workshop on Case Study Methods, Harvard University, October 17–19, 1997, 5.

[104] Andrew Bennett and Alexander L. George, "Process Tracing in Case Study Research," A paper presented at the MacArthur Foundation Workshop on Case Study Methods, Harvard University, October 17–19, 1997, 5.

[105] Andrew Bennett and Alexander L. George, "Process Tracing in Case Study Research," A paper presented at the MacArthur Foundation Workshop on Case Study Methods, Harvard University, October 17–19, 1997, 5.

evidence that the national security decision-making process continued to work as intended in the aftermath of September 11, 2001.

Chapter 1 presented a preliminary view of the policy process during the post-war planning for Operation Iraqi Freedom. The first research task was to trace the policy process, searching for evidence of how the process actually worked and comparing that to the statutory policy process of stakeholder discourse and consensus building described in Chapter 2. The framework for comparison was structured around the stages of policy development identified in Chapter 2: problem definition, agenda setting, identification of desired goals or end states, use of information to develop policy options, evaluation of policy options and implementation plan.

The policy process was considered verified if evidence of stakeholder discourse and consensus building was found at each stage of the policy process. The researcher used an archival review of the literature to search for indicators of discourse and consensus building in each stage of the policy process, as depicted below.

Literature sources included policy documents, congressional testimony and transcripts of public statements pertaining to Iraq post-war planning that were publicly released by the White House, the National Security Advisor and the Departments of State and Defense. These documents were obtained online from the Military Education Research Library Network (MERLN) at National Defense University. MERLN is the home page for Military Policy Awareness Links (MiPAL) that gives researchers direct access to a repository of all publicly available U.S. policy documents on selected topics.[106] The repository also contains public documents on Iraq from the Department of Homeland Security and the Central Intelligence Agency. The specific subject matter of these documents pertains to policy issues other than the development of post-war policy in Iraq and they were not included in the analysis.

To select the documents to be included in the analysis, the researcher first obtained the MERLN list of Iraq policy documents. Next, the researcher limited the scope of review to documents published between the release of the National Security Strategy in September 2002 and the continuation of the national emergency with Iraq declaration by President Bush on July 31, 2003. This ending date was chosen because continuation of the emergency declaration is an official acknowledgment that post-war policy was not being implemented as planned. This limited the initial review to 130 documents, of which the White House released 36, the Department of State released 28, and the Department of Defense released 66.

The researcher next reviewed each of these 130 documents to determine what, if anything, they brought to the understanding of the post-war policy

---

[106] http://merln.ndu.edu.

process. Documents were selected for further review only if their subject matter pertained to development of post-war policy in Iraq. Eighteen documents were selected for further review.

The researcher next conducted four Internet searches of government websites using the Google search engine and the following phrase: Iraq "Pre-War Planning." Searches included the following sites: house.gov, senate.gov, cia.gov and centcom.mil. This search process obtained six additional documents that were not discovered during the MERLN search. Finally, the researcher conducted two final Internet searches using the key words, "Iraq + pre-war + planning" at: http://search.yahoo.com/search/options and http://clusty.com/search?query. This search yielded 3 additional documents that were no longer available on government websites, but had been placed on commercial servers by interested parties. In total 27 public documents published between September 2002 and July 31, 2003 were selected for review.

In addition to government documents published during the established time frame, the researcher reviewed analysis of the pre-war policy process by academics, international relations practitioners and defense policy analysts. This provided a context in which to place the analysis. Many of these sources provided leads to additional information. These sources were obtained through the two Internet searches listed above. Finally, during the Internet searches, nine public documents were discovered that were not published during the time frame of collection. These documents were reviewed and notations made, as they were relevant to the pre-war policy process because they provided historical facts that are noted in the analysis.

TABLE C-4 Indicators of Stakeholder Discourse

Stages of the Policy Process	Indicators of Discourse and Consensus Building
Problem Definition	Shared reality of the post-war process
Agenda Setting	Shared prioritization of necessary tasks for problem resolution
Goals	Shared end state
Option Development	Use of information to develop options rather than verify preconceived opinions
Evaluation of Options	Discussion of trade-offs
Implementation Plan	Participation of all stakeholders in implementation process

Evidence of the policy process was collected through an archival review of these public documents. One benefit of this methodology was that the review of documents was unobtrusive and the method did not influence the process under study. A second benefit was that the public documents presented the formal position of stakeholders as policy decisions unfolded, when many outcomes remained unknown. Analysis by academics, international relations practitioners, and defense policy analysts outside the executive departments (many of which were published after security and stability issues had arisen in Iraq) were integrated in to the summary of analysis in Chapter 4, but were not included in the initial summary of evidence. In this way, the researcher was able to present stakeholder interactions as they unfolded, before integrating them in to discussions that were shaped by known events.

The next research objective was to dig deeper into the dynamics of stakeholder roles and interactions as causal mechanisms in the policy process. Borrowing from Allison and Zelikow, we know the decision makers brought organizational cultures and institutional differences with them to the policy development process. These differences, detailed in Chapter 2, are presented in Table C-5.

The search for the meaning of these institutional differences in the post-war policy process ensued. Did evidence indicate that these differences impacted discourse and consensus building during the policy process? If so, did these differences help or impede problem definition, agenda setting, development of goals, development of options, evaluation of options and implementation?

In Chapter 2 the literature on institutional differences between the Departments of State and Defense was used to design a framework for how institutional differences between these departments might impact their approach to the policy process. That framework is provided in Table C-6.

An archival review of the literature was used to search for the presence of institutional differences and their impact during the decision-making process. When the review uncovered differences in approach to the policy process, the researcher assessed the impact of the differences. Three outcomes were possible for each analysis: either there was evidence that institutional differences supported the policy process, they impeded the policy process, or they had no affect on the policy process. Evidence that differences supported discourse and consensus building was viewed as having a positive effect on the policy process. Evidence that differences created unresolved conflict or withdrawal of either stakeholder from the policy process was considered an indication that differences impeded the policy process.

TABLE C-5 Institutional Differences of the Departments of State and Defense

	Department of State	Department of Defense
Mission	Foreign Diplomacy and Engagement	Defense of Homeland and Vital National Interests
Core Values	Intellect and Individual Strengths	Efficiency, Leadership and Teamwork
Structure	Functional Around Issues of Engagement	Span of Control—Bureaucratic Authority and Accountability
Culture	Think and Analyze	Plan and Operationalize
Use of Information	Inductive—From Concrete to General—Evolving	Deductive—From General to Concrete—Ending
Training	On the Job or Just in Time	Ongoing—Grooming of Leaders

Evidence

One of the most difficult tasks of research is determining what evidence is useful to the analytical process. Since this case study is comprised of an archival review of the unclassified post-war policy literature, it is not a matter of drawing a random sample or conducting interviews to determine what happened during policy meetings. It is a matter of finding well documented and complete sourcing of the unit of analysis.

One limitation of this pursuit is that public documents, primarily testimony and speeches, do not allow the researcher to "listen in" on stakeholder discussions. A second limitation is that the full picture is not available due to security concerns and classification of additional documents. As noted by Allison and Zelikow, in the second edition of *The Cuban Missile Crisis*, many of Allison's observations in the first edition were found to be incorrect 30 years later, when additional documents were declassified and available for analysis. They note, however that the new information did not take away from the original discussion, but enhanced their understanding of the decision-making framework.[107] Similarly, the information necessary for a thorough historical analysis of the pre-war planning for post-war Iraq may not be available for decades. An initial evaluation is still relevant, as it contributes to the development of lessons learned regarding the functioning of the interagency process.

---

[107] Graham Allison and Philip Zelikow, *Essence of Decision: Explaining the Cuban Missile Crisis*, 2nd ed. (New York: Addison-Wesley Educational Publishers, Inc., 1999), vii.

TABLE C-6 Differences in Approach to the Policy Process

	Department of State	Department of Defense
Approaches to the Policy Process		
Problem Definition	Evolutionary and Flexible	Concrete and Doctrine Driven
Agenda Setting	Subject to Change Based on New Information	Part of the Planning Process to Organize, Train and Equip for Troop Deployment
Desired Goal/ End State	Infinite—Always More to be Done	Completion of Strategic Objectives
	Changes As New Information and Possibilities Arise	The Beginning Point for Operational Planning
Policy Option Development	Fluid – Based on International Relationships	Based on Military Doctrine
	Assumes Sustained Engagement	Assumes Imposition of U.S. Will on Others and Departure
Evaluation Criteria	Effectiveness, Equity, Efficiency	Efficiency, Effectiveness, Equity
Implementation	Persuasion/Diplomacy	Decisive Victory/Coercion

The primary source of material for analysis was public documents, published by executive departments and the White House. These included not only public policy statements but also transcripts of open-door testimony to Congress, as well as press releases and transcripts of interviews given to media outlets. These documents were available from the Military Education Research Library Network at National Defense University. The researcher first reviewed the documents for topic relevance. Second, the researcher looked for indicators of discourse and consensus building to verify the policy process. Third, the researcher examined the topic relevant documents for indicators of the impact of institutional differences on the policy process.

Secondary sources were used to provide a context within which to integrate the research results. These secondary sources were not used to provide initial analysis, because most of them were written after security concerns presented in Iraq. As such, their writings and statements reflect historical knowledge that was not available to the stakeholders at the time policy decisions were made. They provide primarily anecdotal information regarding intent of stakeholders and a retrospective view of internal dynamics of executive departments.

Although post-war planning has been very controversial, the researcher attempted a balanced discussion of the policy process. In addition to formal public documents, sources included articles published by academics, international relations practitioners, and defense policy analysts outside the executive branch that describe or analyze the policy process. Information provided by journalists was used to shed light on the policy process, only in so far as it provided first person accounts of the policy process by stakeholders. In this way, every effort was made to separate fact from opinion in the analysis process.

Summary

The content of research questions and their theoretical propositions should have a bearing on the selection of research methods. This research incorporates a qualitative analysis of the interagency policy process for post-war reconstruction and stability operations in Iraq at the conclusion of Operation Iraqi Freedom. The policy process is the unit of analysis (case). It is first examined through the method of process tracing to determine if the policy process was "verified," or worked as statutorily designed. Next, the researcher searched to determine if institutional differences of stakeholders impacted the policy process. If differences impacted the policy process, the researcher assessed if the impact supported or impeded the policy process.

In Chapter 1 the researcher provided a description of the policy development process for post-war operations in Iraq. In Chapter 2, the researcher described the national security decision-making process as it is statutorily designed to work and defined the role of the National Security Council to arbitrate differences between the Departments of State and Defense in the decision-making process.

This chapter provided the framework for analysis of two research hypotheses:

- Institutional differences between the Department of State and the Department of Defense in their missions, core values, structures, culture, use of information, and training, impeded the development of effective post-war policy.
- The National Security Council failed to adequately synthesize interagency discourse to support the policy process.

Chapter 4 contains the results of an archival review of the literature that traced the post-war policy process. This case study approach utilizes process tracing to determine policy verification, or if the policy process worked as it was statutorily designed to work. The results of that analysis are then used as a starting point from which evidence of institutional differences are analyzed to determine their impact on the policy process. Three possibilities exist: the evidence reveals that institutional differences between the executive departments supported the policy process, that institutional differences impeded the policy process, or that institutional differences had no bearing on the policy process.

CHAPTER 4: POLICY ANALYSIS

Overview

The technique of process tracing is used to observe and analyze the decision process from initial conditions to final outcomes.[108] It may be used to discover how independent variables influenced the dependent variable, if they did. It does not provide empirical data or test causation in a manner that would necessarily be generalized to predict future events. It does, however, allow for a comparative view of "process verification," or how the process should work based on prior theory or rule, and "process induction," or how the causal mechanisms are actually observed to have worked.[109] Additionally, process tracing explores the evolution of the policy process by noting evidence of the causal mechanisms (stakeholder roles and interactions) along the way.

This chapter provides analysis resulting from an archival review of public documents that traced the post-war policy process for Operation Iraqi Freedom. Two research objectives are met. First, using the pre-war policy process for post-war planning as the unit of analysis, this case is examined to determine if the policy process worked as it was statutorily designed to work. Second, the results of this process of policy verification are then used as a starting point from which evidence of institutional differences are analyzed to determine their impact on the policy process. Three possibilities exist: the evidence reveals that institutional differences between the executive departments supported the policy process, that institutional differences impeded the policy process, or that institutional differences had no bearing on the policy process.

Chapter 1 provided a preliminary view of the policy process during the post-war planning for Operation Iraqi Freedom. Noted were the planning assumptions: that there would be huge needs for humanitarian assistance, that Iraqis would stick together to run their country, that securing Iraq would be a short-term requirement, and that financing reconstruction efforts would be accomplished through existing allocations and oil revenues, as well as

---

[108] Gary King, Robert O. Keohane, and Sidney Verba. *Designing Social Inquiry: Scientific Inference in Qualitative Research*, (Princeton, NJ: Princeton University Press, 1994), 226.

[109] Andrew Bennett and Alexander L. George, "Process Tracing in Case Study Research," A paper presented at the MacArthur Foundation Workshop on Case Study Methods, Harvard University, October 17–19, 1997, 5.

support from the international community. The post-war realities were: a much smaller need for humanitarian assistance than anticipated, a far greater than anticipated deterioration of Iraq's oil production facilities, and deep division and violence between the Shi'a and Sunni religious groups, and between those groups and coalition forces.

In Chapter 2 the researcher examined the role of institutional differences in the policy process and described the national security decision-making process as it is statutorily designed to work, defining the role of the National Security Council to arbitrate institutional differences between the Departments of State and Defense in the decision-making process. Of particular note were the potential effects of institutional differences and bureaucratic culture on the policy process. The researcher observed that because their missions differ, the Department of State and Department of Defense may not share the same goals, or "end states." Remembering Clausewitz's warning, "The first, the supreme, the most far-reaching act of judgment that the statesman and commander have to make is to establish ... the kind of war on which they are embarking," it seemed that differences in their agendas and goals might impede the policy process.[110]

In Chapter 3 the researcher provided a framework for this qualitative analysis. Initially, an archival review of 27 public documents traced the post-war planning process. Secondary analysis included research and analysis of academics, international relations practitioners, and defense policy analysts, as well as media interviews with stakeholders. These secondary sources provided historical accounts and contextual information regarding stakeholder interactions. They were not used in the initial analysis because most of the secondary sources were written after the beginning of the Iraq insurgency. They contained opinions of stakeholders who knew the policy outcomes before presenting their opinions of the policy process.

This chapter reports the analysis of the post-war planning process. Two research hypotheses were tested:

1. Institutional differences between the Department of State and the Department of Defense in their missions, core values, structures, culture, use of information, and training impeded the development of effective post-war policy.
2. The National Security Council failed to adequately synthesize interagency discourse to support the policy process.

As discussed in Chapter 2, the pre-war policy process for post-war Iraq would be considered verified if it worked as it was statutorily designed to work.

---

[110] Carl von Clausewitz, *On War*, trans. Michael Howard and Peter Parent (Princeton, NJ: Princeton University Press, 1989), 88.

The National Security Council is responsible for arbitrating stakeholder concerns in a consensus building process. Synthesizing discourse is different from arbitrating institutional differences. The NSC's role is to ensure discourse and a synthesis of ideas. It is not to encourage a blending of institutional cultures, structures and missions. In this regard, it would be possible to find significant differences in the stakeholders' approach to the policy process, and still find a synthesis of discourse between them. The researcher would verify the policy process if evidence of stakeholder discourse and consensus building could be found at each stage.

The researcher employed an archival review of the literature to search for indicators of discourse and consensus building in each stage of the policy process, as depicted in Table C-7. The documents were reviewed chronologically, although that did not appear to be important to the overall analysis.

Problem Definition in the Policy Process

The researcher searched for evidence that the Departments of State and Defense shared the same reality of the post-war process. This included a concern for the same post-war possibilities and evidence of joint planning to meet post-war concerns. The following is a synopsis of the evidence.

During a hearing on "The Future of Iraq" by the Senate Foreign Relations Committee on February 11, 2003, Marc Grossman, Under Secretary of State for Political Affairs, defined the problem by stating that the United States "will want to be in a position to help meet the humanitarian, reconstruction and administrative challenges facing the country in the aftermath of combat operations."[111]

TABLE C-7 Indicators of Stakeholder Discourse

Stages of the Policy Process	Indicators of Discourse and Consensus Building
Problem Definition	Shared reality of the post-war process
Agenda Setting	Shared prioritization of necessary tasks for problem resolution
Goals	Shared end state
Option Development	Use of information to develop options
Evaluation of Options	Discussion of trade-offs
Implementation Plan	Participation of all stakeholders in implementation process

[111] Marc I. Grossman, "The Future of Iraq," Hearing of the Senate Foreign Relations Committee, February 11, 2003.

At the same hearing, Under Secretary of Defense for Policy, Douglas Feith, defined the problem in these terms: "It will be necessary to provide humanitarian relief, organize basic services and work to establish security for the liberated Iraqis."[112] In the same hearing, Senator Joseph Biden, Jr. theorized that "maintaining a secure environment after a possible war in Iraq is going to be the sine qua non for any positive change we wish to bring to Iraq. I suspect we'll discover the definition of security will take on a very broad dimension."[113] On February 23, 2003 in a town hall meeting with the Iraqi-American community, Deputy Secretary of Defense, Paul Wolfowitz, stated, "... it is not too early for the rest of us to be thinking about how to build a just and peaceful and democratic Iraq after Saddam Hussein is gone."[114]

On February 24, 2003 a briefing on humanitarian and reconstruction issues was provided to the White House Press Corps. Elliott Abrams, National Security Council Senior Director for Near East and North Africa, noted there were humanitarian issues already present in Iraq and that conflict could make them worse. He specifically referred to food distribution, refugees and loss of electricity. He noted a strategy had been developed through the interagency process to deal with these issues and that the role of the U.S. military was not to take a lead role in humanitarian relief activities, but to facilitate early secure access by civilian relief agencies to fulfill their humanitarian mandates.[115]

Ron Adams, Deputy Director, Pentagon Office of Reconstruction and Humanitarian Assistance, agreed with Abrams stating, "Our job is to operationalize or to implement the plans that are being developed by the interagency process and by our coalition partners in support of the Commander of U.S. Central Command and the coalition forces that would be involved.[116] Joe Collins, the Deputy Assistant Secretary of Defense for Stability Operations, then commented that the Department of Defense was prepared to support humanitarian relief during combat, support reconstruction efforts after combat, and, most importantly, help the Iraqi people prepare for self-government.[117]

At the same briefing, Gene Dewy, the Assistant Secretary of State for Population, Refugees and Migration, acknowledged the humanitarian mission

---

[112] Douglas J. Feith, "The Future of Iraq," Hearing of the Senate Foreign Relations Committee, February 11, 2003.

[113] Joseph R. Biden, Jr., "The Future of Iraq," Hearing of the Senate Foreign Relations Committee, February 11, 2003.

[114] Paul Wolfowitz, "The Future of Iraq," Hearing of the Senate Foreign Relations Committee, February 11, 2003.

[115] Elliot Abrams, "Briefing on Humanitarian Reconstruction Issues," February 24, 2003.

[116] Ron Adams, Briefing on Humanitarian Reconstruction Issues, February 24, 2003.

[117] Joe Collins, Briefing on Humanitarian Reconstruction Issues, February 24, 2003.

and stated: "The center of gravity of the humanitarian effort is the multilateral system."[118]

On February 26, President Bush addressed the future of Iraq in a speech at the American Enterprise Institute. He commented: "Bringing stability and unity to a free Iraq will not be easy.... The United States and our coalition stand ready to help the citizens of a liberated Iraq."[119] In President Bush's message to the Iraqi people, he stated, "We are taking unprecedented measures to spare the lives of innocent Iraqi citizens, and are beginning to deliver food, water and medicine to those in need."[120]

Responses or statements made by the National Security Advisor and staff members of the National Security Council were attributed to the White House. This is because of both the role of the NSA and the fact that the staff of the NSC are assigned to the White House. Table C-8 chart summarizes the evidence related to problem definition.

Analysis of the Problem Definition Stage

Overall, the need to provide stability and humanitarian assistance was the primary theme of policy makers as they attempted to publicly define the problem for development of a post-war policy. Perhaps this is because they were apprehensive of the direct or indirect impact of combat on humanitarian needs. This was alluded to in briefs and testimony as an unknown entity, a qualifier per se of their estimates of needs assessments. For example, Elliott Abrams' statement above reflects a concern that combat could make humanitarian needs much more grave. Public discussions of problem definition in the development of post-war policy indicate stakeholder consensus. However, a review of the agenda setting process reveals a slightly different view.

Agenda Setting in the Policy Process

The researcher searched for evidence that the Departments of State and Defense shared their prioritization of necessary tasks for problem resolution. The public discussions defining the problem of post-war policy seemed to indicate discourse between the departments. Logic would predict that the stakeholders, having similarly defined the problem, would work together to establish a list of priorities that would solve the problem. This process would confirm their shared understanding of the problem.

---

[118] Gene Dewey, Briefing on Humanitarian Reconstruction Issues, February 24, 2003.

[119] George W. Bush, Speech at the American Enterprise Institute on the Future of Iraq, February 26, 2003.

[120] George W. Bush, Message to the Iraqi People, April 10, 2003.

TABLE C-8 Problem Definition for Post-War Policy

	The White House	Department of State	Department of Defense
Problem Definition	Bringing stability, unity and humanitarian assistance to the people of Iraq	Meet the humanitarian, reconstruction and administrative challenges in the aftermath of combat: a multilateral approach	Provide humanitarian relief, organize basic services and work to establish a peaceful, just, democratic and secure Iraq

Both the Departments of State and Defense report interagency involvement in the planning initiatives for post-war contingencies. However, it is noteworthy that what developed was a dual planning process rather than an integrated plan based on stakeholder consensus. This researcher contends that these dual planning initiatives reflect agenda setting, as both groups prepared for their concerns of post-war realities.

The Department of Defense reported as early as July 2002 that six interagency working groups were developed to coordinate post-war planning on the following issues. The Iraq Political-Military Cell was formed to develop the conditions for Iraq's transition to stability and sovereignty. The Executive Steering Group met to discuss strategic planning and policy recommendations for the National Security Council Deputies' Committee meetings. The Humanitarian and Reconstruction Group prepared plans for relief and reconstruction operations. The Energy Infrastructure Working Group designed plans to return Iraq's oil industry to pre-war levels. The Coalition Working Group coordinated military requirements and diplomatic strategy to build coalition support. Finally, the Global Communications Group planned to counter disinformation campaigns.[121] The Department of State participated in each of the interagency planning groups formed by the Department of Defense.

In a separate initiative the Department of State sponsored 17 separate working groups, composed primarily of Iraqis living outside Iraq who integrated ideas and plans for building a new Iraq. This initiative, established in April 2002, became known as the "Future of Iraq Project."[122] Participants in the project worked together to form concepts of governance and discuss the immediate and long range needs of the Iraqi people after regime change. Additionally, Iraq experts, such as Phoebe Marr, participated in the discussions.

---

[121] U.S. Department of Defense, "Pre-war Planning for Post-war Iraq." Available at http://www.defenselink.mil/policy/isa/nesa/postwar_iraq.html.

[122] U.S. Department of State, "Duty to the Future: Free Iraqi Plan for a New Iraq," April, 2003. Available at http://www.usinfo.state.gov.

Although invited, DOD personnel were prohibited by the Secretary of Defense from participating in this initiative.[123] This points to a lack of discourse and consensus building early on in the policy process and reflects intent on the part of the Department of Defense to exclude the Department of State from the policy process.

The Future of Iraq Project working groups included: Democratic Principles and Procedures, Economy and Infrastructure, Defense Policy and Institutions, Education, Public Health and Humanitarian Needs, Civil Society Capacity Building, Transitional Justice, Water, Agriculture and Environment, Preserving Iraq's Cultural Heritage, Public Finance, Oil and Energy, Local Government, Anti-Corruption Measures, Foreign and National Security, Free Media, Migration and Public Outreach.[124]

A comparison of the working groups is provided in Table C-9. The researcher arranged the groups in a manner as to note the corresponding discussions that occurred during the dual planning process. For example, the DOD working group for "Preparations for Relief and Reconstruction Efforts" corresponded to the Future of Iraq Project working groups for "Public Health and Humanitarian Needs, Water, Agriculture and Environment, Migration, Economic and Infrastructure, and Public Finance."

Analysis of the Agenda Setting Stage

Two things stand out when one reviews the functions of these planning groups side by side. The first is that the interagency groups developed by the Department of Defense focused on providing policy recommendations to decision makers, preparing for the worst case scenario with regard to humanitarian issues and destruction of the oil infrastructure, maintaining coalition support for the effort, countering the Arab media, and determining what standards would be used to verify stability and sovereignty, hence an exit strategy. In fact, Under Secretary Douglas Feith testified before the Senate Foreign Relations Committee that "The faster all the necessary reconstruction tasks are accomplished, the sooner the coalition will be able to withdraw its forces from Iraq and the sooner the Iraqis will assume complete control of their country."[125]

Second, the approach of the Department of State was to include free Iraqis in the planning process and to open that process to areas of discussion far beyond the scope of DOD review. State personnel seemed to focus first on the health and safety of Iraqis, then on the long-term tasks of institution

---

[123] David Rieff, "Blueprint for A Mess," *New York Times Magazine*, November 2, 2003.

[124] U.S. Department of State, "Duty to the Future: Free Iraqi Plan for a New Iraq." April, 2003. Available at http://www.usinfo.state.gov.

[125] Douglas J. Feith, Undersecretary of Defense, Testimony before the Senate Foreign Relations Committee, February 11, 2003.

TABLE C-9 Defense and State Working Groups

Topics of Discussion	Department of Defense Interagency Working Groups	Department of State Future of Iraq Project Working Groups
Stability and Governance	Conditions for Stability and Sovereignty	Civil Society Capacity Building
		Defense Policy and Institutions
		Transitional Justice
		Local Government
		Democratic Principles and Procedures
		Foreign and National Security
		Anti-Corruption Measures
U.S. Policy Recommendations	Strategic Planning and Policy	None
	Recommendations to U.S. Administration	
Relief and Reconstruction	Preparations for Relief and Reconstruction Efforts	Public Health and Humanitarian Needs
		Water, Agriculture and Environment
		Migration
		Economic and Infrastructure
		Public Finance
Oil/Energy	Return Iraq's Oil Industry to Pre-War Standards	Oil and Energy
International Aid	Build Coalition Support	Public Outreach
Use of Media	Counter Disinformation of Hussein Regime	Free Media
Education	None	Education
Culture	None	Preserving Iraq's Cultural History

and democracy building. This difference is best described as the difference between DOD preparing to implement a strategic plan and DOS determining how the actual work should be done. An analogy would be the difference between designing a prototype car and determining what should be included in the driver's manual. The differences were not cross-purpose to each other, but focused on different parts of the overall problem.

No evidence was found that indicated the NSC or the National Security Advisor to the President attempted to synthesize these dual planning activities. Additionally, there is no evidence that these differences in approach to agenda setting impeded the development of post-war policy. In fact, had the information produced by the Future of Iraq planning group been integrated into DOD planning activities, it might have strengthened the policy outcome. It was not the differences that impeded the policy process, but the lack of discourse.

Signs of conflict were evident during review of the agenda setting stage. During the February 11 testimony before the Senate Foreign Relations Committee, Under Secretary of State Grossman told the Committee that he and DOD Under Secretary Feith's testimony should be treated as a consultation because some of the policies were still under discussion.[126] He then spoke of the Future of Iraq Project, in evolutionary terms, stating, "I hope you won't be surprised to find that the list of priorities of course tracks with the work we're doing in the program on the future of Iraq. I hope you also won't be surprised that we are working in these areas to set for ourselves very clear benchmarks, very clear timelines and very clear ways to see if this is necessary, if we are succeeding."[127] Grossman's testimony left room for change in plans based on new information. DOS was still working the agenda.

Under Secretary Feith's testimony was far more concrete. He stated, "President Bush directed on January 20th the creation of a post-war planning office. Although the office is located within the policy organization in the Department of Defense, officials detailed from departments and agencies throughout the government staff it. Its job is planning and implementation. The intention is not to theorize but to do practical work."[128] The time for theoretical discussion was over. DOD was moving to convert a strategic plan to an operational plan, and appeared frustrated that DOS was still working the agenda. Again, the two departments were not at cross-purposes, but were working different stages of the policy process.

How did the Department of Defense planners move so quickly through the agenda setting stage? Remembering that the ORHA was established in

---

[126] Marc Grossman, Under Secretary of State for Political Affairs, Testimony before the Senate Foreign Relations Committee, February 11, 2003.

[127] Marc Grossman, Under Secretary of State for Political Affairs, Testimony before the Senate Foreign Relations Committee, February 11, 2003.

[128] Douglas Feith, Under Secretary of Defense, Testimony before the Senate Foreign Relations Committee, February 11, 2003.

January 2003, how did planners so quickly determine the agenda for post-war policy? The DOD began an interagency policy process in July 2002 to coordinate strategic plans and to develop policy recommendations for the National Security Council.[129] The planners focused on humanitarian assistance and infrastructure reconstruction. Little operational planning was done with regard to security and stability. In an interview conducted late in 2003, Feith admitted that "nobody will find a single piece of paper that says: Mr. Secretary or Mr. President, let us tell you what post-war Iraq is going to look like, and here is what we need plans for. If you tried that, you would get thrown out of Rumsfeld's office so fast. If you ever went in there and said: Let me tell you what something's going to look like in the future, you wouldn't get to your next sentence."[130] The time for theoretical discussions was over.

Goals in the Policy Process

Evidence discovered in the February 11, 2003 testimony reveals that the Departments of State and Defense shared the same post-war goals, perhaps. Representatives of both departments presented the same list in congressional testimony. Under Secretary Feith referred to the list as "objectives" while Under Secretary Grossman referred to the list as "guiding principles." The list included:

- Demonstrate to the Iraqi people and the world that the United States aspires to liberate, not occupy Iraq or control their economic resources
- Eliminate Iraq's chemical and biological weapons, its nuclear program and its related delivery systems (DOD included research and production facilities in their description and added "This will be a complex, dangerous and expensive task.")
- Eliminate Iraq's terrorist infrastructure (DOD added that "A key element of U.S. strategy in the global war on terrorism is information about terrorist networks that the coalition acquires through our military and law enforcement actions.")
- Safeguard the territorial unity of Iraq. (DOD added, "The United States does not support Iraq's disintegration or dismemberment.")
- Begin the process of economic and political reconstruction, working to put Iraq on a path to become a prosperous and free country. (DOD added "The U.S. government shares with many Iraqis the hope that their country will enjoy the rule of law and other elements of democracy under a broad-based government that represents the various parts of Iraqi society.")[131]

---

[129] http://www.defenselink.mil/policy/isa/nesa/postwar_iraq.html.

[130] James Fallows, "Blind into Baghdad," *The Atlantic Monthly*, January/February, 2004.

[131] Marc Grossman and Douglas Feith, Testimony before the Senate Committee on Foreign Relations, February 11, 2003.

After laying out these "guiding principles," Under Secretary Grossman stressed the importance of working with a broad interagency representation, as well as allies in the task of locating, securing and disposing of weapons of mass destruction. He also emphasized engagement by the Department of State with other U.S. government agencies, non-governmental organizations, and international organizations to provide humanitarian assistance to Iraqis.

Grossman next addressed reconstruction, testifying that the Future of Iraq Project paralleled the Department of Defense interagency process. This is important because he noted the dual rather than integrated planning process. Grossman was telling Congress there were two perspectives for consideration. As he moved to a discussion of the political future of Iraq, he emphasized discussions of free Iraqis and the importance of practical planning that included their thoughts for what could be accomplished in the aftermath of a change of government in Baghdad. He then provided examples of their work.[132]

By comparison, Under Secretary Feith referred to the list as objectives. He noted a two-part commitment to stay long enough to achieve these objectives, and then to leave once Iraqi officials were able to shoulder the responsible. Feith stressed the need for security to allow reconstruction efforts, and noted that the faster these tasks were completed, the sooner the coalition would be able to withdraw its forces. He then discussed the creation of the Office of Reconstruction and Humanitarian Assistance, to facilitate provision of aid, coordinate relief in Civil-Military Operations Centers, reestablish the UN food program, and integrate these efforts to make them operational. Feith's discussion of elimination of weapons of mass destruction was similar to Grossman. He deviated from Grossman's testimony by including a discussion of the planning for resumption of oil production, although admittedly the organizational mechanisms by which this would be handled had not yet been determined.[133]

In a February 2003 speech before the Council on Foreign Relations, Stephen Hadley, Deputy National Security Advisor to the President, listed the same principles or objectives mentioned by both state and defense personnel. Additionally, he stated, "The goal which we are confident we share with Iraq's people is an Iraq that is whole, free, and at peace with itself and its neighbors; an Iraq that is moving toward democracy in which all religions and ethnic communities have a voice and in which individual rights are protected regardless of gender, religion or ethnicity; and an Iraq that adheres to the rule of law at home and lives up to its international obligations."[134]

---

[132] Marc Grossman, Under Secretary of State for Political Affairs, Testimony before the Senate Foreign Relations Committee, February 11, 2003.

[133] Douglas Feith, Under Secretary of Defense for Policy, Testimony before the Senate Foreign Relations Committee, February 11, 2003.

[134] Stephen Hadley, Deputy National Security Advisor, Speech at the Council on Foreign Relations, February 12, 2003.

In an April 2003 press briefing, National Security Advisor Condoleezza Rice mirrored Hadley's comments, stating, "Our goals are clear: We will help Iraqis build an Iraq that is whole, free and at peace with itself and with its neighbors. It will be an Iraq that is disarmed of all WMD; that no longer supports or harbors terror; that respects the rights of Iraqi people and the rule of law; and that is on the path to democracy."[135] She added that the method of achieving these goals was not yet worked out.[136]

Analysis of the Goal Setting Stage

Did the Departments of State and Defense share a common goal or envision a common end state in the development of post-war policy for Operation Iraqi Freedom? The rhetoric of goal setting between personnel of the Department of State and Department of Defense personnel is very similar and mirrors the discussion of goals by the National Security Advisor and her deputy. Institutional differences can be seen in their testimony, as the difference between guiding principles and objectives is a cultural artifact. Also, we see the Department of State continuing to gather information, rather than developing an operational plan. Meanwhile, the DOD is moving ahead with their objectives. Still, there are more similarities than differences between the statements of the two departments, as noted in Table C-10.

The administration's goals are clear and indisputable. The last two points of comparison reveal a clear difference of perception between the departments as to how the goals might best be accomplished. However, this is not surprising given the roles and missions of the two departments. Although the Central Command operational plan, including the military's assessment and intent for Operation Iraqi Freedom, has not been published for public review, there is little doubt that the Phase IV or transition plans included reinforcement of support for humanitarian operations, support of non-governmental and international organizations in their nation-building efforts, and redeployment of troops. These phrases have become routine in crisis action exercise planning and wargame activities at military schools. Simultaneously, the Department of State viewed post-war efforts as a matter of long-term engagement. The following discussion regarding use of information to develop options provides insight into these differences in perspective.

---

[135] Condoleezza Rice, National Security Advisor, Press Briefing on April 4, 2003.
[136] Condoleezza Rice, National Security Advisor, Press Briefing on April 4, 2003.

TABLE C-10 Comparison of Post-War Policy Goals

Goals/Objectives	Department of State	Department of Defense
We will liberate—not occupy—Iraq	Yes	Yes
We will eliminate WMD and their delivery systems	Yes	Yes
We will eliminate the terrorist infrastructure	Yes	Yes
We will safeguard the territorial unity of Iraq	Yes	Yes
We will work to make Iraq a free and prosperous country	Yes	Yes
We will work with broad representation of Iraqis and international organizations	Emphasis	Not an emphasis
We will provide security to speed reconstruction efforts, and then we will leave	Not an Emphasis	Emphasis

Option Development

The researcher conducted a search for evidence of how options were developed, if at all. This included evidence of the manner in which information was collected, how it was used to narrow the focus of policy options and implementation. Key in this review was how the information was collected and the weight given to that information by the stakeholders. Was there agreement or an acceptance of "ground truth" with which to pursue policy development? Was there an agreement that some things were unknowable, particularly when there was no agreement?

In his February testimony before the Senate Foreign Relations Committee, Marc Grossman testified that each of the Future of Iraq Project working groups was engaged in planning to determine what could be accomplished now, and in the aftermath of a change in government in Baghdad.[137] He stated, "We are listening to what the Iraqis are telling us."[138] The Future of Iraq Project began in

---

[137] Marc Grossman, Under Secretary of State for Political Affairs, Testimony before the Senate Foreign Relations Committee, February 11, 2003.

[138] Marc Grossman, Under Secretary of State for Political Affairs, Testimony before the Senate Foreign Relations Committee, February 11, 2003.

April 2002 and testimony regarding post-war security concerns was presented to Congress by Iraq expert Phoebe Marr in August of that year.[139]

Other than a mention of lessons learned in Afghanistan, there were no indications in the testimony of Douglas Feith of the sources of information used in post-war option development. With regard to the planning activities of the Office of Reconstruction and Humanitarian Assistance, Feith emphasized "The intention not to theorize, but to do practical work."[140]

An exception to the failure to publicly identify information sources is found in Feith's testimony regarding detailed planning for humanitarian relief that included an interagency effort. This implies some level of discourse between stakeholders in policy development. He noted that this working group was linked to Central Command, as well as the United Nations and non-governmental organizations involved in humanitarian relief.[141]

Later in February, Deputy Secretary of Defense, Paul Wolfowitz, discussed with free Iraqis and Iraqi-Americans how they might help the post-war process. He laid out a plan for them to assist the U.S. military as civilians, to be employed by contractors, to serve as translators, or to join the U.S. military. He further stated that this would "take advantage of your professional skills in a wide variety of areas, while also capitalizing on your understanding of local languages and culture."[142] There is no mention of including free Iraqis in the development of post-war options and, as previously mentioned, DOD rejected the work of the Future of Iraq working groups.

An overview of the potential humanitarian issues in post-war Iraq was prepared for Congress and published by the Congressional Research Service just days before the beginning of Operation Iraqi Freedom. This research pertained to food security, sanitation and health, and migration. It further observed that the determination of humanitarian need was an interagency process. The report also noted that DOD was in charge of creating "humanitarian space," and that how the war was fought and for how long would partially determine humanitarian needs.[143]

There is also evidence of detailed pre-war planning by a senior interagency team, which established a baseline assessment of conditions in Iraq and defined relief and reconstruction plans, sector by sector. In testimony before the Senate Foreign Relations Committee, the Director of the Office of

---

[139] Phoebe Marr, Testimony before the Senate Foreign Relations Committee, August 1, 2002.

[140] Douglas Feith, Under Secretary of Defense for Policy, Testimony before the Senate Foreign Relations Committee, February 11, 2003.

[141] Douglas Feith, Under Secretary of Defense for Policy, Testimony before the Senate Foreign Relations Committee, February 11, 2003.

[142] Paul Wolfowitz, Deputy Secretary of Defense, Town Hall Meeting with Iraqi-American Community, February 23, 2003.

[143] Rhoda Margesson and Johanna Bockman, "Potential Humanitarian Issues in Post-War Iraq: An Overview for Congress," Report for Congress, Congressional Research Service, The Library of Congress, March 18, 2003.

Management and Budget, Joshua Bolton, noted that the immediate relief and long-term reconstruction needs were detailed and action plans developed with benchmarks for evaluation at one month, six months, and one year. Bolton said these measures were required by the President, who wanted a means of evaluating the progress of improvement in the lives of the Iraqi people.[144]

Finally, testimony on the financial reconstruction in Iraq, provided to the Senate Banking, Housing, and Urban Affairs Committee in September 2003, provides historical evidence of the reconstruction planning process. John Taylor, Under Secretary of Treasury for International Affairs, stated that late in 2002 Treasury officials began developing a strategy for financial reconstruction which addressed such issues as how to pay Iraqi workers, the currency, the banking system, Iraq's transnational debt, reconstruction costs, and international fundraising efforts. This process included engagement with the World Bank and the International Monetary Fund to create a needs assessment.[145]

Analysis of Option Development

Evidence indicates an extensive process of discourse and interagency cooperation with regard to development of policy options for humanitarian assistance and reconstruction of Iraq's economic institutions. Information was used by stakeholders to develop options that supported policy goals in these areas.

However, no evidence was found that indicated use of information by the Department of Defense to develop post-war security and stability operations, even though that was an emphasis of discussion during the goal setting stage of policy development. This point is critical to the analysis, given that DOD was admittedly responsible for creating the secure "humanitarian space" in which reconstruction plans would be implemented.[146] As noted in Chapter 1, two of the planning assumptions of DOD was that Iraqis would stick together to run their country and securing Iraq would be a short-term requirement. In fact, as predicted by Iraq experts, just the opposite was true and chaos ensued. Although the tendency to ignore information that is inconsistent with one's pre-existing beliefs is not unique to this situation, in this particular case it

---

[144] Joshua Bolton, Director of the Office of Management and Budget, Testimony before the Senate Foreign Relations Committee, July 29, 2003. The interagency group included representatives from the Departments of Defense, State, and Treasury; USAID, CIA; and, from the White House, staff of the National Security Council and the Office of Management and Budget. Additional agencies were called upon as expertise was needed.

[145] John B. Taylor, Under Secretary of Treasury for International Affairs, Testimony before the Senate Banking, Housing, and Urban Affairs Committee Subcommittee on International Trade and Finance, September 16, 2003.

[146] Rhoda Margesson and Johanna Bockman, "Potential Humanitarian Issues in Post-War Iraq: An Overview for Congress," Report for Congress, Congressional Research Service, The Library of Congress, March 18, 2003.

multiplied the problems by creating an environment in which relief and reconstruction efforts were futile.

Evaluation of Options

The researcher next searched for evidence indicating discourse and consensus building between the stakeholders with regard to the trade-offs between
policy options in the decision-making process. Both DOD and DOS agreed that
the degree of humanitarian assistance that would be required was unknown.
Under Secretary of State Grossman testified: "U.S. government agencies are
engaged in planning to meet Iraq's humanitarian needs with an emphasis
on civilian-military coordination. This effort is led by the National Security
Council and the OMB. USAID and State are engaged with non-governmental
organizations and the international organizations that will be important partners in addressing Iraq's humanitarian needs. Civilian and military officials
regularly consult and coordinate plans."[147] He further indicated effort to "think
through" reconstruction needs and objectives, given the many uncertain-
ties.[148] As noted in Chapter 1, coalition forces were over-prepared to provide
humanitarian assistance. Options for security and stability operations were
not developed, thus they were not part of the evaluation.

Under Secretary Feith's testimony provided no evidence of discussions
regarding trade-offs or evaluation of policy options by the Department of Defense
in the decision-making process. And, in a late February briefing, Joseph Collins,
Deputy Assistant Secretary of Defense for Stability Operations concluded "There
are many unknowns. There are many unknown unknowns. And all of this is
complicated by the fact that what happens to the population of Iraq in any contingency that might ensue is, to a large measure, in the hands of Saddam Hussein."[149]

Collins' statement paralleled the views of National Security Advisor
Condoleezza Rice. After the war began, Rice stated that because it was impossible to know what the condition of Iraq would be at the conclusion of Saddam
Hussein's regime, many of the specifics of achieving post-war goals could only
be developed when "Saddam's regime is gone."[150] She further commented that
the President through the Secretary of Defense provided policy guidance for the
ORHA, and that it was being developed and coordinated on an interagency basis.[151]

---

[147] Marc Grossman, Under Secretary of State for Political Affairs, Testimony before the Senate
Foreign Relations Committee, February 11, 2003.

[148] Marc Grossman, Under Secretary of State for Political Affairs, Testimony before the Senate
Foreign Relations Committee, February 11, 2003.

[149] Joseph Collins, Deputy Assistant Secretary of Defense for Stability Operations, Briefing at
the Foreign Press Center Building, Washington, DC. February 28, 2003.

[150] Condoleezza Rice, National Security Advisor, Press Briefing, April 4, 2003.

[151] Condoleezza Rice, National Security Advisor, Press Briefing, April 4, 2003.

Analysis of Option Evaluation

The lack of information, alluded to by Deputy Assistant Secretary Collins and National Security Advisor Rice, seemed to indicate a belief on the part of the Administration that options for some post-war activities could not be developed or evaluated until the fall of the Hussein regime. This view is consistent with Under Secretary Feith's earlier statements that DOD did not plan because the Secretary of Defense did not believe it was possible to plan for an uncertain future.[152]

The discussion to this point reflects the actions of the civilian Department of Defense. Uniformed military personnel evaluated post-war planning, in parallel activities to those of the Departments of State and Defense. Scott Feil, a former Army War College Fellow, testified in February 2003 that the Naval War College, the National Defense University, the Institute for Defense Analysis, the Joint Staff and Joint Forces Command, and the Army War College had held conferences, exercises, and simulations to determine conditions and requirements for success.[153]

Feil noted that the interagency task forces, and the Department of State in particular, had worked diligently to determine requirements, but had not put together a process or plan that could be implemented by the military or a civilian administrator. Similarly, the U.S. Central Command and the Department of Defense had conducted their own planning operations. He noted that each had made formal or informal contact with international organizations and experts, exchanging a great deal of information. He concluded that although the problem had been well defined, the effort to implement procedures and organize resources remained fragmented.[154]

The crux of Feil's testimony was that *simultaneous planning across the realm of stakeholders had occurred, but it had not been integrated in order to form an implementation plan.* Feil also testified that "Post-conflict reconstruction in Iraq can be successful—if success is adequately defined and if the resources match intent. But time is short, the planning process has not kept pace with the military and diplomatic timeline, and the agencies who can resolve some of the outstanding issues are running out of time to do so."[155]

Feil attached to his prepared testimony the results of a two and one half year (2000–2003) study conducted by the Association of the U.S. Army and the Center for Strategic and International Studies. This study focused on the execution of tasks for reconstruction and noted that security was the foundation

---

[152] James Fallows, "Blind into Baghdad," *The Atlantic Monthly*, January/February, 2004.

[153] Scott R. Feil, Testimony before the Senate Foreign Relations Committee, February 11, 2003.

[154] Scott R. Feil, Testimony before the Senate Foreign Relations Committee, February 11, 2003.

[155] Scott R. Feil, Testimony before the Senate Foreign Relations Committee, February 11, 2003.

for post-conflict reconstruction efforts. It provided structure.[156] However, one participant in the study later noted, "If you went to the Pentagon before the war, all the concentration was on the war. If you went there during the war, all the concentration was on the war. And if you went there after the war, they'd say, 'That's Jerry Bremer's job.'"[157] As noted in Chapter 1, Jerry Bremer was the civilian administrator of the Coalition Provisional Authority, who replaced Joe Garner in Baghdad.

The Secretary of Defense prohibited DOD personnel from attending the Future of Iraq meetings. It was not that things were "unknowable." It was that the Secretary of Defense did not believe in planning for unproven contingencies. This is consistent with the Secretary's plan for transforming the military to be organized, trained and equipped to flexibly respond to any role or action. In a speech on transformation of the military in January 2002, Rumsfeld said the military should not continue to plan for threats as it did during the Cold War, but should have forces and capabilities to respond to new and unexpected challenges.[158]

The Implementation Plan

The researcher searched for evidence of discourse and consensus building by all stakeholders in the development of an implementation plan, and for evidence of stakeholder differences. As noted in Chapter 3, a difference in approach to implementation might be Department of State's reliance on persuasion and diplomacy, while DOD relied on decisive victory and coercion.

Under Secretary of State Marc Grossman concluded his February 11 testimony to the Senate Foreign Relations Committee by emphasizing the ongoing consideration and discussion of an implementation plan with free Iraqis, technocrats, intellectuals, allies and Congress. He proposed a three-stage course of implementation: (1) Stabilization by the Coalition military—laying the groundwork, (2) Transition of authority to Iraqi institutions during the development of a democratic Iraq, and (3) Transformation of Iraq, based on a democratic constitution and elections.[159]

This concept of a post-war plan was echoed by Prime Minister Tony Blair, when in testimony before the British Parliament he noted that the process of Iraq's reconstruction would occur in three phases: (1) Coalition forces and the ORHA would first ensure that security and humanitarian needs were met,

---

[156] Scott R. Feil, Testimony before the Senate Foreign Relations Committee, February 11, 2003.

[157] James Fallows, quoting Frederick Barton, "Blind into Baghdad," *The Atlantic Monthly,* January/February, 2004.

[158] Donald Rumsfeld, Secretary of Defense, Remarks delivered at National Defense University, January 31, 2002. Available at http://www.defenselink.mil/speeches/2002/s20020131-secdef.html.

[159] Marc Grossman, Under Secretary of State for Political Affairs, Testimony before the Senate Foreign Relations Committee, February 11, 2003.

(2) An Iraqi Interim Authority would be established to help Iraqis assume more control of their government, and (3) Elections to bring a fully representative Iraqi government.[160] Blair's testimony occurred within days of a meeting with President Bush in Ireland to discuss the coalition's commitment in Iraq.

At the completion of major combat operations in May, another State Department executive provided further insight into the plan. In testimony before the House International Relations Committee, Alan Larson noted that although the primary concern remained the establishment of stability and security, reconstruction activities were beginning. Larson further noted that his department worked with DOD and others for seven months to prepare for humanitarian relief, reconstruction, and institution building in Iraq. According to Larson, the way ahead was to continue the work of State Department employees to support Iraqi efforts to reconstruct their criminal justice institutions, develop a free market economy, establish democratic institutions and protect human rights.[161]

With regard to implementation of post-war policy, DOD Under Secretary Douglas Feith testified that on January 20 the President directed the creation of the Office of Reconstruction and Humanitarian Assistance (ORHA) to plan and implement post-war operations. ORHA would interface with non-governmental organizations and international government organizations and would be responsible for integrating and operationalizing efforts to provide aid, establishing civil-military operations coordination centers, reconstructing Iraq, vetting the Iraqi officials with whom they would work, and eliminating WMD. The responsibility for administering post-war Iraq was directed to the Commander of the U.S. Central Command. Feith noted the chain of command, stating, "… the coalition forces responsible for post-conflict administration of Iraq—whether military or civilian, from the various agencies of the governments—will report to the President, to General Tom Franks, the Commander of the U.S. Central Command, and the Secretary of Defense."[162]

In Feith's prepared statement (although missing from his testimony) he noted that CENTCOM had established a Combined Joint Task Force (CJTF) to be responsible for organizing coalition forces. The CJTF was to work closely with the ORHA to facilitate relief and reconstruction activities. Feith did not disclose the communication lines between the CENTCOM commander and the CJTF or between the CJTF and the ORHA.[163]

---

[160] Tony Blair, Testimony before Parliament, April 14, 2003.

[161] Alan P. Larson, Under Secretary for Economic, Business, and Agriculture Affairs, Testimony before the House International Relations Committee, May 15, 2003.

[162] Douglas Feith, Under Secretary of Defense for Policy, Testimony before the Senate Foreign Relations Committee, February 11, 2003.

[163] Douglas Feith, Under Secretary of Defense for Policy, Prepared testimony before the Senate Foreign Relations Committee, February 11, 2003.

On February 28, 2003, representatives from the Departments of Defense and State, as well as USAID, briefed the Foreign Press Corps on humanitarian relief planning in Iraq. (It is important to remember that the Department of State planners defined humanitarian assistance as an immediate provision of basic aid, while reconstruction operations were defined as long-term projects.) During the briefing, a clear implementation plan for humanitarian assistance was explained by the USAID official. Michael Marx stated 60 individuals had been deployed as part of a Disaster Assistance Response Team (DART) that identified and responded to humanitarian needs while coordinating the U.S. Government's response.[164] A DOD representative echoed the role of the Pentagon and the armed forces to support these operations. Joseph Collins stated the Pentagon was involved in "humanitarian mapping" to develop targeting no-strike lists to minimize damage to infrastructure and protect innocent lives.[165] When questioned how the reconstruction of Iraq would be organized, a Department of State representative explained that those issues had not yet been worked out. He noted that in terms of detailed structural charts as to who would do what, no decisions had been made. He stated there was no framework as to how it would work, but "our position would be to facilitate as much as possible those involvements of a worldwide coalition on that."[166]

Analysis of the Implementation Plan

The evidence overwhelmingly indicated that all stakeholders participated in development and implementation of a pre-war plan to provide humanitarian assistance to Iraqis in the post-war aftermath. The sequencing of implementation was well defined in spite of only vague references to roles, responsibilities, mechanisms of action, and channels of communication between the Department of State and the Department of Defense, Central Command, the Coalition Joint Task Force, and the DOD Office of Reconstruction and Humanitarian Assistance (ORHA).

Although the implementation plan for humanitarian assistance was in place, very little immediate humanitarian assistance was needed in Iraq. Humanitarian assistance was only one part of the overall plan—regardless of which sets of plans one reviewed. The ORHA, which had only been in existence for two months prior to the beginning of the war, was tasked with developing an operational plan to integrate efforts to provide aid, establish civil-military

---

[164] Michael Marx, Disaster Response Team Leader, Office of U.S. Foreign Disaster Assistance, Briefing at the Foreign Press Center Building, Washington, DC, February 28, 2003.

[165] Joseph Collins, Deputy Assistant Secretary of Defense for Stability Operations, Briefing at the Foreign Press Center Building, Washington, DC, February 28, 2003.

[166] Richard Greene, Principal Deputy Assistant Secretary of State for Population, Refugees and Migration, Briefing at the Foreign Press Center Building, Washington, DC, February 28, 2003.

operations coordination centers, reconstruct Iraq, vet the Iraqi officials with whom they would work and eliminate WMD. The implementation plan for security and stability was never revealed. Based on the secondary analysis presented later in this chapter, there probably was not one.

Summary of Initial Analysis

A review of the policy process did not uncover evidence of stakeholder discourse and consensus building at each stage. Although there seemed to be agreement with regard to problem definition, analysis of the agenda setting stage revealed a difference in perspective between the departments. The Department of Defense agenda was based on operational objectives, to do certain things and leave, while the Department of State agenda was to "work" 17 different issues of concern that would lead to the long-term development of democratic institutions in Iraq. There was overlap in the agenda setting stage, as depicted in Table C-7. Even though the opportunities for discourse were not fully utilized, the researcher notes a partial consensus in this stage of the policy process as depicted in Table C-11.

With regard to the development of goals and options, the story is similar. The Department of State and Department of Defense shared the same goals, although for State, they were guiding principles (flexible,) while for Defense they were objectives (much more concrete.) There was confusion with regard to their end state or final outcome. For DOD, the goal was to complete the task and leave. For DOS, it was to stay and work long-term nation building projects. Given their missions, this was not surprising or unreasonable. However, given their missions, the Department of Defense should not have been given the lead in the reconstruction process.

During the option development and evaluation stages of policy development, extensive effort was exerted in post-war planning by a variety of government organizations. However, it was a dual planning system that was not successfully integrated through the interagency process. There is no indication of discourse between State and DOD with regard to issues other than humanitarian assistance. The conflict between State and DOD regarding the use of exiles to develop a new government in Iraq is well known. DOD went to Iraq believing the Iraqis would welcome the United States as liberators.[167] DOS did not make that assumption. The departments used sources of information that supported their opinions. There is no indication their vastly different assumptions were vetted in the interagency process at the National Security Council. The policy process, as statutorily defined, was not verified. A summary of the analysis is provided in Table C-11.

---

[167] United States Department of Defense, Background Briefing on Reconstruction and Humanitarian Assistance in Post-War Iraq. March 11, 2003. Available at http://www.defenselink.mil/news/Mar2003/t03122003_t031bgd.html.

TABLE C-11 Summary of Analysis of the Policy Process

Stages of the Policy Process	Indicators of Discourse and Consensus Building	Indicators of Discourse and Consensus Building
Problem Definition	Shared reality of the post-war process	Yes
Agenda Setting	Shared prioritization of necessary tasks for problem resolution	Partial
Goals	Shared end state	Partial
Option Development	Use of information to develop options	Partial
Evaluation of Options	Discussion of trade-offs	No
Implementation Plan	Participation of all stakeholders in the implementation process	Partial

Evidence from Secondary Sources

One of the most difficult tasks of the initial research was to cite only first person sources, primarily executive departmental personnel responsible for the post-war decision-making process. The review of public documents, tracing the policy process as it unfolded, was conducted in this manner to ensure objectivity of the results. However, additional information was available that shed light on the more extemporaneous thoughts of policy makers, during policy development. This researcher believes this analysis would not be complete without a discussion of information available to the researcher through secondary sources. These sources included analysis by academics, international relations practitioners, and defense policy analysts. Media outlets were used as secondary sources only in so far as they provided direct quotes from stakeholders.

Having previously determined that the policy process was not verified, in that it did not work as statutorily defined, the researcher gleaned additional evidence from secondary sources to indicate how the process broke down, presumably during the agenda setting stage of policy development. These sources contain historical accounts of the events that provide first hand discussion of what went wrong by the stakeholders involved. A synopsis of their retrospective analysis is depicted below.

Lack of Discourse

Jay Garner, the man charged with developing and administering the Office of Reconstruction and Humanitarian Assistance (ORHA) in Iraq, provided his perspective during a July 2003 interview with writers from the *Los Angeles Times*. Garner noted of DOD, DOS, USAID, Agriculture, Treasury, and Justice that, "Each one of them did their own planning … and they did it with the perspective of their own agency. What needed to happen was the horizontal integration of these plans." [168] He noted that Secretary of Defense Rumsfeld put ORHA together for this purpose. [169]

In a 2005 report published by the Hoover Institution, Tommy Franks, the commander of Central Command, commented on the lack of discourse between the Department of Defense and Department of State. He indicated that he wished that Secretary Rumsfeld and Secretary Powell had forced their respective departments to work better together, and he acknowledged the Pentagon's refusal to include the State Department in planning. Franks admitted to some degree of personal responsibility for the lack of discourse. He stated, "Uniformed military planners knew the command arrangements and were aware of the relative marginalization of the State Department in the process. They also knew how important it was that someone has responsibility for these types of political and economic tasks. In that sense, they were too willing to be quiet in the hope that somehow the problem would sort itself out." [170]

Air Force Lt. Col. Karen Swiatkowski, retired, who worked in the Pentagon's Near East Bureau, echoed this view. She noted military planners were allowed little contact with the DOD Office of Special Plans, and they often were told to ignore the State Department's concerns and views. Swiatkowski further explained the extent of the conflict, stating, "We almost disemboweled State." [171] Judith Yaphe, Senior Research Fellow and Middle East Project Director at the National Strategic Studies Institute, also supported this view. She noted "The Pentagon didn't want to touch anything connected to the Department of State." [172]

The work of the Future of Iraq Project at State Department was totally discounted by the DOD planners. David Phillips, a conflict management specialist with the Council on Foreign Relations and participant in the planning process, stated: "The Office of Special Plans discarded all of the Future of Iraq Project's

---

[168] Mark Fineman, Robin Wright and Doyle McManus, "Preparing for War, Stumbling to Peace," *Los Angeles Times*, July 18, 2003.

[169] Mark Fineman, Robin Wright and Doyle McManus, "Preparing for War, Stumbling to Peace," *Los Angeles Times*, July 18, 2003.

[170] Michael E. O'Hanlon, "Iraq Without a Plan," *Policy Review*, The Hoover Institution, January 2005.

[171] Jonathan Landay and Warren Strobel, "Lack of Planning Contributed to Chaos in Iraq," *The Kansas City Star*, July 12, 2003.

[172] David Rieff, "Blueprint for A Mess," *New York Times Magazine*, November 2, 2003.

FIGURE C-4 Breakdown of the policy process.

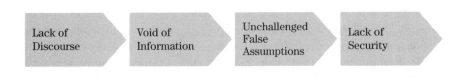

planning. I don't know why."[173] Two participants in the project described the events as follows: Isam Al Khafaji, a moderate Iraqi academic, stated, "What I had originally envisioned—working with allies in a democratic fashion—soon turned into collaborating with occupying forces." [174] He believed the project had been marginalized by the Pentagon's reliance on Ahmed Chalabi and the other Iraqi exiles.[175] Another participant, Feisal Istrabadi, noted "The Pentagon won the war in January and shunted us off to one side on the theory that they could re-invent in two months what we had done in ten months."[176]

Anthony Cordesman, a foreign policy analyst, blamed the lack of discourse on the entity that has statutory authority and accountability to negotiate the policy process. Cordesman stated, "We have to understand that it was the function of the NSC to ensure that the interagency process worked. Failure must be placed at the level of the NSC and the president."[177]

The Void of Information

As earlier noted by Jay Garner, the problem was not that planning did not occur, but that it had not been shared or integrated into an operational plan. General Anthony Zinni (Ret.), a former commander in the region, was critical of the lack of understanding of what was knowable. He stated, "We inherited Baghdad. You can't go in there without a plan, without understanding the scope of the problem: political, security, economic, humanitarian, reconstruction on the ground. We had no plan for that. And it was all knowable."[178] As noted in Chapter 1, General Zinni had previously written a plan for Iraq regime change.

---

[173] David Rieff, "Blueprint for A Mess," *New York Times Magazine*, November 2, 2003.

[174] David Rieff, "Blueprint for A Mess," *New York Times Magazine*, November 2, 2003.

[175] David Rieff, "Blueprint for A Mess," *New York Times Magazine*, November 2, 2003.

[176] Barbara Slavin and Dave Moniz, "War in Iraq's Aftermath Hits Troops Hard," *USA Today*, July 21, 03.

[177] Barbara Slavin and Dave Moniz, "War in Iraq's Aftermath Hits Troops Hard," *USA Today*, July 21, 03.

[178] Union-Tribune's Editorial Board, "Q and A: Anthony Zinni," *San Diego Union Tribune*, April 16, 2004.

Paul Dicker, an Army War College student, reviewed the unclassified information available to planners prior to initiation of combat in Iraq and determined there was ample information to predict a need for additional security forces.[179] The pre-war documentation of potential post-war problems included, but was not limited to the following sources. First, a review, conducted by the Marine Warfighting Laboratory in January 2003, stated the number one critical capability for operational success in Iraq would be the ability to maintain a secure environment, followed by return of basic necessities and return of infrastructure responsibility to Iraqis.

Second, in April 2002 the Future of Iraq Project predicted widespread looting and criminal activity. It recommended security patrols in all major cities to protect the infrastructure. Third, an independent task force sponsored by the Council on Foreign Relations released a report in March 2003, which forecast the need for military forces to sustain a secure environment. Finally, Bathsheba Crocker of the Center for International and Strategic Studies predicted the need for civil policing in January 2003.[180] It should also be noted that Dr. Phebe Marr, an Iraq specialist, testified before the Senate Foreign Relations Committee in August 2002 that: "If firm leadership is not in place in Baghdad 'the day after' Saddam is removed, retribution, score settling, and blood letting, especially in urban areas, could take place."[181]

During the evidentiary search this researcher did not review any documents produced by the intelligence community. One secondary source reports Bill Harlow, a CIA spokesman, stated, "The U.S. intelligence community warned early and often about myriad threats it anticipated at the onset of the war and the challenges likely to erupt in the postwar environment."[182] Harlow also noted that intelligence officials were "utterly consistent in arguing that reconstruction rather than war would be the most problematic segment of overthrowing Saddam's regime."[183]

Evidence of False Assumptions

Larry Diamond, Senior Advisor to the Coalition Provisional Authority (CPA) in Baghdad, provides a personal perspective of events. He opines that

---

[179] Paul F. Dicker, "Effectiveness of Stability Operations During the Initial Implementation of the Transition Phase for Operation Iraqi Freedom," March 19, 2004.

[180] Paul F. Dicker, "Effectiveness of Stability Operations During the Initial Implementation of the Transition Phase for Operation Iraqi Freedom," March 19, 2004.

[181] Phebe Marr, Testimony before the Senate Foreign Relations Committee, August 1, 2002.

[182] Mark Fineman, Robin Wright and Doyle McManus, "Preparing for War, Stumbling to Peace," *Los Angeles Times*, July 18, 2003.

[183] Mark Fineman, Robin Wright and Doyle McManus, "Preparing for War, Stumbling to Peace," *Los Angeles Times*, July 18, 2003.

Administration planners were not willing to commit the resources needed for security, and that they never understood or included the people they sought to liberate in the decision-making process. He further noted that Pentagon planners were "contemptuous of the State Department's regional experts who were seen as 'too soft' to remake Iraq."[184] Diamond claims they ignored the detailed planning of the Future of Iraq Project, which had predicted many of the postwar problems. They did not prepare for the worst, but assumed that Iraqis would welcome U.S. troops as liberators. The plan was regime change, followed by handing the country over to expatriates such as Ahmed Chalabi."[185] General John Keane who retired in July 2003 expressed the view that Pentagon leaders were "seduced by the Iraqi exiles in terms of what the outcome would be."[186]

Even National Security Advisor Condoleezza Rice believed that it was just a matter of bringing in new leadership. She stated, "The concept was that we would defeat the army, but the institutions would hold—everything from ministries to police forces."[187] With regard to the government infrastructure, Rice indicated a belief that: "You would be able to bring new leadership but that we were going to keep the body in place."[188] Jim Dobbins a Rand Corporation analyst, defined the problem as follows: "It's not true there wasn't adequate planning. There was a volume of planning … They planned on an unrealistic set of assumptions."[189]

Lack of Security

Failed planning based on faulty assumptions can directly be tied to an unintended policy outcome—the lack of security in post-war Iraq. A lack of discourse allowed Pentagon officials to ignore information that was inconsistent with their perspective. Anthony Cordesman, a policy analyst with the Center for Strategic and International Studies, noted that policymaker's were not interested in intelligence warnings about post-war difficulties and "may sometimes have discouraged such analysis."[190] The result was a lack of preparation by the uniformed services to adequately secure the country. Maj. General Buford Blound, Commander of the Army's 3rd Infantry Division, noted that "Looting

---

[184] Larry Diamond, "What Went Wrong in Iraq," *Foreign Affairs*, September/October, 2004.

[185] Larry Diamond, "What Went Wrong in Iraq," *Foreign Affairs*, September/October, 2004.

[186] John Keane, Testimony before the House Armed Services Committee, July 15, 2004.

[187] Michael R. Gordon, "The Strategy to Secure Iraq Did Not Foresee a 2nd War," *New York Times*, October 19, 2004.

[188] Michael R. Gordon, "The Strategy to Secure Iraq Did Not Foresee a 2nd War," *New York Times*, October 19, 2004.

[189] Mark Fineman, Robin Wright and Doyle McManus, "Preparing for War, Stumbling to Peace," *Los Angeles Times*, July 18, 2003.

[190] John Diamond, "Prewar Intelligence Predicted Iraqi Insurgency," *USA Today*, October 24, 2004.

wasn't taken into military consideration ... It never came in the order process that it would be a major problem."[191] One army colonel said "We were trying to clear out the bad guys, provide security and restart the government. Nobody ever taught us how to do that."[192]

The policy outcome of this policy failure was massive looting, followed by insurgency. Jay Garner, chief of the ORHA, views the events as follows: "I think that there were Ba'athist Sunnis who planned to resist no matter what happened and at all cost, but we missed opportunities, and that drove more of them into the resistance." He further notes, "Things were stirred up far more than they should have been. We did not seal the borders because we did not have enough troops to do that, and that brought in terrorists."[193] In another interview, Garner expressed his frustration at the instability brought on by a lack of post-war security. He stated, "If you're not there, the vacuum gets filled in ways you don't want."[194] He further noted the planning process was for immediate restoration of government services, but when the ORHA personnel arrived the government was not there any more because of the looting.[195]

The Senior Advisor to the CPA admits, "We just weren't honest with ourselves or with the American people about what was going to be needed to secure the country." He noted that Iraq was a security nightmare that did not have to happen and that nothing else is possible because of the lack of security. He viewed the lack of security as directly affecting coalition goals, stating, "You can't develop democracy without security."[196]

A policy analyst at the Hoover Institution, summarizes the outcome as follows: "Invading another country with the intention of destroying its existing government, yet without a serious strategy for providing security thereafter defies logic and falls short of proper professional military standards of competence. It was in fact unconscionable."[197]

Perhaps the most surprising evidence was the statements of the individual most responsible for DOD's pre-war plans for post-war Iraq. In July 2003, Douglas Feith, Under Secretary of the Department of Defense for Policy, offered: "War, like life in general, always involves trade-offs." He further countered, "It's not right to assume that any in Iraq can be attributed to poor

[191] Barbara Slavin and Dave Moniz, "War in Iraq's Aftermath Hits Troops Hard," *USA Today*, July 21, 03.

[192] Mark Fineman, Robin Wright and Doyle McManus, "Preparing for War, Stumbling to Peace," *Los Angeles Times*, July 18, 2003.

[193] Michael R. Gordon, "The Strategy to Secure Iraq Did Not Foresee a 2nd War," *New York Times*, October 19, 2004.

[194] David Rieff, "Blueprint for a Mess," *New York Times Magazine*, November 2, 2003.

[195] David Rieff, "Blueprint for a Mess," *New York Times Magazine*, November 2, 2003.

[196] James Sterngold, "Stanford Expert Says Iraq Spinning Out of Control," *San Francisco Chronicle*, April 25, 2004.

[197] Michael E. O'Hanlon, "Iraq Without a Plan," *Policy Review*, The Hoover Institution, January, 2005.

planning."[198] A year later, Feith maintained that planners anticipated disorder and looting but determined other risks such as oil field fires, refugees, and hunger were more dangerous. He viewed the situation as a viable trade-off of resources. Feith stated, "Nobody expected this to be immaculate. Everybody expected that this was going to be a war and that there was going to be an aftermath and the aftermath was going to be … untidy."[199]

Summary of Policy Verification

An initial search of primary sources, public documents, revealed a lack of stakeholder discourse and consensus building during all but one stage of the policy process. The researcher searched secondary sources for evidence that would either support or refute this analysis. However, statements of the stakeholders, both State and Defense personnel, confirm the initial finding of a dual planning process that did not integrate discourse to support the policy process.

As noted in Chapter 2, the National Security Council is the official point of discourse between the Secretary of State and the Secretary of Defense in negotiating foreign and military policy.[200] Ideally, interagency teams work within the NSC framework, negotiating and coordinating policy that is administered by the National Security Advisor. In the pre-war planning for post-war Iraq, the policy process broke down during the agenda setting stage, and the National Security Council failed to adequately synthesize interagency discourse to support the policy process.

This lack of discourse allowed the Department of Defense to ignore information that was not consistent with its perspective. As noted earlier, DOD personnel were prohibited from participating in the Future of Iraq Project as early as April 2002. Contemptuous of Department of State experts, Pentagon planners later discarded all information obtained through the Future of Iraq Project. The failure of the NSC to force a synthesis of discussion had a direct bearing on policy outcomes, particularly with regard to security and stability operations.

The Role of Stakeholder Differences in the Policy Process

Chapter 3 presented the methodology for analysis of stakeholder differences in the policy process. It was hypothesized that institutional differences between the Department of State and the Department of Defense in their missions,

---

[198] Jonathan Landay and Warren Strobel, "Lack of Planning Contributed to Chaos in Iraq," *The Kansas City Star*, July 12, 2003.

[199] Mark Fineman, Robin Wright and Doyle McManus, "Preparing for War, Stumbling to Peace," *Los Angeles Times*, July 18, 2003.

[200] U.S. Code, Title 50, *National Security Act of 1947*, Section 101.

core values, structures, culture, use of information and training impeded the development of effective post-war policy.

The first task was to determine if any of these differences were apparent during the review. An evidentiary examination of the literature finds that differences of structure, culture, and use of information did appear during the policy process. The researcher did not find evidence of the other institutional differences mentioned above. This is not to say they were not present, but they were not noted during the archival review of public documents. The following examples depict the institutional differences noted during the policy process.

- Structural differences are noted during the February 11, 2003 testimony of Marc Grossman and Douglas Feith, when they present differing views of the agenda setting process. Feith reveals that five DOD teams are planning for an invasion, task completion, and quick return of the country to Iraqis' authority and accountability. This concept of control is part of the DOD structure. Grossman, on the other hand, notes an extensive network of 17 working groups, and the Future of Iraq Project, designed around the concept of engagement with free Iraqis. He further notes that his testimony should be treated as a consultation, because some policies were still under discussion. This closely parallels DOS's tendency to structure work around functional issues of engagement.
- Cultural differences, particularly relating to the tendency of DOS employees to think and analyze and their DOD counterparts to plan and operationalize, are noted when Feith states that the intention of the DOD planners is not "to theorize, but to do practical work."[201]
- With regard to their use of information, Department of State planners were very inclusive of their sources of information, involving as many individuals as possible in the agenda setting process. The DOD Office of Special Plans excluded even uniformed military planners from providing input.
- Another cultural difference is noted at the goal setting stage of the policy process, when the Department of State refers to the five "guiding principles," as though they are flexible mechanisms that will evolve with time. The same list is referred to by the Department of Defense as objectives, which would be carried out by coalition forces, working in conjunction with the DOD Office of Reconstruction and Humanitarian Assistance. In that same testimony, he provided the authorities and chain of command for the operation.[202]

---

[201] Douglas Feith, Under Secretary of Defense, Testimony before the Senate Foreign Relations Committee, February 11, 2003.

[202] Douglas Feith, Under Secretary of Defense, Testimony before the Senate Foreign Relations Committee, February 11, 2003.

- Another difference is that of DOS's preference for engagement (opening the process) vs. DOD's preference for accountability (closing the process) in their method of doing work. This was evidenced in the goal setting stage when DOS personnel included a broad representation of free Iraqis and international organizations in the planning process. DOD relied on a small number of Iraqi exiles, who emphasized only a minimal need for post-war security. This allowed the military to plan for regime change, a brief occupation, and a quick exit strategy.
- Cultural differences again presented as DOS personnel thought through reconstruction needs, while DOD personnel determined they were unknowable and thus not apt for planning—end of discussion.
- The discussion of an implementation plan revealed additional cultural differences, perhaps based on how the stakeholders viewed their own institutional structures. The Department of State version of an implementation plan was stated in functional terms: stabilization, followed by transition of authority, followed by transformation. DOD's discussion revolved around the creation of the ORHA by the president and the responsibility of the CENTCOM Commander to administer post-war policy. When a State Department official was asked about the organization for reconstruction activities, he noted there was not a framework, but the DOS would "facilitate as much as possible those involvements of a worldwide coalition on that."[203]

It is clear from the review of evidence that institutional differences of the Department of State and the Department of Defense conditioned each organization to approach the policy process in a different manner. As noted in Chapter 3, the DOS tended to be more flexible, open to new information, aware of the importance of sustained engagement, and looking for effective solutions that included the international community. DOD used the planning process to determine strategic objectives and operational plans that were based on chain of command, decisive victory, and departure from the area of responsibility.

The most surprising outcome of this analysis was to search through volumes of documents that revealed ample evidence of institutional differences, to look deeper into stakeholder roles, interactions and the organizational differences, and to determine that ultimately they had no meaning. Although the evidence of differences is clear, and those differences conditioned each organization to approach the policy process differently, *there was no evidence that those differences impacted the policy outcome.* Even when conflict emerged, it does not appear that it affected the policy outcome because it was not negotiated. For example, as noted by Anthony Cordesman earlier in this chapter, the

---

[203] Richard Greene, Principal Deputy Assistant Secretary of State for Population, Refugees and Migration, Briefing at the Foreign Press Center Building, Washington, DC, February 28, 2003.

Pentagon discouraged analysis that was inconsistent with its plans. As noted earlier, General Franks, the Commander of Central Command, admitted the Pentagon refused to include the Department of State in the planning process and discarded plans provided by the Future of Iraq Project.

The evidence supports a conclusion that the differences between these stakeholders, primarily in their organizational cultures, led to differences in their approach to agenda setting, development of goals, development of options, and development of an implementation plan. However, this dual planning process in and of itself did not impede the policy process. The impediment was that the differences in assumptions, arising from the differences in planning, were not synthesized or negotiated in an interagency process. As noted earlier that is the responsibility of the National Security Council and the National Security Advisor to the President. Simply, there is no evidence that the National Security Council or the National Security Advisor attempted to negotiate or synthesize differences with regard to security and stability operations. This is telling because as previously noted, measures were required by the President for humanitarian assistance and reconstruction activities. There is no evidence the same level of oversight was present with regard to security operations.

To explain further, one must look at the alternate hypothesis. If the cultural and institutional differences did not exist, would the stakeholders have produced a different policy product? The evidence portrays a Department of Defense that did not encourage or accept information from other stakeholders in the policy process. The evidence includes a Secretary of Defense who did not believe in planning for unknown contingencies and a planning staff that did not value dissenting views. And, the evidence reveals that the Department of Defense shut out input from the Department of State planning process as early as July 2002. Referring to previous chapters, the DOS Future of Iraq Project began in April 2002, while the DOD planning process began in July 2002. The CENTCOM operational plan was dusted off from General Zinni's tenure as Commander, and while the command waited for the final word from the Pentagon regarding post-war stability operations, major conflict was initiated. As noted earlier, as late as May 2003, the plans were not formalized for post-war action.

Using the logic of Allison and Zelikow, reported in Chapter 2, there is far more evidence to conclude that the policy outcome was what it was because of who came to the game than there is evidence to conclude that the policy process was impeded by organizational differences. In their explanation of who comes to the game, Allison and Zelikow note that in addition to positions, players have personalities, operating styles and histories. They further state, these "peculiarities of human beings remain an irreducible part of the mix."[204]

---

[204] Graham Allison and Philip Zelikow, *Essence of Decision: Explaining the Cuban Missile Crisis*, 2nd ed. (New York: Addison-Wesley Educational Publishers, Inc., 1999), 296–298.

The evidence supports the conclusion that the development of post-war policy was going to be exactly what it was, regardless of meetings, regardless of discourse, regardless of attempts to integrate other players into the discussion. The development of post-war policy was going to be what the Secretary of Defense, who excluded outsiders and other stakeholders from the decision-making process, determined it would be. What is unclear is whether the decisions of the Secretary of Defense were questioned by the National Security Council, the National Security Advisor, or approved by the President. In this regard, only the declassification of presidential documents will provide that information.

With regard to Secretary Rumsfeld, even after the chaos ensued in Iraq, he denied that poor planning had any bearing on the inability of U.S. soldiers to stop the looting. He stated: "Freedom's untidy, and free people are free to make mistakes and commit crimes and do bad things. They're also free to live their lives and do wonderful things, and that's what's going to happen here."[205]

Summary of the Research Objectives

This chapter analyzed the pre-war policy process for post-war Iraq by tracing the stages of the policy process, observing evidence of stakeholder differences and interactions, and searching for indications that the National Security Council arbitrated these differences. Using the pre-war policy process as the unit of analysis, the researcher determined that the process did not work as it was statutorily designed to work, and was not verified. Evidence collected and noted during this review was used as a starting point for analysis of the impact of stakeholder differences on the policy process. The researcher determined that institutional differences, although present during policy development, did not impact the policy process in a manner that affected policy outcomes or implementation plans. Two research hypotheses were tested:

1. Institutional differences between the Department of State and the Department of defense in their missions, core values, structures, culture, use of information, and training impeded the development of effective post-war policy.
2. The National Security Council failed to adequately synthesize interagency discourse to support the policy process.

Hypothesis number one was not supported. Although numerous indications of institutional differences were evidenced, it is impossible to determine that these differences had any impact what so ever in the development of post-war policy.

The evidence supports hypothesis number two, in that the National Security Council did not synthesize interagency discourse to support the policy process.

---

[205] James Fallows, "Blind into Baghdad," *The Atlantic Monthly*, January/February, 2004.

Chapter 5 provides a summary of the findings of this research and places these findings in a theoretical framework that sheds light on the meaning of these conclusions. The researcher also notes the limitations of this study and makes recommendations for further inquiry and analysis.

CHAPTER 5: FINDINGS AND CONCLUSIONS

Overview of Research Objectives and Conclusions

The unit of analysis for this study, the pre-war policy process for post-war Iraq, was submitted to a qualitative analysis using the technique of process tracing. The policy process was primarily managed by the Department of Defense and the policy outcome relied on certain assumptions that later proved to be false. The unintended consequences of the failed policy were a lack of preparation for post-war realities and an insurgency that threatens the reconstruction process.

The post–Cold War trend of using the U.S. military in "other than war operations"[206] has changed the roles and responsibilities of the Departments of State and Defense, executive departments that represent two of the nation's instruments of power. The research explored the national security decision-making process, noting the changing structure of the process and the evolution of civil-military affairs. Institutional differences between the Department of State and the Department of Defense were defined, as was the national mechanism to synthesize discourse between these organizations, the National Security Council. The roles of the President and Congress to oversee the functions of foreign policy and defense were also noted. This contextual framework was used to develop two hypotheses:

1. Institutional differences between the Department of State and the Department of Defense in their missions, structures, core values, culture, use of information, and training impeded the development of effective post-war policy.
2. The National Security Council failed to synthesize interagency discourse to support the policy process.

The researcher incorporated an archival review of public documents to trace the policy process. The researcher first sought to determine if the policy process could be verified, or did it work as it was statutorily designed to work. Did the National Security Council effectively synthesize interagency discourse to support the policy process? Second, the researcher searched for evidence of institutional differences between these executive branch departments to determine if those differences impeded the policy process.

---

[206] Dana Priest, *The Mission* (New York: W.W. Norton & Company, 2003), 41–57.

The researcher determined that the policy process did not work as it was statutorily designed to work and, thus, was not verified. Hypothesis two was supported by evidence of a dual planning process, with very little discourse between the two planning groups.

With regard to hypothesis one, there was ample evidence of institutional differences between the Departments of State and Defense. There was also evidence that these differences conditioned each organization's approach to the policy process. However, in a surprising outcome, the evidence did not support the hypothesis that institutional differences impeded the policy process. This was because the personal characteristics of the Secretary of Defense and his impact on the policy process seemed to outweigh other policy inputs. Donald Rumsfeld closed the Department of State out of the policy process as early as July 2002 and as late as January 2003.

As noted by Allison and Zelikow, the "peculiarities of human beings remain an irreducible part of the mix."[207] Tony Klucking discussed the importance of policy participants in his dissertation. In his analysis of the Defense Reorganization Act of 1986 using Kingdon's policy streams model, Klucking noted that the although the problem, policy, politics process and policy window impact policy development, a fifth component, participants, are too significant to be ignored.[208]

This researcher failed to address the importance of stakeholder values in the analysis process. Values, derived from roles and interests, as well as historical analogies and personal characteristics, may explain how facts are integrated into the decision-making process. Although the researcher considered the role of values when designing the study, she eliminated values as a variable because they are methodologically difficult to prove and because the Iraq case has already been subjected to much discussion of the influence of "neo-conservative" values in the Bush Administration, and hence the policy process. Also, the Iraq policy process was subjected to oversight by many bi-partisan congressional committees that did not find it so objectionable as to impede its implementation.

Two other limitations of the analysis are noted. First, the sources of evidence were incomplete because the researcher did not access classified documents that might have provided additional details of the policy process. Second, the researcher did not have access to the meetings of the working groups and interagency teams, other than through the testimony and historical recollections of stakeholders before congressional committees and the media, respectively. However, this said, the researcher does not believe either of these limitations is significant enough to discount what can be learned by tracing

---

[207] Graham Allison and Philip Zelikow, *Essence of Decision: Explaining the Cuban Missile Crisis*, 2nd ed. (New York: Addison-Wesley Educational Publishers, Inc., 1999), 296–298.
[208] Tony V. Klucking, "Kingdon on Defense: An Analysis of the Policy Streams Approach and a Policy Streams Analysis of the Goldwater-Nichols Act," (Auburn University, 2003), 73.

the public documents available in the ongoing development of post-war Iraq policy. As noted by Allison and Zelikow, as information is declassified, new information will sharpen the analysis.[209] However, immediate lessons learned have practical application in the current environment.

What Went Wrong?

Much of what went wrong in Iraq can be traced to the false assumptions of the DOD planning groups, particularly with regard to Iraqis greeting U.S. forces as liberators, as noted in Chapter 1. Robert Gates, a former CIA analyst and later Director of Central Intelligence, notes that decision makers sometimes attempt to insert their beliefs and values into the information process, and that results in "policy pitfalls."[210] Two of those pitfalls mentioned by Gates were attempts by policy makers to use intelligence to support decisions already made, and labeling information as "incomplete" or "soft" if it didn't agree with the policy makers' policy preferences. There is some evidence of this in the Iraq case, as DOD developed its own intelligence analysis office to review and take another look at the reports of CIA analysts.[211] Its reliance on one source of information, Iraqi exiles, led to false assumptions on the part of the Department of Defense planners. These assumptions, ultimately, led to the lack of preparation by U.S. forces to engage in security and stability operations in Iraq.

Secondly, one cannot ignore the failure of the National Security Council to integrate information and discussions that occurred in the two stove-piped planning processes. Also, there is no evidence to indicate that the National Security Advisor discussed with the President the trade-offs if the DOD security assumptions were wrong. The Secretary of Defense, in effect, circumvented the consensus building interagency process prescribed by law, and the National Security Advisor and the President did not hold him accountable for that circumvention. This entire portion of the national security decision-making process was ineffective.

Third, although DOD was well within its traditional role and mission to enter Iraq to effect regime change, it was not acting in its traditional role when, well before the initiation of combat, it assumed responsibility for the nation-building actions of the Office of Reconstruction and Humanitarian Assistance. Congressional committees heard repeated nondescript testimony from DOD personnel regarding the scope, longevity, and cost of reconstruction operations. Congress has a history of looking the other way with regard to military

---

[209] Graham Allison and Philip Zelikow, *Essence of Decision: Explaining the Cuban Missile Crisis*, 2nd ed. (New York: Addison-Wesley Educational Publishers, Inc., 1999), vi.

[210] Robert M. Gates, "The CIA and American Foreign Policy," *Foreign Affairs*, Winter, 1987/88, 215–230.

[211] Douglas J. Feith, Under Secretary for Policy, DoD Briefing on Policy and Intelligence Matters, June 4, 2003.

plans and in this case they once again did not stop or delay military action until a more detailed plan was developed. The checks and balances system put in place by the founding fathers failed to ensure accountability.

One possible reason for congressional inattention to the matter was that there did not appear to be a central repository of facts regarding post-war planning. For example, testimony before the Senate Foreign Relations Committee might not have been reviewed by the Senate Banking Committee, and so forth. This means that most committees only saw the portion of post-war planning that pertained to their area of concern and were not able to discern that the overall plan was lacking. Two committees, the House Permanent Select Committee on Intelligence and the Senate Select Committee on Intelligence, may have received a more detailed overview of the pre-war planning process. However, the nature of these committees and the classification of testimony before these committees make it impossible to know for sure the complete extent of information that was provided to Congress until those documents are declassified. Based on the experience of Graham Allison and Philip Zelikow in their analysis of the Cuban Missile Crisis, it was thirty years before the final documents were declassified and all the pieces of the official record could be submitted for analysis.

What Does This Mean?

For starters, it is just as important to disprove a hypothesis as to find evidence that supports it, particularly with regard to organizational culture. Much has been made of the institutional differences between the Department of State and Department of Defense. In this particular case, the differences, although obvious and pronounced, did not equate to problems. Instead it was the stovepiped planning processes rather than the differences between the processes that impeded the policy process. Different is okay, not talking about the differences is not!

Second, the national security decision-making process was, for lack of a better term, hijacked by one entity within the Administration. The ability of one group to develop and implement policy without consensus from other stakeholders must be stopped and safeguards must be invented to prevent this from happening again.

Third, new plans for "Joint Operations Concepts" must account for institutionalization of the joint concept. Defense Secretary Donald Rumsfeld recently noted that the 2005 Quadrennial Defense Review must take a broader view of future challenges and give greater weight to the role of other federal agencies, nongovernmental organizations and coalition partners.[212] Joint Operation

---

[212] "Rumsfeld Shifts QDR's Direction, Broadens Focus on Terrorism, WMD," *Inside the Pentagon,* February 10, 2005. Available at http://ebird.afis.osd.mil/ebfiles/e20050211351214.html.

Concepts dictate that each command headquarters will have a Joint Interagency Coordination Group to harmonize campaign planning and achieve a unity of effort between civilian and military departments and agencies.[213] Additionally, plans are being discussed to implement a 2000 finding by the Center for the Study of the Presidency, which recommended additional synergy between commanders and state department personnel. These recommendations included:

- Joint education and training mechanisms for future leaders
- Strengthening regional cooperation, beginning with relationships in Washington
- Deployment of State Department's regional expertise to the field
- Establishment of a Regional Planning Center, staffed by both state and defense personnel
- Deployment of both a flag officer and an equivalent civilian to support both the regional commander and the regional assistant secretary of state.[214]

Finally, the Department of State is developing a new Reconstruction and Stability Office to assist in future activities. Although these reform measures may be helpful, creating new mechanisms are not meaningful if the constructs are not institutionalized in the concept of operations.

In March 2004, the Center for Strategic and International Studies released a report entitled: "Beyond Goldwater-Nichols: Defense Reform for a New Strategic Era." In this report they noted little unity of effort in planning and conduct of interagency and coalition operations resulted in inadequate capacity for complex planning. They recommended that the NSC should establish an office for stability operations and that an entire new agency should be established to meet this need. The report is summarized by the researcher as, "We've done joint, but we still lack effectiveness."

Recommendations for Further Study

As planning documents are declassified, many others will review the pre-war planning process for post-war Iraq. This researcher has several recommendations for those reviews. First, the planning process for humanitarian assistance is well documented, and so it should be used as a point of comparison only in future studies. This is because it does not add anything to the discussion. Both DOS and DOD planning groups identified the concern for humanitarian relief in their problem definitions and this is one of the areas in which the stakeholders

---

[213] U.S. Army, "Draft Blueprint for Future Joint Operations Could Be Ready in April," February 9, 2005. Available at http://www.InsideDefense.com.

[214] Center for the Study of the Presidency, "Forward Strategic Empowerment: Synergies between CINCs, the State Department, and Other Agencies," August, 2000.

seemed to engage in discourse and consensus building. Far more is to gain from deep analysis of the areas in which discourse and consensus building did not occur, and perhaps comparing the planning process for humanitarian assistance, which worked well in comparison to these failures. This researcher opines that the post-war humanitarian assistance planning process worked as it should because the planners had agreement on pre-war assumptions.

Second, the researcher recognizes the invaluable resource of minutes for the working group meetings. When it becomes possible to access those minutes, a Freedom of Information Act (FOIA) request is in order. Once in hand, the minutes should be subjected to a content analysis of words and phrases. It is believed by this researcher that they may shed additional light on linguistic patterns that can be used to assess future planning activities of the stakeholders.

Finally, it would be interesting to compare the post-war planning process for Operation Enduring Freedom with that of Operation Iraqi Freedom. The same set of actors showed up for the process. One operation succeeded and the other was problematic. What made the difference?

BIBLIOGRAPHY

Abizaid, Lt. Gen. John. CENTCOM Operation Iraqi Freedom Briefing, March 23, 2003. Available at http://www.globalsecurity.org/wmd/library/news/iraq/2003/iraq-030323-centcom02.htm.

Abrams, Elliot. Senior NSC Director for Near East and North Africa, Briefing on Humanitarian Reconstruction Issues, February 24, 2003.

Adams, Ron. Deputy Director, ORHA, Briefing on Humanitarian Reconstruction Issues, February 24, 2003.

Allison, Graham. "Conceptual Models and the Cuban Missile Crisis," *American Political Science Review*, Vol. 63: (3), 1969.

Allison, Graham, and Philip Zelikow, *Essence of Decision: Explaining the Cuban Missile Crisis*, 2nd ed., New York: Addison-Wesley Educational Publishers, Inc., 1999.

Armitage, Richard L. Prepared Statement before the Senate Committee on Foreign Relations, May 18, 2004.

Bennett, Andrew, and Alexander L. George, "Process Tracing in Case Study Research," A paper presented at the MacArthur Foundation Workshop on Case Study Methods, Harvard University, October 17–19, 1997.

Berger, Peter L. and Thomas Luckman. *The Social Construction of Reality: A Treatise in the Sociology of Knowledge.* New York, NY: Anchor Books, 1966.

Biden, Joseph R. Jr., Senator, "The Future of Iraq," Hearing of the Senate Foreign Relations Committee, February 11, 2003.

Blair, Tony. Prime Minister of Great Britain, Testimony before Parliament, April 14, 2003.

Bolton, Joshua. Director of the Office of Management and Budget, Testimony before the Senate Foreign Relations Committee, July 29, 2003.

Burkhart, Ross E., and Michael S. Lewis-Beck, "Comparative Democracy," *American Political Science Review*, Vol. 88, 1994.

Bush, George W. Message to the Iraqi People, April 10, 2003.

————. Speech at the American Enterprise Institute, February 26, 2003.

Center for the Study of the Presidency, "Forward Strategic Empowerment: Synergies between CINC's, the State Department, and Other Agencies," August, 2001.

Chairman of the Joint Chiefs of Staff, "Theater Security Cooperation Planning," Draft, Joint Publication 5-0, Doctrine for Planning Joint Operations, December, 2002.

Clark, Robert P., Jr., *Development and Instability, Political Change in the Non-Western World*. Hindale, Illinois: The Dryden Press, 1974.

Clausewitz, Carl von. *On War*, Edited and translated by Michael Howard and Peter Parent. Princeton, NJ: Princeton University Press, 1989.

Collins, Joseph. Deputy Assistant Secretary of Defense for Stability Operations, Briefing on Humanitarian Reconstruction Issues, February 24, 2003.

————. Deputy Assistant Secretary of Defense for Stability Operations, Briefing at the Foreign Press Center Building, Washington, DC, February 28, 2003.

Conlin, Christopher C. "What Do You Do for an Encore?" *Marine Corps Gazette*, September, 2004.

Cummins, Chip. "Export, Storage Troubles Snarl Iraq's Oil Industry," *The Wall Street Journal*, May 7, 2003.

Dahl, Robert A. *On Democracy*. New Haven: Yale University Press, 1998.

DeLeon, Peter. "Models of policy discourse: Insights versus prediction," *Policy Studies Journal*, Vol. 26, 1998.

Dewey, Gene. Assistant Secretary of State for Population, Refugees and Migration, Briefing on Humanitarian Reconstruction Issues, February 24, 2003.

Diamond, John. "Prewar Intelligence predicted Iraqi Insurgency," *USA Today*, October 24, 2004.

Diamond, Larry. "What Went Wrong in Iraq," *Foreign Affairs*, September/October, 2004.

Dicker, Paul F. "Effectiveness of Stability Operations during the Initial Implementation of the Transition Phase for Operation Iraqi Freedom," March 19, 2004.

Eland, Ivan. 'Turning Point' in the War in Iraq: But Which Way Is It Turning?" November 19, 2003. Available at http://www.independent.org/tii/antiwar/e111903.html.

Fallows, James. "Blind into Baghdad," *The Atlantic Monthly*. January/February, 2004.

Feil, Scott R. Testimony before the Senate Foreign Relations Committee, February 11, 2003.

Feith, Douglas J., Under Secretary of Defense for Policy. DoD Briefing on Policy and Intelligence Matters, June 4, 2003.

————. Testimony before the Committee on International Relations, U.S. House of Representatives, May 15, 2003.

————. "The Future of Iraq," Hearing of the Senate Foreign Relations Committee, February 11, 2003.

Fineman, Mark, Robin Wright and Doyle McManus, "Preparing for War, Stumbling to Peace," *Los Angeles Times*, July 18, 2003.

Friedrich, Carl. "Public Policy and the Nature of Administrative Responsibility," in *Public Policy*, Carl J. Friedrich (Vol. Ed.), Cambridge, MA: Harvard University Press, 1940.

Gates, Robert M. "The CIA and American Foreign Policy," *Foreign Affairs*, 66: (2), (Winter, 1987/88).

Gordon, Michael R. "The Strategy to Secure Iraq Did Not Foresee a 2nd War," *New York Times*, October 19, 2004.

Greene, Richard. Principal Deputy Assistant Secretary of State for Population, Refugees and Migration, Briefing at the Foreign Press Center Building, Washington, DC, February 28, 2003.

Grossman, Marc I., Under Secretary of State for Political Affairs, "The Future of Iraq," Hearing of the Senate Foreign Relations Committee, February 11, 2003.

Hadley, Stephen. Deputy National Security Advisor, Speech at the Council on Foreign Relations, February 12, 2003.

Hartwick, Douglas A. "The Culture at State, the Services, and Military Operations: Bridging the Communication Gap," National Defense University, 1994.

Hass, Richard N. "Defining U.S. Foreign Policy in a Post–Cold War World," U.S. Department of State, 2002.

Jefferies, Chris. "Bureaucratic Politics in the Department of Defense: A Practitioner's Perspective." *Bureaucratic Politics and National Security*, Edited by David C. Lozak and James M. Keagle, Bolder, CO: Lynne Rienner, 1988.

Joint Pub 3-0, Doctrine for Joint Operations. Washington, DC: Joint Chiefs of Staff, 2001.

Katz, Stanley N. "Gun Barrel Democracy? Democratic Constitutionalism Following Military Occupation: Reflections on the U.S. Experience," *Princeton Working Papers*, No. 04-010.

Keane, John. Testimony before the House Armed Services Committee, July 15, 2004.

King, Gary, Robert O. Keohane, and Sidney Verba. *Designing Social Inquiry: Scientific Inference in Qualitative Research*. Princeton, NJ: Princeton University Press, 1994.

Klucking, Tony V., "Kingdon on Defense: An Analysis of the Policy Streams Approach and a Policy Streams Analysis of the Goldwater-Nichols Act." Washington, DC: Storming Media, 2003, 73.

Landay, Jonathan, and Warren Strobel, "Lack of Planning Contributed to Chaos in Iraq," *The Kansas City Star*, July 12, 2003.

Larson, Alan P. Under Secretary for Economic, Business, and Agriculture Affairs, Testimony before the House International Relations Committee, May 15, 2003.

Lijphart, Arend. "Comparative Politics and the Comparative Method," *American Political Science Review*, Vol. 65: (3), 1971.

Lin, Ann Chih. "Bridging Positivist and Interpretivist Approaches to Qualitative Methods," *Policy Studies Journal*, Vol. 26: (1), 1998.

Lindblom, Charles E. "The Science of Muddling Through," *Public Administration Review*, Vol. 19:(2), 1959.

Madison, James. *The Federalist Papers*, as accessed on December 15, 2004. Available at http://www.federalistpapers.com.

Marcella, Gabriel. "National Security and the Interagency Process: Forward Into the 21st Century," *Organizing for National Security*, Carlisle Barracks: Strategic Studies Institute, November, 2000.

Margesson, Rhoda, and Johanna Bockman. "Potential Humanitarian Issues in Post-War Iraq: An Overview for Congress," Congressional Research Service, The Library of Congress, 2003.

Marr, Phebe. Testimony before the Senate Foreign Relations Committee, August 1, 2002.

Marx, Michael. Disaster Response Team Leader, Office of U.S. Foreign Disaster Assistance, Briefing at the Foreign Press Center Building, Washington, DC, February 28, 2003.

Metz, Steven, and Raymond Millen. "Insurgency and Counterinsurgency in the 21st Century: Reconceptualizing Threat and Response," Strategic Studies Institute monograph, November, 2004.

Miles, Matthew B., and A. Michael Huberman. *An Expanded Sourcebook: Qualitative Data Analysis*. Thousand Oaks, CA: Sage Publications, Inc., 1994.

Moe, Terry M. "The New Economics of Organization," *American Journal of Political Science*, Vol. 28, 1984.

O'Hanlon, Michael E. "Iraq Without a Plan," *Policy Review, No. 128*, Stanford University, The Hoover Institution, December, 2004 and January, 2005.

Otterman, Sharon. "Grand Ayatollah Ali al-Sistani," *Middle East Information Center*. January 16, 2004. Available at http://middleeastinfo.org/article3861.html

Parsons, Wayne. *Public Policy*, Northampton, MA: Edward Elgar Publishing, Inc., 2001.

Patton, Michael Quinn. *Utilization Focused Evaluation*, Thousand Oakes: Sage Publications, 1996.

Priest, Dana. *The Mission*. New York: W.W. Norton & Company, Inc., 2003.

Princeton University Press, "The Role of Theory in Comparative Politics: A Symposium," *World Politics*, Vol. 48: (1), 1995.

Rice, Condoleezza. National Security Advisor, Press Briefing on April 4, 2003.

Rieff, David. "Blueprint for A Mess," *New York Times Magazine*, November 2, 2003.

Rife, Rickey. "Defense Is from Mars, State Is from Venus," Army War College: Carlisle Barracks, 1998.

Ross, Karol G., and Gary A. Klein, Peter Thunholm, John F. Schmitt and Holly C. Baxter. "The Recognition-Primed Decision Model," *Military Review*, July/August, 2004.

Salid, Roshan Muhammed. "Al-Zarqawi: America's new bogeyman," *Al Jazeera*, July 1, 2004.

Scott, Richard. *Institutions and Organizations*. Thousand Oaks: Sage Publications, 2001.

Simon, Herbert A. "The Proverbs of Administration," *Public Administration Review*, Vol. 19, 1946.

Slavin, Barbara, and Dave Moniz, "War in Iraq's Aftermath Hits Troops Hard," *USA Today*, July 21, 2003.

Snyder, Jack. "Military Bias and Offensive Strategy," *The Ideology of the Offensive: Military Decision Making and the Disasters of 1914*, Cornell Studies in Security Affairs, 1984.

Sorenson, David. Lecture at Air War College, August 2, 2004.

Sterngold, James. "Stanford Expert Says Iraq Spinning Out of Control," *San Francisco Chronicle*, April 25, 2004.

Taylor, John B. Under Secretary of Treasury for International Affairs, Testimony before the Senate Banking, Housing, and Urban Affairs Committee Subcommittee on International Trade and Finance, September 16, 2003.

United States Code, Title 10, *The Goldwater-Nichols Department of Defense Reorganization Act of 1986*.

United States Code, Title 50, *National Security Act of 1947*, Section 101.

United States Department of Defense, Background Briefing on Reconstruction and Humanitarian Assistance in Post-War Iraq, March 11, 2003. Available at http://www.defenselink.mil/news/Mar2003/t03122003_t031bgd.html.

United States Department of Defense Directive 5100.1, 1947.

United States Department of Defense. "Pre-war Planning for Post-war Iraq." Available at www.defenselink.mil/policy/isa/nesa/postwar_iraq.html.

United States Department of State, "Department Notice," July 10, 2003.

United States Department of State, "Duty to the Future: Free Iraqi Plan for a New Iraq," April, 2003. Available at http://www.usinfo.state.gov.

United States Department of State, *FY 2004–2009 Department of State and USAID Strategic Plan*, August 20, 2003.

Union-Tribune's Editorial Board, "Q and A: Anthony Zinni," *San Diego Union Tribune*, April 16, 2004.

Ware, Michael. "The Enemy with Many Faces," *Time*. September 27, 2004.

The White House. *The National Security Strategy of the United States of America*. September 17, 2002.

Wilson, James Q. *Bureaucracy: What Government Agencies Do and Why They Do It*. New York: Basic Books, 1989.

Wolfowitz, Paul. Deputy Secretary of Defense, "The Future of Iraq," Hearing of the Senate Foreign Relations Committee, February 11, 2003.

————. Town Hall Meeting with Iraqi-American Community, February 23, 2003.

Wright, Deil S. *Understanding Intergovernmental Relations*. Belmont, CA: Brooks/ Cole, 1988, excerpts reprinted in *Classics of Public Administration*, Jay M. Shafritz and Albert C. Hyde (eds), Orlando, FL: Harcourt Brace & Company, 1997.

Yin, Robert K. *Case Study Research: Design and Methods*, 2nd ed., Thousand Oaks, CA: Sage Publications, 1994.

http://defense.iwpnewsstand.com/insider.asp?issue=02092005

http://merln.ndu.edu

http://news.bbc.co.uk/1hi/world/middle_east/3770065.stm

http://www.csis.org/isp/gn

http://www.defenselink.mil/policy/isa/nesa/postwar_iraq.html

http://www.defenselink.mil/speeches/2002/s20020131-secdef.html

http://www.intelligence.gov/1-relationships.shtml

http://www.jfcom.mil/about/fact_jiacg.htm

http://www.state.gov

http://www.usembassy-israel.org.il/publish/peace/peace1.html

http://www.whitehouse.gov/nsc/history.html

Index

Boxes, figures, and tables are indicated by *b*, *f*, and *t* following the page number.